W9-DGT-157

Managed Mental Health Care

Mental Health Practice Under Managed Care
A Brunner/Mazel Book Series

S. Richard Sauber, Ph.D., Series Editor

The Brunner/Mazel Mental Health Practice Under Managed Care Series addresses the major developments and changes resulting from the introduction of managed care. Volumes in the series will enable mental health professionals to provide effective therapy to their parents while conducting and maintaining a successful practice.

Mental Health Practice Under Managed Care, Volume 8

Managed Mental Health Care

Major Diagnostic and Treatment Approaches

Edited by

S. Richard Sauber, Ph.D.

Brunner/Mazel
A member of the Taylor & Francis Group

Library of Congress Cataloging-in-Publication Data

Managed mental health care : major diagnostic and treatment approaches
/ edited by S. Richard Sauber.
    p.   cm. — (Mental health practice under managed care : v. 8)
  Includes bibliographical references and index.
  ISBN 0-87630-812-4 (pbk.)
  1. Managed mental health care.   2. Psychotherapy.   I. Sauber, S.
Richard.   II. Series.
  [DNLM: 1. Mental Disorders—therapy.   2. Mental Disorders—
diagnosis.   3. Managed Care Programs—United States.   4. Mental
Health Services—United States.   W1 ME9268 v.8 1997 / WM 400 M266
1997]
  RC480.5.M323   1997
  362.2'0425—dc21
  DNLM/DLC
  for Library of Congress   97-1084
                                                                       CIP

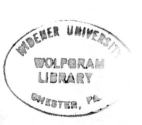
DISCARDED
WIDENER UNIVERSITY

Copyright © 1997 by Brunner/Mazel, Inc.

All rights reserved. No part of this book may be reproduced
by any process whatsoever without the written
permission of the copyright owner.

Published by
BRUNNER/MAZEL, INC.
A member of the Taylor & Francis Group
1900 Frost Road, Suite 101
Bristol, Pennsylvania, 19007

Manufactured in the United States of America

1 2 3 4 5 6 7 8 9 0 BRBR 9 0 9 8 7

WIDENER UNIVERSITY
WOLFGRAM
LIBRARY
CHESTER, PA.

Contents

Contributors

Darren W. Adamson, Ph.D., L.M.F.T., CEAP
Director of Corporate Health Resources and Vice President of EAP Services for Mesa Mental Health. Dr. Adamson is licensed as a Marriage and Family Therapist in New Mexico and Utah and is a Certified Employee Assistance Professional. He is a member of EAPA and AAFMT.

Daniel L. Araoz, Ed.D.
Holds Diplomates in Counseling and Family Psychology with the American Board of Professional Psychology; Professor of Mental Health Counseling at C.W. Post Center of Long Island University and Director of the Long Island Institute of Erickonsian Hypnosis.

Dennis A. Bagarozzi, Ph.D.
Director, Georgia Preferred, Inc., a private group mental health service organization. Dr. Bagarozzi has coauthored six clinical textbooks and published over 75 journal articles. He is on the editorial board of numerous journals, and is the Section Editor of Family Measurement Techniques of the *American Journal of Family Therapy.*

William L. Buchanan, Ph.D.
Director of Child and Family Psychology and Neuropsychology for the Group Affiliated Psychological and Medical Consultants in Gainsville, Georgia. He is coauthor of the *Dictionary of Family Psychology and Family Therapy,* published by Sage in 1993.

Marie A. Carrese, Ph.D.
Associate Professor of Counseling at York College of the City University of New York and in independent practice on Long Island, New York.

James W. Croake, Ph.D., ABPP
Professor of Psychology and Psychiatry in the Department of Psychiatry at the University of Washington Medical School, Seattle, and the University of Southern Alabama College of Medicine, Mobile.

Michael D. Gardner, Ph.D.
Clinical Supervisor for LDS Social Services in Washington, D.C. and Facility Staff at Virginia Tech and Frederick Community College. Dr. Gardner is the former coordinator of the Employee Assistance Program for Intermountain Health Care.

David A. Gross, M.D.
Co-director of the Palm Beach Evaluation Treatment Center and Medical Director for the Center for the Treatment of Phobias and Anxiety Disorders in Delray Beach, Florida. Formerly, Dr. Gross was the medical director of Fair Oaks Psychiatric Hospital, Delray Beach, Florida. Dr. Gross has published extensively in psychiatric journals and taught psychosomatic medicine and consultation–liaison in psychiatry at the Yale University School of Medicine.

Luciano L'Abate, Ph.D.
Professor Emeritus of Psychology, Georgia State University, and Director of the Multicultural Services at the Cross Keys Counseling Center in Conley, Georgia.

Judith A. Lewis, Ph.D.
Director of the Addictions Studies Program at Governors State University, University Park, Illinois, and director of Curriculum and Instruction at the Illinois Addiction Training Center at Governors State University.

Mark Mays, Ph.D., J.D.
Faculty in the Department of Psychiatry at the University of Washington Medical School and the Washington State University, as well as on the Law Faculty of Gonzaga University Law School. Formerly, Director of Psychological and Educational Services on a closed panel of a large health maintenance organization in Spokane, and former President of the Washington State Psychological Association.

Andrew Rosen, Ph.D., ABPP
Board-certified diplomate in Clinical Psychology, Co-Director of the Palm Beach Evaluation Treatment Center, and Executive Director of the Center for the Treatment of Phobias and Anxiety Disorders in Delray Beach, Florida.

S. Richard Sauber, Ph.D., ABPP
Editor of the Managed Care Book Series and Editor-in-Chief of the *American Journal of Family Therapy*. He is the author of seven books in the field and Executive Editor

of the *Treatment and Statistical Manual of Behavioral and Mental Disorders, First Edition* (in progress). Dr. Sauber is the Director of the Human Resources Consultation Service in Boca Raton, Florida.

Len Sperry, M.D., Ph.D.
Professor of Psychiatry and Director of the Division of Organizational Psychiatry and Corporate Health at the Medical College of Wisconsin. Dr. Sperry is the author of 25 books and more than 200 journal articles.

Henry I. Spitz, M.D.
Clinical Professor of Psychiatry, Columbia University, College of Physicians and Surgeons, and Director of the Postgraduate Group Psychotherapy Training Program at Columbia-Presbyterian Medical Center, New York, Dr. Spitz also is in practice in New York City.

Preface

The chapters in the handbook were organized and written to assist the provider who may be struggling to understand the ideological considerations of managed mental health care. We need the practical tools necessary to survive in this new world of the big business that has organized health care delivery systems. The contents are presented in such a way as to include the basic chapter headings of nosology, such as anxiety disorders; therapy; specialized programs, for example, employee assistance programs; and populations at risk. Essentially, the authors have integrated the basic knowledge in the professional literature in each of these diagnostic categories and treatment approaches with concepts according to managed care theory and practice.

This book contains the basics for the busy practitioner, and should stimulate our curiosity to expand our interest and motivation for retraining in this new approach to delivery systems. Reading the chapters contained in this handbook will provide an overview and whet the appetite of those who wish to specialize in any of these areas before beginning further reading of the complete text on each subject matter offered in this series. Once the clinical provider understands how to meet the needs of both the customer and the managed care company, then the therapist needs to master brief therapeutic interventions, especially crisis-intervention, group therapy, and computer-assisted therapy, which may be the primary treatment modes of the future. The most common presenting problems may be classified as anxiety, depression, adjustment disorders, and marital/family conflicts.

It also is essential for clinicians to understand employee assistance programs and how these services are now being organized under the control of managed care companies. After all, the employers of these employees are paying the bill, and they are beginning to assert requirements in terms not only of cost, but also of making a difference in the productivity of the workplace.

A new opportunity exists for mental health professionals to become acquainted with these kinds of patients' needs and to provide therapeutic intervention within the managed care framework for service delivery, whether the mode is carve-outs, carve back-ins, or integrative approaches within primary health care.

This handbook and the series offer a unique contribution to our field, given its state of flux. The trouble with the future is that it usually arrives before we are ready for it. We have to stop grieving for what was and move from denial to anger to acceptance to cooperation! Managed care is here to stay, and indemnity plans are disappearing rapidly. We no longer have professional autonomy; this luxury is being replaced with the payor or, in "the integrative system," the *case manager*. Our old-boy referrals have been made obsolete by price-based and utilization-based networks. We were comfortable with obedient patients, who are becoming more informed patients and thus empowered consumers. The days of the "righteous" provider have passed, the patient is questioning, and the managed care customer is right. Private practice has been of the mom and pop mentality, now resembles the supermarket, which soon will be the concept of a mall. Before there was no utilization review, now there is third-party utilization review, and eventually we will have internal network review. The movement is from retrospective to concurrent to prospective.

The failure of health care legislation has propelled many monumental changes in the delivery of mental health services. The position of the current Congress is for the development of states' initiative for their own health care systems. We can expect and are witnessing the introduction of different mental health models, from independence to integration in the stages of health care evaluation (see Table 1).

This will determine how behavioral and primary health care will be offered and state policy will dictate the role of the provider and how to finance and deliver mental health services. During the 1990s, privatization of the health industry began with capitation to shift the risk and cost overruns associated with free care upon demand to private corporations as a way to finance care for indigent and disabled persons and for illegal aliens. This approach has come a long way since Congress passed the Health Maintenance Organization Act in 1973, and then strengthened it in 1976 and 1981.

"We are witnessing the passing of an era."

We are now faced with control of mental health by business managers

TABLE 1

Stages of Health Care Evolution

	Stage One *Fragmented Delivery and Care*	Stage Two *Developing Coalitions*	Stage Three *Formal Networks*	Stage Four *Managed Delivery and Care*
Employers	Purchase from major indemnity insurers	Form coalitions to increase purchasing clout	Incentivize employees to select HMOs	Contract directly with integrated systems
HMOs	0–10% market share Growth of several small HMOs	11–30% market share Emergence of larger HMOs	31–50% market share Emergence of dominant HMOs	50% + market share Dominance of regional mega-HMOs
PPOs	Emergence of PPOs	Proliferation of PPOs	PPOs reduce panels	PPOs act like HMOs
Hospitals	Academic/teaching hospitals still rule	Reduction of bed capacity	Development of PHOs	Integration of PHOs with MCOs and payors
Physicians	Solo/independent practice	Formation of IPAs (no UR)/Develop prepaid groups to serve HMOs	IPAs institute UR management/Group consolidation	Consolidation into mega-multispecialty organizations
Providers	Independent providers	Loosely aligned provider networks	Risk-bearing formal provider networks	Strong provider-payor alliances

Source: Rehnwall, P. (1995) *Contracting & Capitation Strategy.* Nashville, TN: Business Networker.

and investors, the exploitation of inexpensive labor in the form of reduced provider fees, and the use of lesser-credentialed counselors and mental health technicians, standardized cookbooks of care where covered lives are channeled through predetermined treatment; mass delivery vehicles, such as group therapy; computerized assessment and treatment checklists; routine dispension of psychotropic medications by nonpsychiatric physicians; mergers and acquisitions leading to semi-monopolies; and a mass exodus by private practitioners out of the profession. This text and the other books in the series are written as survival guidebooks to help prepare practitioners to provide managed behavioral health care therapy during this transition to the industrialization of health services.

S.R.S.

1

Introduction to Managed Mental Health Care: Provider Survival

S. RICHARD SAUBER, Ph.D.

Viewed by many as the solution to America's health care crisis, managed health care is spawning a revolution in the delivery of mental health services. Whether managing care or managing costs, providers must learn how to manage themselves and their professional skills in order to survive. There is increased employer interest in how health care dollars are spent. New financial arrangements between insurers and providers have reshaped clinical practice to focus on the goals of efficacy and efficiency in behavioral health care.

Practitioners now have to comply with rigorous cost-containment measures and third-party treatment decisions. As a means of controlling costs, short-term treatment and group therapy have replaced traditional long-term analysis. Alarmingly, the dictates of managed care may lead to increased liability for practitioners. Economic survival almost compels single practitioners to join group practices and multidisciplinary groups.

Managed health care is dramatically changing the dynamics of psychological treatment. This handbook examines the complexities of managed care and its ramifications for the mental health field. This introductory chapter focuses on the following topics: the history of managed care; the impact of managed care; the therapist's role in cost containment; accepting change; detriments of managed care; recommendations for improvement; and survival tactics.

Subsequent chapters have been organized to guide providers struggling to understand managed care. They provide the practical tools needed to survive in this new world of big business and organized health care delivery systems. This book helps the clinical provider understand how to meet the needs of both the patient and the managed care company when it comes to the most common basic diagnostic categories: anxiety, depression, adjustment disorders, and marital and family problems. In order to survive, the therapist has to master brief therapeutic interventions, especially group therapy, which will be the primary treatment mode of the future.

It also is essential for the clinician to understand employer assistance programs and how these services are now being organized under the control of managed-care companies. After all, it is the employers of these patients who are paying the bills. It is necessary to teach these employers that mental health benefits are cost-effective. Studies show that depression and other mental disorders cost society billions of dollars annually. A large percentage of that cost is attributable to absenteeism and lost productivity in the workplace. It is important to convince employers that effective psychological treatment can improve health, increase well-being, and actually lower medical expenditures. (See Appendix I, "Mental Health is Cost-Effective," and Appendix II, "The Economics and Effectiveness of Inpatient and Outpatient Mental Health Treatment" at the end of this chapter.)

In the past, a small number of specialized, nonmainstream mental health caregivers provided personal injury and worker's compensation services. The two services differed in terms of the amount of regulation and fee caps, with worker's compensation being much more rigid. These specialized services are now coming into the mainstream under managed care control. Thus, there are new opportunities for the mental health therapist to become acquainted with these kinds of patients and to provide mental health services that fit with the managed care requirements.

HISTORY OF MANAGED CARE

To understand managed care, it is necessary to understand the history of health care in the United States. Prior to World War II, health care was relatively inexpensive. Most Americans did not have health insurance; they simply paid the family doctor or the hospital when they needed treatment. After the war, medical treatments and the quality of new procedures began to improve greatly, but progress did not come cheap. People realized that they needed some sort of coverage for medical bills, and many employers began to offer health coverage. This worked well for awhile.

Back in the old days, people had a family doctor who knew them and understood their health care needs. But as families grew and moved about, many people found themselves on their own in a confusing world of specialists and ever-changing diagnostic procedures. Many people received care they may not have needed. Costs skyrocketed. Managed care was devised to attack these problems.

The first companies to offer managed mental health care were founded in the 1970s, although attempts to allocate and coordinate the use of resources for mental health services can be traced back to the 1960s in both the public and private sectors. The landmark Community Mental Health Act of 1963, which established a system of community mental health centers (CMHCs), primarily served the needs of America's newly deinstitutionalized chronically mentally ill population. The CMHCs sought to develop a continuum of services for their consumers, focusing on adequate, if not optimal, care with emphasis on outpatient community-based services. A new group of specialists emerged. These community psychiatrists, community psychologists, and community mental health workers, who were employed in community settings, became accustomed to managing minimal public resources to benefit clients most in need of mental health care—a preventive and public health population-based approach.

In the 1960s and 1970s, employers became increasingly aware of the negative impact of alcohol abuse and other personal problems on the productivity of their employers. Some responded by implementing employee assistance programs (EAPs), which originated in earlier employer-sponsored worker-assistance programs for alcoholism. These early programs identified employees in need of mental health or substance abuse services, ensuring appropriate referral to treatment resources. Employers benefited from the cost savings associated with maintaining a healthier work force.

During the late 1970s and 1980s, indemnity insurance coverage for mental health disorders expanded as society became more accepting of psychotherapy and substance abuse rehabilitation. Employers relied on retrospective reviews or, more effectively, on concurrent review processes to validate the need for clinical services for their employees. These processes were often ineffective because neither the providers nor the reviewers of care had the opportunities or incentives to implement treatment plans cooperatively. Employers and benefit consultants believed that providers based treatment planning on benefit maximums rather than on clinical necessity. For example, if the benefit plan allowed for 30 days of inpatient substance abuse care per year, providers often requested 28, 29, or 30 days of inpatient treatment. Some employers responded by restricting or reducing benefits or implementing excessive deductibles for mental health care. An inevitable outcome of this dynamic is that employers might unintentionally deny access to care for employees with clinically significant disorders. To overcome this problem, employers began exploring other approaches to "insuring" care as the costs of mental health care, especially that portion associated with inpatient psychiatric or substance abuse services, skyrocketed in the 1980s.

Many employers turned to health maintenance organizations (HMOs), which have grown steadily in the past decade. Through a gatekeeping system of primary care physicians, management strategies and protocols, management information systems, and capitated financing arrangements, these complex, highly regulated entities served as a partial solution to providing health care to employees. Companies involved with managed mental health care grew as the HMO industry expanded, providing specialized benefit management and clinical services to HMO enrollees. These companies funded their operations through a capitation arrangement with their HMO customers, assuming risk for all mental health care. The capitation form of prospective payment means that a single payment is made for each individual enrolled, regardless of whether that patient requires considerable treatment, a minimal treatment, or no treatment at all.

Several managed mental health care (MMHC) organizations established clinic systems throughout the nation to serve HMO populations (see Figure 1.1, Winegar, 1992).

The latest generation of MMHC systems is the employer-sponsored mental health care provider network (Winegar, 1992). This new benefit

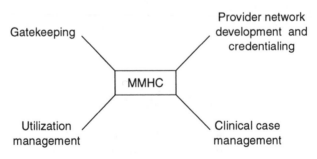

FIGURE 1.1

Model for MMHC organizations.

design is called a network-based product. Consumers are given incentives to use network providers and facilities through reduced out-of-pocket expenses or richer benefit levels. These coverage plans may still provide limited benefits for non–network-delivered services. Benefit designs are sometimes called point-of-service (POS) products, because the consumer determines whether to make use of a network-affiliated professional or facility.

In contrast to traditional indemnity insurance plans, MMHC systems customarily provide utilization review of inpatient care costs to both in- and out-of-network facilities. Reluctant to offer HMO plans (with their reduced choice of providers) alone, these network-based benefit plans provide easy entry into managed-care systems for a growing number of employers who seek increased accountability and cost containment while preserving employee choice of service providers.

By eliminating HMO or indemnity insurance involvement in the mental health care benefit area, employers may also carve out the mental health/substance abuse benefit and contract directly with the MMHC firm through either a capitated arrangement or an administrative-service-only fee arrangement. The capitated arrangement shifts financial risk from the employer to the provider group. The guaranteed cost arrangement offers employers the obvious benefit of having predictable expenses over the life of the agreement. The administrative-service-only arrangement offers less predictability, although performance penalties may be built into agreements with MMHC firms. These agreements allow employers to benefit from the discounted fee arrangements with providers, attractive hospital per diem rates, group practice associations, and other fiscal management strategies associated with existing MMHC operations.

IMPACT OF MANAGED CARE

Managed care can affect a mental health practice in several ways. Polonsky (1993) outlines several basic factors.

- *Short-term psychotherapy.* Managed care emphasizes short-term psychotherapy. Traditionally, many patients have been viewed as unsuitable for short-term therapy. Practicing under managed care means fitting almost every patient who comes through the door into the short-term model. There are potential legal consequences to any treatment planning decision.

- *Third-party control.* A third party, the managed-care company, is now involved in the relationship. This third party is in the driver's seat and ultimately controls the number of sessions available to the patient and the focus of treatment.
- *Privacy violations.* In order to make decisions about treatment planning, managed-care companies need documentation. Providing documentation to managed-care companies raises issues in regard to violations of privacy and the possible consequences of this information being passed on to large corporations and insurers.
- *Quality of service.* Competent professionals realize that taking workshops and classes on managed care is essential. Continuing education in the fields of short-term therapy, group therapy, cognitive-behavior therapy, and alcohol and drug counseling is also important.
- *Patient consent.* It is necessary to inform patients before or during their initial office visit about both the benefits and limitations of their health plans. Managed care organization plans provide a specified number of visits. Additional visits need prior authorization. Clinicians have to be sensitive about delving into issues that require long-term care. Practitioners should advise patients that additional visits may not be authorized. It is advisable to have patients sign a consent form describing the nature and limitations of therapy allowed under their plan.
- *Record keeping.* Therapists should keep records of patients referred by managed-care companies on file. If continued treatment has been denied, they should document that they made an appeal to the managed-care company on behalf of the patient. They should also keep on file releases signed by the patient allowing communication with the managed-care company.
- *Confidentiality.* It is wise to let patients know about the limits of confidentiality at the beginning of psychotherapy. Once reports are sent to the managed-care company, the clinician cannot guarantee the sanctity of information leaving his or her office. Therapists should review treatment planning reports with their patients, and have patients sign forms indicating that they have read and understood the reports. Therapists should outline the advantages and disadvantages of the treatment approach to the patient.
- *Medically necessary treatment.* If the managed-care company denies treatment, the clinician is ethically and legally obligated to appeal and should keep documented evidence of that appeal. The model of service for managed-care organizations is brief therapy. The purpose of care is to resolve symptoms delineated in the latest edition of the *Diagnostic and Statistical Manual of Mental Disorders*

(DSM) and to protect the welfare of the patient. Covered benefits do not include growth-oriented counseling or psychology, relationship problem solving, or psychodynamic therapy aimed at resolving childhood conflicts.

- *Termination of a treatment relationship.* Both patients and therapists have the right to end a therapeutic relationship. The therapist has an additional responsibility to ensure that the patient who is in need of psychological intervention has continued professional support.
- *Realistic goals.* Therapists should prepare patients for short-term therapy or a specific number of visits during the first session. They should clarify goals of treatment and what can and cannot be accomplished in the limited time available. The clinician should be careful not to get into emotional areas or explore problems that cannot be resolved in the number of sessions allowed.

The practice and business of psychotherapy in a cost-conscious era derive from four assumptions, which, Bernstein (1993) believes, reflect the reality of the times in which we live: (a) universal access to health care is an essential goal; (b) rising health care costs are a significant problem; (c) current scientific knowledge of health clearly and inexorably intertwines physical and mental health, and any health care program must incorporate both; (d) the practice of psychotherapy is different and separate (although not unrelated) to the business of psychotherapy, and both must be considered as we formulate a constructive response to the current health care issues.

THE THERAPIST'S ROLE IN COST CONTAINMENT

What is clear is that a new focus on cost containment is here to stay, and given the global economy, it will continue to be an important focus long into the foreseeable future. However, the best approach to cost containment is yet to be determined, and it is critical that health care professionals play an active and constructive role in developing a response to economic realities.

Defining Medical Necessity

Reimbursement for medical treatment is based on "medical necessity," which is currently interpreted as "functional necessity." This interpretation creates problems in mental health treatment. Consider the mental health patient who has moderate to severe anxiety symptoms, but who had always coped with the anxiety and functioned adequately in a career and relationships. Perhaps that patient seeks treatment now because the anxiety has worsened. It may take many therapy sessions before the patient becomes aware of having been the victim, for example, of incest. However, under the criteria of medical necessity, this patient would likely not be authorized for reimbursement for extended treatment for two reasons: first, because the patient is functioning satisfactorily, if not happily; second, because the therapist would be unable to document the incest until long after the treatment reimbursement was denied if the patient remained in therapy. Employee health contracts appear to maintain levels of benefits as long as reviewers deem the treatment necessary. Managed care adopts the position that long-term or more intense work is an indulgence motivated more by therapists' greed than by clinical rationale. This is only one reason why it is so important for mental health practitioners to be actively involved in defining the yardstick by which psychotherapy is determined to be necessary.

Improving Diagnostic Skills

The managed-care process is motivated predominantly by economics, not diagnostics. Economic decisions are not clinical decisions. Under current conditions, psychologists must try to make the best clinical decisions they can within the parameters of the allowed insurance benefits, economic times, and personal financial needs of the individual and his or her family.

Given the expense of long-term treatment, it is necessary to focus on improving diagnostic skills to determine when such treatment is indicated. What managed-care companies know but do not publicly acknowledge is that it is not the long-term care that really is the big expense—it is the 30-day psychiatric hospitalization and substance abuse inpatient rehabilitation.

Publicizing Mental Health Benefits

Mental health professionals must widely publicize the central importance of mental health as a barometer and contributor to physical health (See Appendixes I and II at the end of this chapter). This involves collaboration with politicians, employers, employees, unions, and insurance companies to ensure that the best possible treatment choices remain available for each patient within the context of finite economic resources. Remember that managed care's mandate is to ensure cost containment. It is the therapist's responsibility to make sure that sound clinical decisions are not overrun by the need to contain costs. It is important to educate managed-care and insurance administrators, employers, employees, and union officials as to the appropriate utilization of all forms of psychotherapy and the necessity that mental health services be provided by highly skilled and trained professionals. Otherwise, paraprofessionals, nonprofessionals, and mutual help support groups will provide the service at managed care's cost-cutting prices. If psychologists do not accomplish this, they will be likely to see further erosion of their field, and the future devaluation of psychotherapy. Managed-care and insurance companies will conclude that therapy can always be delivered in reduced amounts of time by people with less training for less payment.

Managed care organizations and the government assert that extreme controls are necessary, rather than applying the principles of the free-market place. The justification is outlined in Table 1.1 with the reasons why health and mental health care does not follow the laws of supply and demand.

Only 6% of the population was enrolled in some kind of fee-for-service indemnity health care plan in 1995. The death of such plans has been swifter than expected. Managed indemnity plans have grown. These plans feature some kind of prospective review of provider network requirements. Health maintenance organizations (HMOs), whose health care providers are employed by the health insurance company, preferred provider organizations (PPOs), where only "referred providers" are on the approved and fully reimbursable provider list, and new

TABLE 1.1

Reasons Why Health Care Does Not Follow the Laws of Supply and Demand

- Consumers don't shop for mental health care based on price.
- Mental health care is not advertised by price.
- From the consumer's perspective, indemnity insurance distorts mental health care price.
- There is a lack of universally accepted treatment standards and diverse treatment providers.
- There is a special nature to the patient–provider relationship.
- Consumers lack knowledge about mental health care services. They must trust the provider for treatment recommendations and quality assurance.

Adapted from William M. Mercer, Inc. (1991). Integrated health plans for managed care in the 90s. In *Driving down health care costs: Strategies and solutions* (pp. 14-1–14.30). New York: Panel Publishers, Inc.

point-of-service (POS) plans, where providers contract directly with payers who have been preapproved as cost-efficient and qualified providers, have also multiplied.

Meanwhile, there is an oversupply of mental health professionals. This oversupply, of course, is not in relation to demand but rather to reimbursement. Reimbursement by managed-care groups to individual psychotherapists is now at a record low. For example, psychotherapy reimbursements are under $25 per session in major marketplaces such as Los Angeles and San Francisco.

Instead of fee-for-service arrangements, insurers are increasingly moving to capitation plans that reimburse providers on the basis of a set fee per case or per a particular client population. Providers share some limit of the risks in providing care. If clients require a greater level of services than expected, the provider may not receive additional reimbursement.

Many plans severely limit mental health coverage as well. The HMO Act allowed HMOs to establish a different level of benefits for those seeking mental health or chemical-dependence treatment. Employee Retirement Income Security Act (ERISA) legislation preempts state laws governing health insurance, including state-managed mental health benefits and provider freedom-of-choice laws. Although some 37 million Americans are insured, Washington Business Group on Health president Mary Jane England, M.D., has estimated that there are 58 million Americans who are underinsured for mental health and chemical-dependence treatment.

Provider groups must be able to integrate the functions of a managed-care company so as to render managed care obsolete. They must be able to:

- Plan treatment prospectively
- Have a network of multidisciplinary providers who can provide a continuum of care in a variety of settings
- Carry out the necessary administrative functions
- Demonstrate results and cost efficiency.

ACCEPTING CHANGE

For those who remain committed to private, solo practice, it will be very difficult and challenging to continue achieving past economic and clinical objectives in the new environment of contracted service delivery systems. Getting on particular provider lists may remain problematic.

Negotiating better contracts with insurers is difficult, if not impossible, for independent providers. Independent outpatient mental health providers typically discount their "usual and customary fee" by 25 to 30 % just to get a contract from a managed-care firm.

Many therapists find it difficult to accept the changes that managed care has wrought in mental health treatment and refuse to become acclimated to these changes. There are four specific "future neuroses," to which therapists, according to James Shulman, fall prey (1994). The first neurosis is *future phobia*, the fear of making decisions, which is most evident in avoidant behavior. The second neurosis is *paradigm paralysis*, the inability to shift point of view, thus restricting flexibility to make changes. (See Chapter 2, "The Paradox of Change.") The third neurosis is *infor-mania*, the constant need for more information to avoid appearing ignorant. Always seeking information limits creativity and decision making. The last neurosis is *reverse paranoia*, the belief that the therapist is following someone else, hoping that the someone is or will be the leader of change. This neurosis stifles self-reliance—not only does it cause the refusal to take leadership, but also stunts the ability to have a vision.

To be in a position to take advantage of the new options, mental health professionals must overcome their future neuroses and participate in the change. The first step is to improve the quality of mental health care in the following ways.

1. Availability: better access to services
   a. Geographic convenience of providers/referrals
   b. Availability on a 24-hour basis
   c. Immediate handling of emergencies
   d. Urgent services provided the same day
   e. Convenient and timely appointments
   f. Timely response to clients' phone calls and correspondence
   g. Timely provision of reports to support medical and other services
   h. Negotiations with payers for off-plan services when in a client's best interest
   i. Obtaining authorizations to facilitate rather than impede treatment

2. Focus: targeted treatment
   a. Inclusion of comprehensive biopsychosocial assessments
   b. Assignment of appropriate level of care based on level of functioning
   c. Solution-focused therapeutic interventions
   d. Participation of client in treatment plan development

e. Involvement of family, employer, and other support systems in treatment where appropriate
f. Therapeutic assignments to maximize treatment gains
g. Treatment in least restrictive safe settings

3. Consistency: solid practice management
   a. Well-organized and documented clinical records
   b. Efficient clinical and office management systems, including data reporting and billing
   c. Accessibility of client billing and case records to external review

4. Satisfaction
   a. High satisfaction (90% level of service, treatment results, follow-up, accessibility, support services, etc.) as measured by surveys of:
      (i) Clients (patients)
      (ii) Employers and/or health plans
      (iii) Primary care physicians
      (iv) EAP of employer
      (v) Providers
      (vi) Staff members
      (vii) Others, including referral, families
   b. Absence of complaints, litigation, and other changes made by clients, providers, and others

5. Outcome
   a. Demonstration that treatment was effective—that is, that it has resulted in:
      (i) Symptom relief
      (ii) Improvement in general level of functioning
      (iii) Improvement in specific level of functioning representing problems and diagnoses
      (iv) Improvement in general health
   b. Demonstration that treatment was efficiently provided in a reasonable number of visits or days, at an appropriate level
   c. Demonstration that services were cost-effective, reducing other costly medical or social problems, amount paid for the results produced

The contrast between managed care and independent private practice offers such divergence that it is easy to understand why professional practitioners have a difficult time becoming service providers. Sykes-Wylie (1994) defines managed care as a corporate, privately run (although often government-regulated) system of health care that coordinates and delivers an entire range of medical and, sometimes, mental health services to a prepaid population. At the same time, this corporation also manages the costs of providing that care. By both selling the "product" and paying the overhead of producing it, the managed-care company theoretically operates under the same incentives as a wholesaler or producer who stays in business by both controlling expenses and maintaining high enough quality to attract customers. Typically, a managed-care company stays within budget by screening medical and mental health services, restricting or denying access to those considered unnecessary or inappropriate, and getting providers to agree to reimbursements below what they could get in the free market.

Most therapists grew to professional adulthood during the Golden Age of private practice when the term "rich therapist" was not an oxymoron. Many thrived in the benign climate of a medical system where practitioners of all specialties had a rare degree of autonomy. They were able to contract privately with individual clients of their own choosing, to set their own fees, to decide on treatment, and to determine the scope and depth of treatment, as well as the time and reasons for its termination.

Some therapists will undoubtedly remain in private practice, although they will probably work longer hours for fewer dollars. Some will join the favored few doing what is now referred to as "boutique therapy"—uninsured, long-term, client-paid psychotherapy for those few souls who can still afford it. But almost everybody else, if they are still in the field at all, probably will join the ranks of managed care providers.

DISADVANTAGES OF MANAGED CARE

There are many critics of managed mental health care. All mental health professionals share a common predilection for what Charles and Beverly Browning, in their book *How to Partner with Managed Care*, called the "three Is" of managed care—intrusion, invasion, and inquisition.

Karen Shore is a New York therapist and organizer of a consumer therapist advocacy group called the Coalition of Mental Health Professionals and Consumers. She compares the managed health care industry to a "totalitarian regime, subjugating patients and therapists and depriving them of freedom and democratic process." Therapists who refuse to disgorge quantities of highly sensitive personal information about clients to reviewers, or who ask for more sessions than the company approves, are susceptible to being blacklisted, says Shore. "A tremendous fear permeates the system, and therapists who do more intensive psycho-dynamic or behavioral work, who argue with reviewers or file appeals of refusals, are kicked out of networks."

This aggressive micromanagement and obsession with cost-cutting characterizes what James Shulman calls the managed care "reign of terror," which began during the mid-1980s when medical costs soared out of sight. According to Shulman, a psychologist and CEO of INTER-ACT Behavioral Healthcare Services, insurance companies compete fiercely for business from employers anxious to reduce budget-breaking health care expenses. These companies ruthlessly prune benefits and deny claims to produce programs that look more cost-effective to their corporate buyers. The priority result has become management of costs, not care.

Under this form of legalized managed care, writes Shulman in the September 1993 issue of *The Ohio Psychologist*, reviewers deny payments for spurious or inappropriate reasons and often refuse to negotiate regarding care, prices, or alternative service delivery systems. Practitioners who refuse to comply with the terrorist-style tactics are "rubbed out" as providers. For survival, many providers adopt compliance, becoming hostages, and thus learn to play the games, accept the prices, and follow the rules. There is one major difference between a terrorist and a managed-care company, Shulman points out: "You can negotiate with a terrorist," at least sometimes.

Managed-care companies relentlessly underbid one another in esti-mating costs of services. They pressure staff members and affiliated providers to focus their best efforts on the corporate bottom line rather than on the welfare of their clients. "When you are being forced to get good numbers on quarterly and even monthly statements, while management is slamming you for being over budget by 10 percent, and in the meantime, the managed care supervisor you reported to last week is gone this week, it's difficult to serve the client very well. And when you have insecure, paranoid and depressed therapists working with insecure, paranoid and depressed clients, it's a nightmare" (Shulman, 1994).

Managed care curtails a practitioner's freedom to decide unilaterally when to see clients, which ones and how many to see, and how much to charge. Instead, treatment decisions must be made in cooperation and coordination with other providers within fairly strict parameters of time, cost, and theoretical orientation. This effectively eliminates long-term, analytically oriented therapy.

The most radical change in store for therapists will be the need to justify what they do with an unprecedented precision and specificity. Therapists, according to Sykes Wylie (1994), are held to almost no objectively measurable external standards for deciding what is wrong with the client, what to do about it, how long it should take to do it, when it can be considered done, and how anybody knows if it is done.

The boundaries of psychological diagnosis and treatment have become so porous and malleable, some say, that every life problem has become a disease, and for every disease there is an expensive, time-consuming, idiosyncratic ad hoc remedy. Critics of therapy's lackadaisical attitude toward accountability also argue that for decades, fundamental clinical decisions have been made virtually by professional fiat, derived only from the in-house rules of a professional guild and the clinical intuition of the individual practitioner. A common complaint is that the same client will receive entirely different diagnoses, modes of treatment, and prognoses for improvement, depending on whether the therapist is a behaviorist, a cognitive psychologist, a structural-strategic family therapist, a Freudian analyst, a biologically oriented psychiatrist, or a Jungian archetype finder. Nor are there common measures for determining appropriate fit between any one of these models and any particular problem—the client shows up for a virtual blind date between his or her presenting complaint and the therapeutic modality of the clinician who happened to get called first.

From now on, however, therapists will have to demonstrate what good matchmakers they are, convincing corporate buyers—the economic "parents" of the client—that the "dates" they arrange between clients and treatment almost always lead to successful (although intentionally brief) marriages. Therapists, in other words, will have to demonstrate in advance that a particular client exhibits the specific functional impairments that make him or her a good candidate for a standard treatment regimen that has already worked in numerous other, similar cases. Now, assigning categorical diagnoses will be much less important than measuring specific symptoms along a continuum of functional impairment. For instance, is she failing to hold a job? Is he too depressed to pay attention to his kids? Is the child suddenly failing school? Therapists must then indicate a specific treatment for resolving a specific problem and address the identified impairment. In other words, practitioners will have to demonstrate the level of impairment, the intensity of treatment, and the expected time it will take in each case. Therapists will no longer get away with saying that therapy is necessary "to improve the client's self-esteem" or "to work on characterological issues" or justify asking for more sessions because "the client seems to be feeling better."

RECOMMENDATIONS FOR IMPROVEMENT

A small but growing body of evidence suggests that managed care is no magic solution for escalating costs, at least not over the long run.

It may even increase expenses by adding bureaucracy to an already bloated system. This bureaucracy sets up obstacles for doctors and patients. These obstacles not only are burdensome, but they often interfere with needed treatment. In plans that encourage the use of a limited circle of physicians, the sickest patients may get the worst care. The bottom line is that managed care often buys little in the way of savings but may cost dearly in terms of quality of care—occasionally with tragic results.

Some suggestions for correcting a few managed-care flaws are as follows:

- Managed-care firms should end micromanagement of individual cases and concentrate instead on setting rational guidelines for care. Only therapists who routinely go beyond those guidelines should be policed closely.
- Companies should simplify the appeals process, especially for severely ill patients.
- Plans should be paid a flat rate per patient, rather than a fee for each visit or procedure, so as to encourage economy. But plans should pay more for patients who require more care because of age or illness. That would reduce the incentive to undertreat or turn away more disturbed people.
- Plans should put more emphasis on quality by rewarding therapists not only for holding costs down, but also for keeping patients satisfied.
- Finally, the patients or employers who pay the bills should get a greater cut of any cost savings, perhaps through a year-end rebate.

Without these changes, critics say, managed care is one cost-busting reform that we just cannot afford.

Managed-care companies seek to sign contracts not so much with individual providers as with integrated systems of care. These systems provide a continuum of care that includes acute beds, day treatment, outpatient care, and comparable services for substance abuse.

Treatment is based on medically necessary criteria and patients are expected to be treated at the right level of care. Utilization review is a critical part of these systems of care as managed-care companies move from micromanagement of cases to a more extensive profiling of providers. On the outpatient side, there is even more emphasis on brief treatment, crisis management, and group therapy for specific clinical problems. In general, there is a differentiation between what is critically needed and what is not. Only treatment that is effective will be supported.

SURVIVAL TACTICS

What does all this mean for providers and what should they be doing to ensure survival in the future health care systems? Since isolated office practice will probably be limited to a small percentage of providers, Bender (1994) advises practitioners to align themselves with a larger system, such as a multidisciplinary group, hospital-based system, or national organization. There is a need for more focused treatment.

The focus in the future will be on efficiency, medical necessity, and amelioration of symptoms. Documentation will clearly state the clinical condition, the treatment approach, and the expected impact of therapy. It will be essential to measure the outcomes of treatment functionally.

In addition, as the DSM (now in its fourth edition) has become more sophisticated with regard to diagnosis, there will be a need for concurrent treatment strategies that will be connected to diagnosis in terms of functional impairments and symptoms. This will become clearer as managed care companies utilize *The Treatment and Statistical Manual of Behavioral and Mental Disorders, First Edition.* This book offers a taxonomy of therapeutic interventions. It will be important to analyze clinical orientation and to be able to clearly enunciate it in relation to pathological conditions. In essence, a degree and a license will no longer ensure an opportunity to practice. Specific clinical skills, treatment, and effectiveness will be examined in the interest of provider selection for therapeutic efficiency.

Participation in multispecialty mental health groups offers clinicians the following advantages:

- The opportunity to gain access to large patient populations as a defense against exclusion from networks and carve-outs.
- The assurance of a sizable enough population of patients to justify the overhead associated with providing the wide range of services necessary while benefiting from economies of scale.
- The availability of office support services that have become necessary in current practice but that are often too expensive for solo practitioners.
- Utilization reviews that can be built into the system, eliminating the cumbersome process of dealing with external reviewers who serve as watchdogs.
- The ability to ensure that patient care is clinically rather than fiscally managed and that the clinical perspective maintains precedence.
- At least some protection against the continued erosion of autonomy and control that most practitioners are currently experiencing.

- The ability to make peer clinical and emotional support available to providers as part of the delivery system.

Therapists can take a number of steps to position themselves in the arena of managed health care. They are as follows:

- Think in terms of prospective not retrospective.
- Focus on maximizing the mental health benefit.
- Develop a proactive approach when involved in the case UR process.
- Develop a long-term outlook when dealing with managed-care organizations.
- Became involved with the managed care organization beyond the scope of the contract.
- Support the channeling and certification process established by the network.
- Establish a predictable billing structure and case review practices.
- Develop a strong continuum of care.
- Make sure that your current credentialing is sufficient.

Positioning ourselves includes attitude change and receptivity to consider the advantages that managed care offers us. The following list of 10 variables comes from Browning and Browning, *How To Partner With Managed Care*, pp. 29–30 (1994).

1. Without some form of external fiscal control, mental health insurance benefits could become but a happy memory of the good old days.
2. For those clinicians who adjust their attitudes and join the "team," the managed care case managers can become a source of success to a private practice, acting as a kind of "referral broker" to that clinician.
3. Managed care may, in fact, help us manage to provide better care to our patients; getting our sights clearly fixed on objectives, goals and outcomes rather than on insights or awareness for their own sakes.
4. The ongoing interactions with our case manager colleagues can help us clinically by linking treatment methodology tightly to diagnosed maladies with another professional to discuss and review the case.
5. Time-limited, focused treatment can help encourage us to help our patients build a support network upon which to depend, separate from reliance on the therapist alone.

6. Short-term, result-oriented counseling tends to be exciting, challenging, and fast-paced. This may keep us from getting bogged down, stuck, or having long periods when the patient does not progress or improve.

7. Accountability to produce measurable results requires us to re-examine our training and literature regarding "Brief Psychotherapy." Managed care may force us to rethink our clinical skills beyond old learnings of graduate school.

8. Time-limited and controlled intervention may help some patients escape the unsuspected snare of addiction to psychotrophic medication administered as an adjunct to their ongoing, long-term therapy. It has too often been the sad truth that long-term treatment results in long-term drug dependence.

9. For far too long our profession has been too fuzzy and less than precise as clinicians have prided themselves in being "eclectic"; meaning (in our opinion) "if it feels good, do it." Perhaps the external accountability for outcome will refine what we do and bring us closer to a true science of human healing and recovery.

10. Last and perhaps least in terms of how much it holds our interest, is the economic advantages derived by our participation in helping to reduce the drain on the health dollar to American business. We are in truth members of a much larger "team" or system, and if we can build a healthier economy as well as healthier patients, then the whole system should benefit.

Managed-care companies have struggled with, and sometimes differed over, the way to best manage mental health services. These companies realize that mental health clinicians are endless fine-tuners. Resolution of the problem that caused the patient to seek care often leads to the treatment of related problems. Treatment of diagnosable illness gives way to the treatment of marriage and family problems, of social or job dissatisfactions. Therapists know how easy it is to play games in attempts to curtail utilization of outpatient services by insisting on DSM-IV non-V code diagnosis, or by insisting that benefits be available for couples therapy but not for marriage counseling.

Managed-care companies have responded by establishing aggressive utilization review procedures to offset "extra" services when benefits must have a cost limit to them. (See Appendix II, at the end of the chapter "Standards of Mental Health Reviewer Practice.")

Thus, managed care has spawned a revolution that is greatly affecting the delivery of mental health services. Therapists must discover how to master the new techniques, learn to comply with the new rules, and help to initiate necessary changes if they hope to survive:

As practitioners, we first need to approach our outpatient treatment within the framework of managed care, which requires us to review the severity of illness and the intensity of service criteria for outpatient psychotherapy. The next step is to select the type of psychotherapy and form the nature of treatment that will be provided, given the categories of many of the MCO's to include crisis resolution, symptom alleviation, therapeutic stabilization, personality change, and major improvement in adaptation of our choices. The severity of illness criteria relates to the patient: (1) having a DSM-IV disorder that is amenable for treatment, (2) exhibiting a distress or dysfunction that does not require inpatient residential or partial hospitalization treatment, and (3) demonstrating motivation to comply with treatment. The intensity of service criteria includes such treatment as individual, family, couple, and/or group therapy.

Crisis Resolution Psychotherapy

The goal of crisis resolution psychotherapy is to stabilize the patient and return him or her to the level of mental functioning that was experienced before the crisis. The crisis may be an abrupt or substantial change in behavior brought on by a specific cause, and it can result in impaired functioning or an increase in personal stress. A mental disorder significantly alters normal life functioning and is brought on by a severe stressor. The Global Assessment Functioning (GAF) as indicated on the GAF scale most frequently is 31 to 50 when a patient is in a crisis situation. The intensity of service may require daily therapy sessions in order to maintain the patient and/or family and to restore the patient to a level of functioning that does not require hospitalization.

Symptom Alleviation

Symptom alleviation is the goal of any psychotherapy aimed at improving the patient's mental condition and level of functioning when experiencing symptoms such as anxiety, panic attacks, depression, or hallucinations.

If we can confirm the following conditions, the patient will meet the severity of illness criteria for outpatient symptom alleviation:

1. The patient has sufficient mental capacity to benefit from therapy. The Global Assessment of Functioning most frequently is 41 to 80.

2. The patient has demonstrated the necessary judgment of insight and capacity for integration by successfully establishing interpersonal relationships, tolerating and revealing feelings, and assuming responsibility for behavior change.

If these conditions exist, the patient will require up to one therapy session per week for up to 12 months or up to two sessions per week for the first six weeks.

Therapeutic Stabilization

Therapeutic stabilization is the goal of psychotherapy aimed at helping a patient to maintain an improved level of functioning. As part of the treatment, the therapist may: offer the patient reassurance of instructions, correct reality distortions, promote change in the patient's environment, or provide a model for healthy interpersonal relationships. If we can confirm the following, then the patient meets the severity of illness criteria for outpatient therapy and stabilization: the patient has sufficient mental capacity to benefit from therapy. The Global Assessment of Functioning most frequently is 21 to 60. The intensity of service criteria requires up to one therapy session per week for up to six months or up to two sessions per month for up to twelve months. Many patients can be maintained therapeutically on a more flexible schedule, such as one session per month or whenever the patient requires a session needed to deal with a temporary destabilization.

Major Personality Change

When psychotherapy is used to remove or modify disturbed patterns of behavior arising from intrapsychic conflict and maladapted learning, the goal of treatment may be characterized as major personality change. The severity of illness criteria for outpatient major personality change includes the following:

1. The patient has sufficient mental capacity to benefit from therapy. The Global Assessment of Function most frequently is 51 to 70.
2. The patient has demonstrated the necessary judgment, insight, and capacity for integration by successfully: assuming responsibility for behavior change, tolerating and revealing feelings, and establishing relationships.

3. The patient understands that the symptoms indicate intrapsychic conflict and maladapted responses to particular stresses in situations. The patient meeting the criteria for the intensity of service generally consists of one or two sessions of therapy per week for up to two years. However, a rationale should be provided to explain why brief, focus treatment is not an effective alternative.

AT-RISK CONTRACTING

We are now experiencing a transition to at-risk contracting which is population-based care. This approach offers providers the opportunity of more autonomy and control while at the same time increasing risks in the financial, legal, clinical, and ethical areas. This phase is requiring behavioral health care delivery system managers to shift their focus and structure of clinical, administrative, and financial arrangements from past ways of providing mental health care. Only large provider groups will be able to compete and service these populations; thus providers need to consider joining and affiliating with those entities that have already or will begin to dominate the marketplace with managed behavioral programs and services for the approximately 50 percent of the 178 million privately insured Americans. Those of you who will staff these centers are advised to be receptive to skill-building and educational channels in order to stay ahead of or at least maintain your capabilities with the massive and rapidly changing ways of care and financial management (Frank et al., 1994).

REFERENCES

American PsychManagement (1991). Clinical Criteria: Standards of mental health reviewer practice. 4–37. Arlington, VA: Value Health.

Bartlett, J., Prest, S., & Soper, M. (1991). *Cigna level of care guidelines for mental health and substance abuse.* Philadelphia, PA: Cigna Corp.

Bender, P. (1994). Behavior health managed care in the future: The provider's role in it. *Provider,* p. 1.

Browning, B. & Browning, C. (1994). *How to partner with managed care.* Los Alamitos, CA: Duncliff's International.

Charter Medical Clinical Documentation for Managers, *Managed Healthcare Handbook Glossary of Terms.* Presentation 2/26/93 at Charter Hospital in West Palm Beach, Florida.

Frank, R. J., McGuireitig, Regier, P. A., Manderscheid, R. and Woodward, A. (1994). Expenditure patterns for mental health and substance abuse: Implications for health reform. *Human Affairs,* I, 337–342.

Joint Commission for the Development of the Treatment and Statistical Manual of Behavioral and Mental Disorders, Inc. (in progress, 1997). *Treatment and statistical manual of behavioral mental disorders,* First Edition.

Mercer, William M. (1991). Integrated health plans for Managed care in the 90's. *In driving down health care costs: Strategies and solutions.* New York: Panel Publishers.

Rice, David & Polonsky, Ira (1993). *How to write treatment planning reports for managed care companies. Part II Axis II Disorders.* Oakland, CA: Professional Health Plan Publishers.

Shore, Karen (1993). Mental health in the Clinton plan: Corporate dictatorship in therapy. *Health/PAC Bulletin,* 28–30.

Shulman, James M. (1994). Dealing with the certainty of increasing or overcoming the future neuroses. *Bulletin of Independent Practice,* 121–122.

Sykes-Wylie, M. (1994). Endangered species. *Networker,* 20–33.

Winegar, N. (1992). *The clinician's guide to managed mental health care.* N.Y.: The Haworth Press.

APPENDIX I

Mental Health Benefit Is Cost-Effective

Why Should Employers Be Concerned About Mental Health?

Twenty-eight million American adults have serious mental disorders other than substance abuse. These mental illnesses cost society an estimated $129.3 billion annually, about half of which is attributable to lost productivity in the workplace.

In any one-month period, almost eight million people experience depression at an estimated annual cost of $16 billion; $10 billion of which is money lost in absenteeism and lost productivity.

Mental illness, including depression, can be as functionally disabling as a serious heart condition, and more disabling than other chronic physical illnesses, such as lung or gastrointestinal problems, angina, hypertension, and even diabetes.

Standard prevalence estimates of primary care patients with diagnosable mental disorders range from 15% to 40%.

Patients with diagnosable mental disorders have been shown to average twice as many visits to their primary care physicians as those without mental disorders.

Medical Savings Stemming from Mental Health Treatment

Besides improving health and increasing well-being, evidence has accumulated to show that psychological treatments actually can lower medical expenditures.

Medicaid patients hospitalized for physical ailments and provided mental health interventions realized average cumulative savings of $1,500 over a subsequent $2^1/_2$-year period. The cost of the mental health intervention was entirely paid for (i.e., totally offset) by these savings. Patients hospitalized without physical ailments who received mental health treatment realized savings ranging from $296 to $392, depending on the severity of the diagnosis.

A three-year study of over 10,000 Aetna beneficiaries showed that after initiation of mental health treatment, client medical costs dropped continuously over 36 months. The health costs of one mental health treatment group fell from $242 the year prior to treatment to $162 two years posttreatment. Other subject groups demonstrated similarly dramatic offset effects, leading the researchers to conclude that a decrease in total health care costs can be expected following mental health interventions even when the cost of the intervention is included.

Research on 20,000 enrollees in the Columbia (Md.) Medical Plan, showed that untreated mentally ill persons increased their medical utilization by 61% during a one-year period. In contrast, the mentally ill who received psychological treatment increased their medical expenditures by only 11% during the same period. A mental health comparison group averaged a 9% increase (Hankin, 1983). Three hundred veterans who received abbreviated mental health treatment following a history of excessive medical health utilization were able to reduce outpatient medical visits by 36%. Control groups, who received no psychotherapy, actually increased outpatient medical utilization.

In other studies, which included elderly subjects, even modest psychological interventions were shown to reduce hospital stays approximately 1.5 days below the control group's average 8.7 days.

APPENDIX II

Economics and Effectiveness of Inpatient and Outpatient Mental Health Treatment*

I. MOST MENTAL HEALTH EXPENDITURES ARE FOR INPATIENT TREATMENT—THE TREATMENT TYPE PRIMARILY RESPONSIBLE FOR RISING MENTAL HEALTH COSTS

- Approximately 70% of all mental health costs are for inpatient treatment.
- In 1981, inpatient treatment accounted for 83% of total mental health expenditures under the Medicare program.
- In 1985, the states spent 65% of their mental health agency budgets on inpatient care, 19% on ambulatory care, 5% on residential programs, and the balance on research and administration.
- Blue Cross/Blue Shield and other indemnity insurance plans spend two thirds of their mental health budgets for inpatient care.
- In fiscal year 1989, CHAMPUS spent over $500 million of $630 million total mental health expenditures on inpatient care.
- A recent study of expenditure and utilization patterns for mental illness and substance abuse services under private health insurance found that inpatient substance abuse services grew 30% between 1986 and 1988 and adolescent inpatient mental health treatment grew 65%.
- The cost of inpatient psychiatric services under CHAMPUS increased 128% between fiscal year 1986 and fiscal year 1989—an increase $2\frac{1}{2}$ times the increase for outpatient psychiatric services.
- In 1989, over 128,000 children were treated in short-term, nonfederal general hospitals at an estimated cost of over $1.5 billion.
- Psychiatric hospitalization results for less than 1 % of the general population but accounts for half or more of the total cost of treatment.

II. MUCH OF THIS INPATIENT TREATMENT CAN BE AS EFFECTIVELY DELIVERED IN OUTPATIENT SETTINGS

- A study of alcoholics was conducted to determine the relative efficacy of inpatient treatment, outpatient treatment, and combination

* Prepared by the American Psychological Association, 1993.

inpatient–outpatient treatment. Six months after treatment, the patients revealed a 67% abstinence rate with no significant differences by treatment setting.

- Twenty-six controlled comparisons of treatment settings for alcohol abuse have consistently shown no overall advantage for residential over nonresidential settings, for longer over shorter inpatient programs, or for more intensive over less intensive interventions.
- Studies suggest at least 40% of the hospital placements of children are inappropriate, either because they have been hospitalized too long or because they never should have been hospitalized at all.
- In a review of reported outcome studies, Herz (1982) concluded that adult partial hospitalization was as effective or more effective than inpatient hospitalization in symptom reduction and community functioning.
- A retrospective study of behaviorally disordered adolescents discharged from a comprehensive residential or partial hospitalization program found that successful follow-up patients were most likely day students rather than residential students.

III. OUTPATIENT TREATMENT IS LESS COSTLY THAN INPATIENT TREATMENT

- After data analysis, one company found that the benefit design encouraged the use of inpatient services rather than less expensive and often more appropriate outpatient services. The individual would pay $2,750 for $3,750 worth of outpatient care in comparison with paying $1,000 of the total comparable inpatient charge of $9,349. Based on historical data, shifting affective psychoses cases that could have been appropriately treated in the outpatient setting would have produced over $41,000 in savings over the two-and-a-half year period.
- A retrospective study of the records of an intensive outpatient community support and treatment program found substantial decreases in hospital costs as a result of clients' participation in the program. Savings in hospital costs alone were $8,006 per client and the cost of initial commitments was reduced by 80 %. Even when the cost of the program itself was included, annual savings from decreased hospitalizations were $272,767.
- In Maine, intensive home-based services for emotionally or behaviorally disturbed children prevented placement in residential treatment settings in 76 to 95% of the cases and saved between $3,000 and $12,000 per family.

- After the creation of an interagency system of care, state hospitalizations of children in Ventura County, California, fell by 25%, saving an average of $428,000 annually.
- In a cost–benefit analysis of outpatient psychosocial rehabilitation for frequent psychiatric recidivists, the average number of hospital days declined from 87.1 to 36.6, resulting in an annual savings of over $5,000 per client following outpatient treatment.
- A comparison of the financial costs during the first year of treatment of patients receiving home-based psychiatric treatment and patients receiving hospital-based treatment was conducted using two estimates of personnel and operating costs. Under both cost models, hospital-based treatment was more expensive: 64.1% more expensive in one case and 108.9% more in the other.
- In 1987, substance abuse treatment costs per patient per year were:
  $3,000 = outpatient methadone maintenance
  $2,300 = outpatient drug-free
  $14,600 = nonhospital residential drug-free.
- Costs for adolescent treatment range from $1,100 for intensive in-home crisis services per episode to $52,300 for residential treatment facilities per episode.
- A 12-day stay in a community hospital costs about $4,000; that amount would cover the cost of a halfway house plus regular outpatient treatment at a mental health center for about 100 days.

APPENDIX III

Standards of Mental Health Reviewer Practice*

Standard I: Theory

Process criteria

The reviewer:
• examines basic clinical information regarding the nature of the patient's illness.
• utilizes theory and critical thinking to apply the relevant clinical criteria.

Outcome criteria

• Certification decisions are based on scientific application of clinical criteria.

Standard II: Data Collection

Process criteria

The reviewer:
• informs the provider of their mutual roles and responsibilities in the review process.
• uses clinical judgment to determine what information is needed.

Outcome criteria

• The data are synthesized and recorded in a standardized format.

* As proposed by American Psychmanagement, Inc., in October 1992.

Standard III: Diagnosis

Process criteria

The reviewer:
- establishes DSM-IV diagnosis on all five axes.
- collects sufficient data to verify a diagnosis by DSM-IV criteria.

Outcome criteria

- DSM-IV diagnosis is confirmed with the provider.
- Diagnoses are recorded in a manner that facilitates planning and research.

Standard IV: Planning

Process criteria

The reviewer:
- collaborates with the provider in establishing appropriate treatment plans based on severity of illness and intensity of treatment.
- collaborates with the provider in identifying appropriate treatment goals within the benefit design.
- collaborates with the provider to appropriately utilize the peer advisor for cases that lie outside of the clinical criteria.
- re-reviews as clinically indicated to establish clinical status, goal achievement, and appropriate dispositional planning.

Outcome criteria

- The review is recorded to reflect collaboration, treatment plan design, goal identification, criteria application, and utilization of peer advisor.
- Reviewer record shows evidence of review and monitoring of dispositional planning.

Standard V: Intervention

Process criteria

The reviewer:
- acts to ensure that the health care needs of the patient are met through high-quality, cost-effective treatment in the least restrictive environment.
- acts as the patient's/family's advocate, when necessary, to facilitate the achievement of health.
- reviews and collaborates with providers to achieve the appropriate clinical outcomes within the benefit design.
- respects the nature of the therapeutic relationship.
- acts to ensure the confidentiality of patient information.

Outcome criteria

- A record of the reviewer's interventions is derived through the reviewer's documentation.
- Patients/families/providers report that they have been assisted/supported through the review process.
- Reviewer's documentation and actions protect the patient's confidentiality.

Standard VI: Evaluation

Process criteria

The reviewer:
- pursues validation of clinical information, suggestions, and new information.
- evaluates impressions and criteria application with peers and in supervision.
- applies recommended strategies to the review process.

Outcome criteria

- The review process and application of criteria are revised on the basis of the evaluation of clinical outcomes.
- Quality of care is reflective of cost-effectiveness.

A complete review requires application of all the following.
1. DSM-IV diagnostic criteria
2. Severity of illness criteria
3. Intensity of treatment criteria

Psychiatric criteria

Address areas related to:
1. Chronic conditions (nonacute)
2. Admissions in lieu of incarceration/legally mandated admissions
3. Inappropriate use of level of care to access benefit
4. Admissions for alternate living arrangements/lifestyle changes
5. Passes while in acute care/AWOL
6. Suicidality/homicidality assessment
7. Perseverance of severe symptoms despite aggressive intervention
8. Nonresponders to conventional treatment
9. Concomitant medical conditions (Axis III)
10. Length of stay related to program design
11. Treatment refusal

Chemical abuse criteria

Address areas related to:
1. Prior attempts rehab/failure to comply/rehab failures
2. Dual diagnosis or medical complications (Axes I, II, and III)
3. Support system assessment (Axes IV and V)
4. Prolonged withdrawal
5. Accessibility issues
6. Program model assessment
7. "Fear of relapse" issues
8. Detox regimen when evidence of withdrawal, which is life-threatening

OUTPATIENT CRITERIA

Initial Review

The following criteria are the basis for evaluating the medical necessity, appropriateness, and quality of the outpatient treatment services. After the initial number of contract specific visits, which do not require

precertification, outpatient treatment must meet all criteria in Section
A—Level of Functioning, at least one criterion from Section B—Functional Deficits, and all criteria in Sections C, D, and E in order to receive
certification without peer review.

A. Level functioning
   1. A condition diagnosed on Axis I or II of the DSM-IV.
   2. Reasonable expectation that the person is capable of making
      change as a result of the proposed treatment plan.
   3. Global Assessment of Functioning (GAF) of 70 or less, supported
      by the clinical data.

B. Functional deficits
   1. Evidence of *symptoms and/or behavior that produces identifiable
      impairment* (e.g., in performance on the job or in school; in
      meeting marital/parenting and/or social/interpersonal responsibilities; and/or in self-maintenance capacity).
   2. Potential for more serious illness without remediation of current condition.
   3. Readily identifiable potential for decompensation or life-threatening behaviors.
   4. Readily identifiable potential for loss of impulse control.

C. In addition to meeting the above criteria, the following must be met.
   1. Information, including mental status examination, current and
      prior mental health and chemical abuse history, psychological
      and laboratory/test results (if performed) must fit documented
      DSM-IV diagnosis.
   2. Impairments in central life role functions must correlate with
      DSM-IV diagnosis.
   3. If patient meets the criteria for psychoactive substance use disorder, treatment is being provided in a specialized chemical dependency program or organized aftercare program and involves
      regular attendance at appropriate community support groups.
   4. Patient is receiving medication and/or has been evaluated by a
      psychiatrist for a DSM-IV classified disorder generally considered
      to have biologically treatable causes and/or amenable to use of
      psychotropic medications.
   5. If patient is a minor, evidence of parental involvement in the
      treatment plan appropriate to the age and developmental level
      of the patient.
   6. Evidence of appropriate medical evaluation and/or treatment
      for concomitant medical conditions.
   7. Evidence that patients receiving psychopharmacotherapy are

reevaluated by a psychiatrist at least every three months and that, for those receiving neuroleptics, AIMS examinations are performed at six-month intervals.

8. Evidence that collateral contacts/support groups (families, social services agencies, AA, NA, CA, ACOA, OA, etc.) are utilized where appropriate.

9. Comprehensive treatment plan matches DSM-IV diagnosis(es), level of severity, and symptom(s) and/or behavior(s) that produce identifiable impairment.

D. In addition to meeting the above criteria, the proposed treatment *must not include:*

1. Psychotherapy solely for DSM-IV condition for disorder not considered amenable to this form of treatment alone.
2. More than one session per day with any one therapist.
3. More than one session per day per modality.
4. Same modality of treatment more than twice per week other than for crisis intervention, acute stabilization, and/or to prevent hospitalization.
5. Individual sessions that exceed 60 minutes in duration.
6. More than one therapist providing the same modality of treatment concurrently.
7. V-code diagnosis as sole or primary diagnosis.
8. Treatment services that are primarily educational or vocational in nature.
9. Psychopharmacotherapy by a nonphysician therapist.
10. Psychiatric services provided by a nonpsychiatrist M.D. or D.O., other than for medication monitoring.
11. Services provided that are beyond the therapist's scope of training.
12. Chronic condition without evidence of change resulting from proposed treatment.

E. If the request is for treatment *more than once per week,* the following criteria must be met.

1. Clinical data to support a diagnosis on Axis I or II *other than* 309.xx (Adjustment Disorders) except 309.21, Separation Anxiety Disorder, and 309.89, PTSD.
2. Global Assessment of Functioning of less than 60.
3. Patient must demonstrate level of central life role dysfunction that clearly supports the need for more intensive therapy. The more intensive the services that are requested, the more severe the level of dysfunction that should be documented.

OUTPATIENT CRITERIA

Concurrent Review

The following criteria are the basis for evaluating the medical necessity, appropriateness, and quality of the outpatient treatment services. Outpatient treatment must meet all criteria in Section A—Level of Functioning, at least one criterion from Section B—Functional Deficits, and all criteria in Sections C, D, and E in order to receive certification without peer review.

A. Level of functioning and B. Functional deficits.

B. In addition to meeting the above criteria, the following must be met.
   1. Adequate explanation of failure to achieve psychotherapeutic and/or psychopharmacological objectives, as evidenced by changes in treatment plan.
   2. Information, including mental status examination, current and prior mental health and chemical abuse history, and psychological and laboratory/test results (if performed) must fit documented DSM-IV diagnosis.
   3. Impairments in central life role functions must correlate with DSM-IV diagnosis.
   4. If patient meets the criteria for psychoactive substance use disorder, treatment is being provided in a specialized chemical dependency program or organized aftercare program and involves regular attendance at appropriate community support groups.
   5. Patient is receiving medication and/or has been evaluated by a psychiatrist for a DSM-IV classified disorder generally considered to have biologically treatable causes and/or to be amenable to use of psychotropic medications.
   6. If patient is a minor, evidence of parental involvement in the treatment plan appropriate to the age and developmental level of the patient.
   7. Evidence of appropriate medical evaluation and/or treatment for concomitant medical conditions.
   8. Evidence that patient receiving psychopharmacotherapy is reevaluated by a psychiatrist at least every three months and that, if receiving neuroleptics, AIMS examinations are performed at six-month intervals.
   9. Evidence of collateral contacts/support groups (families, social services agencies, AA, NA, CA, ACOA, OA, etc.) are utilized where appropriate.

10. Comprehensive treatment plan matches DSM-IV diagnosis(es), level of severity, and symptom(s) and/or behavior(s) that produce identifiable impairment.

C. In addition to meeting the above criteria, the proposed treatment *must not include:*
   1. Deterioration in GAF and/or central life role function assessment ratings without change in treatment plan.
   2. Psychotherapy solely for DSM-IV condition for disorder not considered amenable to this form of treatment alone.
   3. More than one session per day with any one therapist.
   4. More than one session per day per modality.
   5. Same modality of treatment more than twice per week other than for crisis intervention, acute stabilization, and/or to prevent hospitalization.
   6. Individual sessions that exceed 60 minutes in duration.
   7. More than one therapist providing the same modality of treatment concurrently.
   8. V-code diagnosis as sole or primary diagnosis.
   9. Treatment services that are primarily educational or vocational in nature.
   10. Psychopharmacotherapy by a nonphysician therapist.
   11. Psychiatric services provided by a nonpsychiatrist M.D. or D.O., other than for medication monitoring.
   12. Services provided that are beyond the therapist's scope of training.
   13. Chronic condition without evidence of change resulting from proposed treatment.

D. If the patient has been in treatment *more than once per week* and/or has been *seen weekly for more than one year,* he or she must also meet the following criteria.
   1. Clinical data to support a diagnosis on Axis I or II *other than* 309.xx (Adjustment Disorders) except 309.21, Separation Anxiety Disorder, and 309.89, PTSD.
   2. Global assessment of functioning of less than 60.
   3. Patient must demonstrate level of central life role dysfunction that clearly supports the need for more intensive therapy. The more intensive the services that are requested, the more severe the level of dysfunction that should be documented.

CHEMICAL ABUSE STRUCTURED OUTPATIENT CRITERIA

Initial Review

The following criteria are the basis for evaluating the medical necessity, appropriateness, and quality of the outpatient SOPS treatment services. SOPS treatment must meet all criteria in Section A—Level of Functioning, criteria from Section B—Functional Deficits, and all criteria in Sections C, D, and E in order to receive certification without peer review.

A. Level of functioning
   1. A psychoactive substance abuse condition diagnosed on Axis I of the DSM-IV.
   2. Reasonable expectation that the person is capable of making a change as a result of the proposed treatment plan.
   3. Global Assessment of Functioning (GAF) of 70 or less, supported by the clinical data. If patient is being evaluated for an intensive phase of SOPS treatment, GAF should be 60 or less.

B. Functional deficits
   1. Evidence of *symptoms and/or behavior that produces identifiable impairment* (e.g., in performance on the job or in school; in meeting marital/parenting and/or social/interpersonal responsibilities; and/or in self-maintenance capacity).
   2. If being considered for intensive phase of SOPS, patient must demonstrate level of central life role dysfunction that clearly supports the need for more intensive therapy. Examples would include serious impairment in role function and no prior chemical abuse treatment, dangerous drug-seeking behaviors, and denial of problem in spite of significant impairment in social or occupational functioning. The more intensive the services that are requested, the more severe the level of dysfunction that should be documented.

C. In addition to meeting the above criteria, the following must be met.
   1. Treatment is being provided in a specialized chemical dependency program or organized aftercare program and involves regular attendance at appropriate community support groups.
   2. If patient is a minor, evidence of parental involvement in the treatment plan appropriate to the age and developmental level of the patient.

3. Evidence that collateral contacts/support groups (families, social services agencies, AA, NA, CA, ACOA, OA, etc.) are utilized where appropriate.
4. Comprehensive treatment plan matches DSM-IV diagnosis(es), level of severity, and symptom(s) and/or behavior(s) that produce identifiable impairment.
5. Evidence of appropriate medical evaluation and/or treatment for concomitant medical conditions.
6. Evidence of urine/drug screen monitoring as part of the treatment planning.
7. Evidence of appropriate evaluation and/or treatment planning for concomitant DSM-IV disorders.

D. In addition to meeting the above criteria, the proposed treatment *must not include:*
1. Psychotherapy solely for DSM-IV condition for disorder not considered amenable to this form of treatment alone.
2. V-code diagnosis as sole or primary diagnosis.
3. Treatment services that are primarily educational or vocational in nature.
4. Psychopharmacotherapy by a nonphysician therapist.
5. Psychiatric services provided by a nonpsychiatrist M.D. or D.O., other than for medication monitoring.
6. Services provided that are beyond the therapist's scope of training.
7. Chronic condition without evidence of change resulting from proposed treatment.

CHEMICAL ABUSE STRUCTURED OUTPATIENT CRITERIA

Concurrent Review

The following criteria are the basis for evaluating the medical necessity, appropriateness, and quality of the outpatient chemical abuse treatment services. Outpatient treatment must meet all criteria in Section A—Level of Functioning, at least one criterion from Section B—Functional Deficits, and all criteria in Sections C, D, and E in order to receive certification without peer review.

A. Level of functioning
1. A condition diagnosed on Axis I of the DSM-IV (not in full remission).

2. Reasonable expectation that the person is capable of making change as a result of the proposed treatment plan.

B. Functional deficits
   1. Evidence of *symptoms and/or behavior that produces identifiable impairment* in performance on the job or in school; in meeting marital/parenting and/or social/interpersonal responsibilities; and/or in self-maintainance capacity.

C. In addition to meeting the above criteria, the following must be met:
   1. Adequate explanation of failure to achieve psychotherapeutic and/or psychopharmacological objectives, as evidenced by changes in treatment plan.
   2. Impairments in central life role functions must correlate with DSM-IV diagnosis.
   3. If patient meets the criteria for psychoactive substance use disorder, treatment is being provided in a specialized chemical dependency program or organized aftercare program and involves regular attendance at appropriate community support groups.
   4. Involvement or evidence of attempts to involve community and social support systems in treatment.
   5. If patient is a minor, evidence of parental involvement in the treatment plan appropriate to the age and developmental level of the patient.
   6. Evidence of appropriate medical evaluation and/or treatment for concomitant medical conditions.
   7. Evidence of urine/drug screen monitoring as part of the treatment planning.
   8. Evidence of appropriate evaluation and/or treatment for concomitant DSM-IV disorders.
   9. Evidence of collateral contacts/support groups (families, social services agencies, AA, NA, CA, ACOA, OA, etc.) are utilized where appropriate.

D. In addition to meeting the above criteria, the proposed treatment *must not include*:
   1. Deterioration in GAF and/or central life role function assessment ratings without change in treatment plan.
   2. V-code diagnosis as sole or primary diagnosis.
   3. Treatment services that are primarily educational or vocational in nature.
   4. Psychopharmacotherapy by a nonphysician therapist.

5. Psychiatric services provided by a nonpsychiatrist M.D. or D.O., other than for medication monitoring.
6. Services provided that are beyond the therapist's scope of training.
7. Chronic condition without evidence of change resulting from proposed treatment.
8. Individual therapy in the absence of a structured program.

E. If the patient has been in treatment *more than one year,* must also meet the following criteria.
1. Patient must demonstrate level of central life role dysfunction that clearly supports need for more extensive therapy for chemical dependency. There should be a clear expectation that the patient is capable of making further change in the chemical dependency issues as a result of the extended treatment. Treatment focus on such areas as character disorders, other DSM-IV conditions, or codependency should not be the focus in ongoing chemical dependency treatment. The more extensive the services that are requested, the more severe the level of dysfunction that should be documented.

2

The Paradox of Change:
Better Them Than Us!

LUCIANO L'ABATE, Ph.D.

To my mind, the most important development in psychoanalysis in recent years has been the growing recognition that intrapsychic phenomena must be understood in the context of the larger interactional systems in which they take form (Stolorow, 1991, p. 17).

After defining what is meant by change, this introductory chapter argues that five minimally necessary and possibly insufficient conditions necessary for change are (1) admitting the existence of problematic issues, problems, or symptoms that are not changing for the better; (2) allowing for external intervention to help change existing dysfunctional patterns; (3) receiving positive, direct and indirect communications about a client's sense of importance; (4) hoping that change is possible and that it can take place, if it is wanted and worked for; and (5) establishing a sense of control where controls have been either defective or missing.

Change in this chapter does not mean change just for clients. It also means change for the profession of psychotherapy. Why? We have to change in order to be a part of the managed care network, thus becoming "managed care providers." Psychotherapists want to help people change, but can they help change themselves as professionals? We cannot forget that "them" is "us." How do psychotherapists change themselves as people and as professionals? They supposedly know how to change themselves as people by putting themselves in the role of clients and making the psychotherapeutic experience part of their training. However, how many psychotherapists do put themselves in that position? Furthermore, how do psychotherapists change as professionals? How does a profession change its practices, if that change is possible at all? This argument begs the question "How is this change to take place?" In this chapter, various hypotheses will be advanced about helping clients change and bringing about change in the profession of psychotherapy. If change is good for clients, should not change be good for the profession? On the other hand, could it be that the field of psychotherapy is as deeply entrenched as most dysfunctional people, even to the point of denying its dysfunctionality?

Years ago, Rogers (1957) considered three necessary and sufficient conditions for change: empathy, warmth, and unconditional regard. Rogers' original considerations need further expansion by bringing up additional, also necessary, and probably insufficient, conditions for personal and professional change that he did not consider. His original conditions may have been necessary *then* from a monadic, humanistic viewpoint, but they seem rather insufficient *now* in view of further developments in the field of psychotherapy that stress attention to contextual factors. The three *sine qua non* conditions stressed by Rogers may be necessary and sufficient for certain individuals, but seem limited and limiting in view of further developments in marital and family therapy. They may be necessary, but they are definitely insufficient in helping severely dysfunctioning individuals, deeply entrenched conflictful couples; and dysfunctional families (L'Abate, 1986; Liddle, 1992; Stolorow, 1991). With character disorders, for instance, these qualities may be counterproductive. The client may be suspicious of these qualities as being too seductive and too manipulative. We know, of course, that these stylistic qualities do not work at all with schizophrenics.

Rogers' conditions refer to the style of the therapist, but have little if anything to say about structuring skills in psychotherapy. *Style* represents those relationship skills that are fundamental in starting the process of therapy. Structuring represents the *method* that is necessary to help people change, independent of the therapist's style. Both skills are necessary to help people change, especially couples and families. Hence, professional change will mean not only reconsidering style as a necessary but insufficient condition for psychotherapeutic change, but also reconsidering method as another necessary but insufficient condition to obtain change. Whether style and method together become sufficient to deal with human problems remains to be seen. We and our clients need both style and method to obtain results. While issues of style are so personal that they remain outside of the purpose of this chapter, issues of theory and method will be considered as being important for personal and professional change.

WHY CHANGE?

Why should change take place when it is not wanted? There are reluctant clients who do not want change even though other family members and professionals see the need. Why should the field of psychotherapy change when it sees no need for it? It is necessary from the outset to deal with denial as the major defense against change. How do psychotherapists deal with denial in their clients? The answer, of course, is: "In various ways." They first look at the roots and rationale for the denial. What prompted this individual, couple, or family to deny the referral problem, and, by extension, possibly the reality and painfulness of the situation? Underneath the denial there may be fear of the unknown, hopelessness, a threat to feelings of self-worth and self-esteem, and inadequacy. The process of denial, then, has little to do with any rational basis, but it has a great deal to do with an emotional one. By the same token, the fear of change in the psychotherapy profession is no different from the same fear of change in clients. We are not dealing with rationality. We are dealing with emotionality, an aspect that cannot be dealt with rationally. However, if professional change does not take place inside the psychotherapy profession, eventually it will be forced from the outside. Change is now being mandated through a variety of mechanisms, such as reductions in and restrictions on insurance and third party payments, managed care, and even elimination of mental health benefits if deemed too expensive and too inefficient (Giles, 1993; Goodman, Brown, & Deitz, 1992; Ridgewood Financial Institute, 1993; Winegar, 1992).

Wanting to Change

Hence, we have to ask ourselves: "How does change come about?" "Why and when do people want change?" There are at least three reasons for people to want change. The first reason is *necessity*. Change is wanted when the costs of staying the same are higher than the costs of changing. When faced by choices such as hospitalization, incarceration, divorce, or financial or emotional bankruptcy for self or for loved ones, and there is no other alternative but therapy, then people may accept the inevitable choice that seems less costly than others. In spite of this argument, of course, many dysfunctional people still refuse help, no matter how serious the consequences may be.

The second reason is *conflict*. When conflict, either internal or external, is too high, and, again, too costly, then people will consider cheaper alternatives. As Averill and Nunley (1992) concluded: "Of all the sources of novelty, perhaps none is more important than conflict" (p. 242). Whether change in therapy can be equated to novelty remains to be seen. However, the psychotherapy profession will not change unless there is sufficient conflict, both internal and external to the profession, to warrant a more effective course of action. The issue here, of course, is what that course of action should be.

The third and last reason for change is *coercion*. Although none of us, as people and as professionals, consider coercion in positive terms, if change does not take place from inside a profession, then it may be mandated by the outside. This coercion is already taking place. Many insurance companies demand accounting of treatment and severely limit the number of sessions available to their (our) clients. Mental health benefits, seen as too expensive by many insurance companies, are being written off from other health benefits. How can psychotherapists help when clients tell them from the outset that their insurance contracts limit the number of therapy sessions available? Should psychotherapists send clients away or should they consider more cost-effective, helpful strategies? Psychotherapists will have to learn to rely on group techniques more than on individual ones. The latter will become the luxury of those who can afford them, regardless of insurance benefits. Furthermore, in addition to learning to rely more on group techniques and less on individual ones, psychotherapists will need to enlarge their professional repertoire to include new ways of helping. They will have to use two other medias of intervention that, thus far, have been given short shrift by the psychotherapeutic community; that is, the written and nonverbal (see Table 2-1 on p. 52). Is that enlargement to other media too painful to consider? Are psychotherapists so rigid and entrenched in their practices that they cannot add a few new skills to their traditional (mostly verbal) repertoires?

What Does Change Mean?

If we have learned anything about changing in the last generation of practice and research in the field of psychotherapy (Ehrenwald, 1991; Freedheim, 1992), then we should be able to summarize what change means. For change to take place, four minimum components seem necessary. They may well be insufficient. Change takes place when there is a *new* response that is also *positive* and *strong* enough to be incorporated in one's repertoire by making a distinct difference and giving *direction* to one's life (Prochaska, DiClemente, & Norcross, 1992). Thus, novelty, positiveness, strength, and direction describe, at least in part, the process of change. A new experience becomes positive to the extent that the professional helper affirms the client's individual worth directly and indirectly, by, among others, listening and complimenting efforts to change. Meeting regularly with a professional listener and helper is a new and positive experience that becomes strong enough in its weekly repetition.

The first component of *newness* or *novelty* is defined by any experienced attitude, feeling, or behavior that was not previously present in the past and that becomes available in a person's emotional, cognitive, and behavioral repertoire. This new experience is, therefore, *different* from past ones—even if it had been potentially available, it had not been used heretofore. This is a new experience for those who have not been listened to in their past lives. Talking about him- or herself to someone who listens and who seems to care, who responds to inner feelings, is a new, positive, and exciting experience, in a way that may not have been in times of past experiences. In the client's past, feelings and subjective perceptions may have been discounted and even punished.

The second component of change requires a new response to be of a *positive* nature, defined as self-enhancing and rewarding behavior that does not damage anyone else. After all, a person can change for the worse by either doing nothing or by using negative means. A new positive behavior is one that helps someone feel good, enhanced, and whole as a human being, and hurts no one. This sense of positivity is achieved through (1) hearing someone in authority affirming the validity of a client's perceptions as determined by attendant feelings, and (2) having an affirmation of the validity and importance of past, painful experiences that have been negatively influential in his or her life. These two aspects (regularity of meetings and talking), in and by themselves, may be sufficient to make a difference in someone's life. Positive affirmation and reframing can be a new experience where negativity may have been the hallmark of past experiences.

As Cantor and Kihlstrom (1987) suggested, effecting change is based on avoiding what they called old scripts and learning new ones (pp. 227–234), while persisting in efforts to change and reflecting on the self. Persistence means frequent repetition, practice, and rehearsal that may increase the habitual preeminence of this new behavior, a third component of change characterized by *strength*. This quality of strength is added when a person's perceptions and experiences are affirmed and validated *repeatedly*. Strength also means any behavior that is forceful, intense, and powerful enough to make a difference in how someone is going to live the rest of his or her life. This difference is seen in Rogers' "corrective emotional experience," so-called peak experiences, or even routine repetition and repetitive practice of new and positive behaviors.

These three components of change can be reframed as being based on *frequency and duration* of appointments and positive affirmations, and on *intensity* in the emotional experience of meeting with someone to share intense and painful feelings and emotions. A fourth component of *direction* is necessary to find out how we learn from past experiences to change our lives toward more rewarding and realistic goals. It is possible to have novelty, positiveness, and strength, but without direction as to how to use these components they could lead us around in circles, as in a maze, without pointing energy and efforts toward rewarding goals.

Thus, the psychotherapeutic experience allows for the acquisition and emission of new responses that were not experienced or present in a client's past repertoire, either emotively, cognitively, or behaviorally. For instance, preset appointments help achieve some sense of regularity, predictability, and stability, where none was present in the past. This regularity is important to establish or reestablish a sense of control where controls, in the past, either were not present or, at best, were weak and inadequate.

Given these components of change, why are so many people (professionals are people too!) afraid of it? Among the many possibilities that come to mind, the following are derived from clinical practice: (1) change so defined is too demanding of a person's limited resources; thus (2) change is a threat that may prove his or her "badness," "craziness," or inadequacy, with the threat of possible banishment and hospitalization; (3) the inability to change in general is a lifelong pattern that has in itself produced and propounded the problem, as seen in addictions, borderline cases, and psychoses; (4) rejection of treatment is part of a pattern of overall denial of dependency and a proclamation of independence that does not allow the consideration that the human condition is characterized by interdependence—so-called independence does not exist because we are all, in one way or another, interdependent on one another; and (5) the loss of power, especially in dyadic and family relationships, where the one who has the most power combined with little on no responsibility, stereotypically the man, sees change as a threat to that position. No wonder that men are the ones who are most threatened by change and who find it most difficult to accept psychotherapy as a benign process.

Hence, change is no different from other behavioral dimensions of (1) *duration,* as seen in the length of a therapy session and a sequence, however short or long, of sessions; (2) *frequency* of positive experiences, the peak experiences that take place inside and outside the therapist's office, or rate of appointments, if these can be equated to frequency of positive experiences; (3) *intensity* of depth and strength in the experience; and (4) *direction,* which is just as important as any other component. All four components intermingle in the therapeutic experience.

THE NECESSARY (BUT INSUFFICIENT!) CONDITIONS FOR CHANGE

The foregoing definition of change, a process characterized by novel, positive, frequent, intense, and focused behaviors, is independent of the process necessary, to obtain change. If we have learned anything from systems thinking, it is that the first condition necessary for change in any system, be it physical, human (individual, dyadic, or multirelational, like a family), philosophical, or otherwise, is to admit that it needs external intervention. It can no longer cope or survive with its existing resources. *Calling a professional and asking for help is the first step in producing change.* Sometimes this step may be all that is necessary. The admission in itself may provoke a critical reexamination of the system's assets and liabilities that may prompt and provoke a change. Most therapists are aware of many potential clients who have called for help and who, when called back for their failure to follow through with the initial call, indicated how they no longer needed the sought-after help. After the initial call, apparently they came up with some new conclusion about or solution for their problem. These people may be a minority. Nevertheless, they suggest that the admission of the problem is the first step toward its solution. Admission of one's weakness, as indicated even by a simple phone call, takes a lot of strength and may lead toward a reexamination of one's way of living. Very dysfunctional systems may be too weak and unable to ask for help, as in the case of addictive, borderline, criminal, and psychotic systems.

Thus, a necessary condition for change in an ailing, dysfunctional system is to ask for and obtain external intervention. In the most frequent functional conditions, this intervention may consist of talking with a friend or family member, reading a self-help book, going to a concert, meditating and reflecting, taking a trip, or attending a lecture.

What happens when we are confronted by more dysfunctioning conditions? Here we need to differentiate among degrees of dysfunctionality. For instance, most shy individuals could learn from an assertiveness training workshop or similar social skill training. People who are not only shy but also withdrawn and fearful, however, will need more than preventive, psychoeducational preventions (Anderson, Reiss, & Hogarty, 1986; L'Abate, 1990; Lieberman, DeRisi, & Mueser, 1989; McFarlane, 1991). They may need therapeutic interventions in their various compositions (individual, group, marital, or family).

The second condition necessary for change in any system is for intervention to take place from outside that system. As much as we may dislike mechanical metaphors or analogies, we must realize that just as any dysfunctioning machine or motor needs a mechanic and a possible change or realignment of defective parts, so do human systems. We all need outside intervention to change. Even a small cut, if unwashed and ignored, may fester and deteriorate into a dangerous infection. Why should we think that human systems are any different from or better than physical systems to the extent that both types need external intervention to change? We readily admit to a machine's needing an external replacement or adjustment to keep on working. However, we are not willing to admit the same principle for ourselves. For instance, cliches such as "Marriages are made in heaven" testify to the same kind of fatalistic and optimistic thinking. Somehow, no matter how terrible things are, relationships (and individuals) will fix themselves by themselves and without external intervention. Behind this thinking there are apathy, helplessness, and a tremendous fear of change and of confronting the unknown ("The devil I know is better than the devil I don't know!").

There is no dysfunctioning system, physical or human, abstract or concrete, that can adjust, fix itself, and survive from the inside. We may not like the analogy of psychological systems with physical ones. However, we may need to ask what makes us think that psychological systems are any better than physical ones. What evidence do we have that dysfunctioning psychological systems have a greater or different ability to fix themselves than do physical systems? A great deal of this thesis relies on the nature of external intervention. It would not need to be only psychotherapy. Any kind of positive, external intervention or service of sufficient intensity and regularity may produce change. This change may take place provided that it matches the immediate and transcendent needs of clients and that clients themselves are able and willing to absorb and assimilate it for the better. This optimal match has been the goal of psychotherapy theory and research since its very outset.

The third necessary condition is to give clients a sense of importance or status, as in resource exchange theory (Foa, Converse, Tornblom, & Foa, 1993; Foa & Foa, 1974). This sense of importance is basic to the establishment of intimate human relationships, and to exchanges with those relationships (L'Abate, 1994). Without the establishment of this sense of importance, it would be difficult to help people who want our help. How is this sense of importance communicated? It is communicated both directly and indirectly, verbally and nonverbally. It is communicated directly by (1) listening to someone's problems and plight; (2) affirming the validity of someone's perceptions, and (3) asserting the seriousness of the problem as perceived by the person reporting it. It is communicated verbally by reframing positively the request for help. ("Only people who care for themselves ask for help." "You must care a lot about yourself [or each other] if you were strong enough to ask for help;" "You must be very strong because mostly strong people ask for help, weak people are too weak to ask.") It is communicated indirectly and nonverbally by therapists behaving with clients as if the clients were guests in their therapists' offices and accepting the clients' plights as if they were the therapists' own.

The fourth condition necessary for change is to give a sense of hope that through appropriate help, change for the better can and will take place. Thus, the client must be reassured that admitting a problem and asking for help, regardless of the objective seriousness of the problem, are relevant and important to the professional helper. Furthermore, the subjective acceptance of the seriousness of the problem itself, rather than its objective outcome, is necessary to give reassurance that the problem can be solved and that change will bring about such a solution. ("This is a very serious problem, but with your help, I think we can work on it.")

The fifth necessary condition for change is to give clients a sense of control and mastery over their lives (Deci & Ryan, 1987; Gibbs, 1982, 1989; Horvitz, 1990; Hunt, 1971; Langer, 1983; Rodin, Schooler, & Schaie, 1990; Wegner & Pennebaker, 1993). People want help because their lives or someone in their lives is out of control. However, how is a sense of control and mastery to be achieved? The references cited here concerning this topic focus on dialectical or empirical aspects of control. They do not give any hint or suggestion as to how to help people reestablish a sense of control and mastery over their lives. Past behavioristic positions have simplistically stressed the importance of immediate consequences and contingent reinforcements. However, these positions have been shown to be practically, philosophically, and empirically limited in helping complex human systems. We are controlled by external reinforcements as well as by internal emotional attitudes and cognitions that direct our behavior above and beyond immediate and concrete reinforcements. Many people work for internal and abstract, if not transcendental, reasons. Behavioral positions deal strictly with the output of behavior, not with the input, and in that regard they remain incomplete and wanting. Control is achieved when access, input, and the beginning of any behavior sequence, *as well as* the exit, output, and end of that sequence, are regulated. It is just as important to help people establish a sense of control at the input, from the beginning of the undesirable behavior ("If you want to stop it, start it") as well as at the output, its end (L'Abate, 1986, 1994).

How is control established in real life? In actual, everyday reality, control consists of beginning a behavior, such as going to work at a certain, predetermined time, and leaving work at a given, preestablished time. Employers control their employees by requiring them to show up at an established time and to leave at another predetermined time. If employees are late, they have to come up with a good excuse, and if they want to leave earlier, they also have to come up with a good reason. In certain cases, employees are penalized for any deviation from the agreed-upon norm of preestablished starting and ending times. Thus, control is established through regulation of inputs (entrances, beginnings, accesses) as well as outputs (exits and endings).

This real-life analogy is also a rationale for establishing controls during the process of psychotherapy. We give our clients a preset time, and thus appointment time and duration are established in a predictable, regular, and repeatable sequence. Sometimes this sequence may not be sufficient, or it may be too expensive or too lengthy. Consequently, it may be necessary to require a parallel process of homework meetings and written assignments at preset, prearranged times to increase repetitive predictability and establish regularity (L'Abate, 1986, 1992). The quality of *regularity,* established as well by a person's brushing her teeth three times a day, having meals, and going to and coming home from work at the same time every day, helps create a sense of control. The establishment of regularity over the beginning and end of any behavioral sequence, plus directions as to what should happen in between, *is* control. Very likely, without a sense of repetitive regularity, such a sense of control would not be established.

The regularity of therapy appointments has a great deal to do with a client's establishing or reestablishing a sense of mastery and control over his or her life. Regularity of therapy appointments is doubled by requiring clients to have regular home meetings to match and parallel the frequency of therapy sessions. This practice of regular home meetings, although based on personal impressions, whether required of individuals, couples, or families, seems to produce a faster increase in a sense of mastery than just the regularity of therapy sessions alone. Once this double regularity (at home and in the therapist's office) is accepted and agreed upon from the outset of the therapeutic relationship (through a written contract), it is incumbent on the therapist to administer sufficient written homework to make sure that the therapy hour is even more effective and productive by enlarging and strengthening the sphere of therapeutic influence from the therapy office to the home (L'Abate, 1986, 1990, 1992). More about the nature of these homework assignments in Chapter 6 of this volume.

THE CONTEXT OF CHANGE: THE MAGICAL NUMBER 3

Once we define *what* change consists of and we specify the conditions necessary for change, we beg the question of *where* change is to take place. The answer to this question can be found, in part, in Stolorow's quotation at the beginning of this chapter—in larger interactional systems. As soon as we answer in this fashion, however, we have to define what these systems consist of. We assume without questioning that change needs to take place within intimate relationships and within the individuals who determine these relationships. Furthermore, we need to specify that change should be in relationships that matter; that is, in enduring, committed, close, and prolonged relationships that are based on interdependence. This specification is not sufficient because these relationships are embedded in a cultural context that needs specification as well. Contextually, dysfunctionality takes place at various individual, dyadic, or multirelational levels, especially in the family as a whole unit of interacting personalities. One cannot change at the individual level without impinging on and influencing change in those who live close by or who are related by blood, legal, or emotional ties.

A more comprehensive viewpoint, above and beyond interdependent relationships, would need to pinpoint where change is to take place, once we consider larger interactional systems as representing the context for change. Once we break down the rather general and encompassing term "context" into three specific settings, we obtain a matrix of three larger interactional systems that would include (1) communication media through which we exchange resources, either nonverbal, spoken, or written, (2) settings; and (3) resource modalities (Figure 2-1).

Communication Media

The three media of communication, as summarized in Table 2-1, are fairly well defined inside and outside the therapy office. Ideally, there

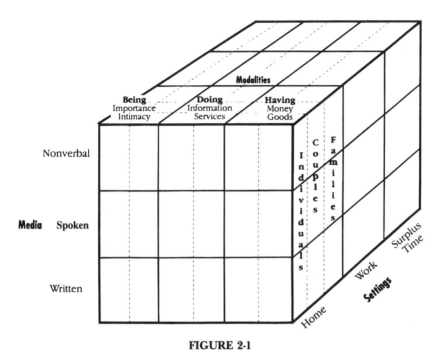

FIGURE 2-1

The Context of Change.

should be an isomorphic process going on between the therapist's office and the other three settings—home, work, and leisure. As Table 2-1 shows, thus far therapists have used one-third of the three available communication media. The traditional overreliance on the spoken medium at the expense of the other two has severely curtailed the options available to us and to our clients. In the future, *change for therapists will include learning how to use judiciously the other two media of communication, nonverbal and written, in addition to the spoken. Once these two media are added to the therapeutic armamentarium, the other change will be consist of decreasing the number of individual sessions and increasing group, couple, and family sessions.* Once these two changes are in place, it will be easier to help more people for each unit of the therapist's time than ever before. In addition to the three media mentioned here, there is the kinesthetic medium that is just as important as the other three media, but is included along with the nonverbal.

Settings

We may assume that the family is the primary setting, but that is not necessarily the only setting that affects the client. The family setting

TABLE 2-1

Media of Communication and Functions of Intervention Settings

Media of Communication	Functions of Intervention Settings	
	Inside Therapist's Office	*Outside Therapist' Office*
Spoken	Evaluation Emotional Support Confrontation of Issues Motivation for Change Generalization to Outside	Dialogue with: self, partner, relatives, family of origin, friends, children, and coworkers
Nonverbal	Awareness Exercises Nonverbal Communication Calistenics, Aerobics Dance, Art, Play Biofeedback Kinesiology	Sports and Exercise Nutrition–Diet Vitamins Meditation
Written	Toward a Classification of Writing	

Structure	Content	Goal	Format
Open Focused Guided Programmed	Traumatic vs. Trivial	Cathartic vs. Prescriptive	General vs. Specific

From L'Abate, 1994. Most of the foregoing verbal functions can also take place without face-to-face contact between therapists and clients. For instance, they can take place long distance through the written modality, depending on the client and the situation.

may be the most immediate and major focus of therapy. However, there are other settings, each with its own peculiar and specific task demands, that influence clients' lives. There are work and surplus time activities, for instance, that have a great deal of influence—in some cases, they have more influence than either family or work settings. Witness the influence of religion, for instance, and sport addictions, such as running, that in some cases are stronger in their influence than either family or work settings (Yates, 1991). Surplus time is included in whatever time is left after home and work responsibilities are done. This time includes transitory settings, such as banks, bars, beauty salons, houses of worship, grocery stores, hospitals, libraries, schools, stadiums, sport arenas, and shopping malls. These settings are necessary for enjoyment and survival, but they do not have the permanency and primary survival value of home and work. Surplus time also includes transit settings that are necessary to go from one setting to another. These settings include airports, bus stations, cars, highways, roads, trains, and hotels.

Resource Modalities

While the three communication media and three settings may be obvious, the three modalities mentioned here may not be as explicit. These modalities were derived from resource exchange theory (Foa, Converse, Tornblom, & Foa, 1993; Foa and Foa, 1974). This theory posited that six resource classes are exchanged (given and received) between and among individuals. These classes are status, love, information, services, goods (or possessions), and money. The six classes can be condensed into three modalities. The first modality consists of being or *presence*, being emotionally available to self and to important others. It combines status and love, renamed, respectively, as the attribution of importance to self and intimacy. The latter is defined as the ability to share joys and pleasures, as well as hurts and fears of being hurt. The second modality consists of doing or *performance*, combining information with services. The third modality consists of having or *production*, combining money with possessions. The combination of performance and production defines the concept of power (L'Abate, 1994).

Hence, personality can be defined interpersonally through competences in being, doing, and having (L'Abate, 1986, 1994). The two major dimensions of interpersonal living would be *presence* and *power*. Presence, the ability to love, is nonnegotiable in its receptive aspects, but it can be negotiated in its expressive ones. We do not need to argue about our subjectively receptive feelings of love for someone. However, we may need to negotiate how those feelings are expressed to accommodate to that someone's needs and wishes. Power, on the other hand, is negotiated in functional relationships and nonnegotiable or poorly negotiated in dysfunctional ones. Thus, the theory's major assumptions lie in the ability to love and the ability to negotiate. These abilities are lacking in our clients in one way or another. Ultimately, these two are the abilities that need to be taught to them, directly or indirectly, if we therapists know how. If we do not, how can we help our clients?

From this vantage point, then, therapy means helping individuals, couples, and families change their concerns with performance and production to concerns about presence and the ability to love. Admittedly performance and production are necessary for survival, but they are not sufficient for full enjoyment as well as survival. Dysfunctional individuals need help to increase presence; that is, they must learn to become more emotionally available to themselves and to important others. Changes need to be made in how clients prioritize the relative values of media, modalities, and settings. By changing one part, change may reverberate to other parts of the context thus defined, producing the so-called ripple effect so dear to systems thinking.

Given three communication media, three settings where exchanges take place, and three exchange modalities, we now have constructed a framework of larger interactional systems that defines the overall context of change (see Figure 2-1). Once we have this definition of context, then we can specify in greater detail one of the major maxims of systems thinking, namely, that *change in one part of this context may affect other parts of the same context.* Interconnectedness and wholism are useful systems concepts that are represented concretely by the analogy of the ripple effect. However, compared with the rest of systems thinking, this proposal, as summarized in Figure 2-1, shows some advantages over traditional systems thinking that were not possible heretofore. This proposal includes manageably *finite* and *limited* processes rather than infinite and unlimited ones. Consequently, these processes are more *specific* and *detailed* in comparison with rather general, undefined, and vague concepts of systems thinking. They are also more *concrete* than the abstract notions of systems thinking ((L'Abate & Colondier, 1987; Merkel & Searight, 1992; Searight & Merkel, 1991). Consequently, because of these characteristics—finiteness, specificity, and concreteness—this proposal is more verifiable than systems thinking, which, as a whole, is difficult to evaluate and verify.

CHANGE FROM CLIENTS TO PROFESSIONALS

The process of change for our clients should possess the same components for psychotherapists. We psychotherapists, however, are at least as resistant to change as some of the clients we want to help, if not more so. For instance, how does the principle of external intervention apply when the ailing system is an organization, or, at even a higher supraordinate level, a whole profession? What will it take for the entire profession of psychotherapy to acknowledge the need for external intervention? The first necessary step for external intervention to take place, of course, lies in the profession itself acknowledging and admitting the need for change. Without this initial acknowledgment and admission there would not be room or reason for external intervention to take place. The admission of a need for external help, however, can only take place if and when the profession admits to the need for change, but "what change?"

Professional change will take place when psychotherapists start implementing new, positive practices with sufficient intensity and strength to make a difference for themselves and for their clients. The major change will be in terms of cost-effectiveness; that is, greater effectiveness in clinical procedures, more clients per unit of therapist's time, and consequently, lower costs for clients. This is a direction quite different from existing practices, where cost-effectiveness and accountability, among other criteria, are not even addressed and are, in fact, avoided, if not scorned. This change, of course, implies frequently using new, positive, and powerful practices that have not been used in the past, as suggested earlier.

Admitting that the field of psychotherapy may need change, a position that many therapists would not be willing to accept, of what would this change consist? How can this change take place if the therapeutic community denies that it needs change? It takes conflict and pain to ask for change and help from the outside. After all, the field of psychotherapy is by now (1) well *institutionalized* to the point of being a tax-deductible item in the formal IRS tax returns; (2) quite *successful* in providing a fairly good living and important status for most of its competent practitioners; (3) fairly *organized* in various, large, and growing professional mental health organizations and disciplines; (4) largely *spread out* and still *growing* among various mental health disciplines; and (5) sufficiently *pervasive* at all private and public levels of enterprise. With all these positive qualities, how can one argue for dysfunctionality and the need for change?

It would be necessary to make the unpopular and questionable case for change in the same term that it would be made for any change-resistant human system that is receiving rewards for its dysfunctionality. Addicts, for instance, strongly deny their need for therapy because they do not want change to take place. As long as their addiction gives them pleasure that they would not receive otherwise, why should they change? By the same token, the psychotherapeutic community would resist and attack any position that would speak to its supposedly sick or seemingly unhealthy condition, when so many rewards, as listed above, are available.

What are the characteristics of an unhealthy organization? How can a case be made for dysfunctionality in what seems an otherwise very healthy, successful, and well-functioning profession? Whoever is willing to make this case runs the risk of professional retribution, even rejection and banishment. In spite of possibly disastrous consequences, this chapter will make a proposal for change at the professional level. This proposal derives from what we know about changing clients, whether this knowledge is relevant to changing a profession or not. As Liddle (1992) notes:

> For clinicians to change their personal practice model in a way that would incorporate empirical values requires not only new information, examples to learn from, and new modes of thinking but also a way of dealing with the emotional aspects of a change of this nature (p. 256).

Research, however, is not a characteristic of a profession, and it is very doubtful whether it will ever be. Research is mostly an academic pursuit based on transcendental determinism and objective, public, and intersubjective demonstrability. A profession usually is based on dialectical immediacy and private, personal profitability (L'Abate, 1986, 1994; Stricker, 1992). Hence, we are faced by two quite different value systems. The sooner we accept them as being almost mutually exclusive, the better off we shall be. There may be a few professionals who are able to balance and integrate both value systems. However, these few may not be greater than 3 to 5% of the whole psychotherapy profession. How can a small minority influence change for the majority? That task is clearly unrealistic and bound to fail.

If we change our traditional clinical and professional practices and the analogy of a ripple effect is valid, then we should be able to change ourselves as people at home, at work, and in leisure time activities. If flexibility (rather than rigidity) is the characteristic of a functional system, should this quality reflect itself in everything we are, do, or have? If we are indeed open to change, should psychotherapists not be more amenable to change than even their clients? By enlarging personal and professional repertoires should psychotherapists not be able to help a wider number of clients? If psychotherapists do not change, how can they expect their clients to change? One of the few examples of professional change over time, derived from self-critical feedback, is the one illustrated by the work of Selvini-Palazzoli (Selvini-Palazzoli, Cirillo, Selvini, & Sorrentino, 1989). Of course, there may be other examples of which this author is not aware.

SHORTCOMINGS IN THE PROFESSION OF PSYCHOTHERAPY

As traditionally practiced through the spoken medium, there are many shortcomings in the profession of psychotherapy that are either denied or swept under the rug of avoidance and even arrogance. Among those that come to mind are (1) a proliferation of therapeutic approaches, a number ranging into the hundreds; (2) immediate denial of negative feedback—whoever is foolish enough to raise criticisms about the status of the psychotherapy profession (to provide negative feedback) is either ignored or personally criticized for whatever arguments are used to bolster such criticisms; (3) entrenchment and rigidity in its practices, because of their undeniable and evident success—if a good living is to be made in this practice, why change it?; (4) conflicts, splits, disagreements, and division (a) among theoretical positions, many of them with mutually antagonistic clinical practices; (b) in the failure of evaluation to direct practice, where most research on diagnostic and evaluative instruments takes place without treatment, and where treatment takes place without evaluation; (c) in the failure of research to direct evaluation and practice; (d) between research and practice through avoidance of evaluation of outcome as standard operating procedures; (e) in the unbridled and uncritical acceptance of untested and untestable therapeutic gimmicks and gurus; (f) in the adoption of techniques on the basis of their seductive appeal or the charismatic influence of their leader rather than their proven usefulness; (g) in the avoidance of joining and integrating with preventive, psychoeducational approaches; (h) in an obsessive avoidance of empirical verifiability and professional accountability; (i) in the traditional overreliance on the spoken medium with parallel underreliance on both nonverbal and written media; and (j) overreliance on individual approaches rather than using groups, couples, and families, making therapy more expensive than it needs to be.

The best example for the denial of reality that surrounds the profession of psychotherapy is the trend toward skyrocketing costs in physical and mental health, with little attention paid by the profession to cost-effectiveness and accountability in treatment (L'Abate, 1990, 1992). If these trends persist—and there is no evidence to show that they will not—ultimately psychotherapeutic practices, as currently exist, will be insufficient to deal with many ills of our society and to provide adequate services for those who need them. Considering the millions of people needing help, half a million therapists and counselors will not be enough. Psychotherapy based on the spoken word is a drop in the bucket, and an expensive drop at that! Furthermore, as long as we limit ourselves to the spoken word and fail to use the other two media available to us, we will fail to find out which medium is best for which group of people. As a result, our clinical practices are destined to remain static and unchanging (L'Abate, 1990). Yes, we are a much-needed profession, well established in the mainstream of American culture. If psychotherapists can add to the tremendous strides made in the last quarter of a century and to the assets we have accumulated over the same period, we will increase the relevance of psychotherapy manyfold over what has been accomplished thus far.

THE CHALLENGE OF MANAGED CARE

Managed care in mental health care is here to stay, whether therapists like it or not. Therapists are going to face being questioned about their practices, demonstrating their results, and defending their fees (Giles, 1993; Goodman, Brown, & Deitz, 1992; Ridgewood Financial Institute [RFI], 1993; Winegar, 1992). The issue of effectiveness, and especially cost-effectiveness, is now becoming paramount: "Clearly, the ability to measure the clinical effectiveness of psychotherapy is emerging as an important marketing tool for both medical care companies and therapists" (RFI, 1993, p. 34). Cost containment and continuous quality improvement will become standard criteria of evaluation. Therapists will need to "establish standard clinical problem-solving methods that can be measured against treatment outcomes" (RFI, 193, p. 34).

As Goodman, Brown, and Dietz (1992) summarize these issues:

> "Private practice" is becoming an endangered species. Unless mental healthcare practitioners can articulate what they are doing for their patients and also convincingly explain why they are doing it, purchasers and providers [of mental health insurance] are going to be increasingly unwilling to pay for their services. If mental healthcare services are too subjective to quantify, they "may well be too subjective to pay for" ... Practitioners are being asked to articulate their clinical rationale for the recommended treatment, and, for the first time, to provide the supportive, convincing clinical evidence that is the basis for that treatment decision—what is known as "articulating the process of care." Clinicians are not systematically educated about the value of articulating and documenting their own (usually intuitively accurate and preconscious) thought processes. Instead, they are trained to make the expedient, though tunneled, leap from diagnosis to treatment with nary a glance into the chasm of treatment choices and alternative care options that have become the focus of today's external reviewers (p. 15).

Winegar (1992) warned therapists who fail to heed the call for managed care, cost containment, and cost-effectiveness:

Those professionals who fail to understand these revolutionary changes will see their ability to provide services to their clients and to control their professional futures greatly diminished. Those who do understand these changes, and understand that all practitioners in the coming years will be involved in this revolution, will not only exercise more control over their practices and professional lives, but prosper and grow in this era of change. (p. 1)

The above indicates that these changes are mandated from outside the profession, leaving no choice to psychotherapists but to change if they want to survive. Thus, the dreaded danger of external coercion, the demand for accountability that was scorned by most therapists in the past, and an emphasis on pragmatic demonstrability rather than dialectical aesthetics will stress the role of the therapist as a scientist rather than as an artist. Style alone will no longer be sufficient to demonstrate results. What method(s) are used and what results are obtained will be the bottom line of clinical practice. Therapists will have no choice but to use additional media of communication and more cost-effective group compositions. This conclusion also means that therapists will have to start using objective evaluations on a pre-posttreatment basis, learning to rely on writing as a cost-effective medium of communication not only with their clients, but also with the insurance providers.

A PROPOSAL FOR PROFESSIONAL CHANGE

Among all the many cost-effective possibilities that will be considered in this book, change in the psychotherapy profession can and will take place by (1) enlarging our psychotherapeutic practices from overreliance on the spoken word and adding the nonverbal and written media to our mostly spoken interventions (Bloom, 1992; L'Abate, 1986, 1990, 1992; Pennebaker, 1990), as shown in Table 2-1; (2) enlarging our composition to include individuals in groups, couples, and families, and to spend less time in individual face-to-face contact; (3) requiring evaluation at the outset and reevaluation at the end of the treatment process as standard operating procedure, a process that clinical psychologists were trained to do but that was forgotten in the immediate heat of helping clients and making a living; and (4) submitting our results to the scrutiny of professional peers or review boards.

These are four practices to which the psychotherapy profession is strongly resistant on the basis of a variety of relevant and irrelevant arguments. Ultimately, as discussed above, the decision to change and to incorporate new or more cost-effective practices is being mandated by health providers, because change in current therapeutic practices will not take place otherwise. Initial resistance to the use of writing in psychotherapy practice, either by itself or in conjunction with verbal and nonverbal media, is inevitable. Reliance on the nonverbal and written media as additions or as alternatives to the spoken medium is going to increase slowly but inevitably. While the nonverbal medium includes so many techniques (Table 2-1), making it difficult to compare it with the other two media, the spoken and written media can be compared in terms of their respective advantages and disadvantages (L'Abate, 1994). While both spoken and nonverbal media may require direct, face-to-face contact with a therapist or trainer, writing does not require this contact. It allows therapists to work from a distance, a practice that may have its advantages and disadvantages (L'Abate, 1992; L'Abate & Platzman, 1991). This topic will be discussed in greater detail Chapter 6 in this volume and, eventually, in a separate volume (L'Abate & Baggett, 1997).

Enlarging Psychotherapeutic with Preventive Practices

By enlarging and expanding therapeutic practices, we should be able to solve a much wider range of problems than by relying only on the spoken word. For instance, by introducing nonverbal approaches we may help individuals whose intellectual and educational functioning is lower than ours, and who are not as comfortable relying on the spoken word as we are. This population could include clients of lower socioeconomic status or those who have character disorders and are action rather than introspection oriented. We are so used to relying on the spoken word that we tend to forget that there are many other people who are not as comfortable with it as we are.

In addition to the above changes, therapists may consider enlarging their practices by supervising selected middle-level professionals or lower-level paraprofessionals in the use of psychoeducational, social skills training programs that, as a whole, have been used in preventive programs and not in psychotherapy as traditionally practiced (Anderson, Reiss, & Hogerty, 1986; Gordon & Gordon, 1981; L'Abate, 1990; Liberman, DeRisi, & Mueser, 1989; McFarlane, 1991).

Enlarging Group Composition and Comparing Cost Efficiency Among Compositions and Media

Cost efficiency must include the group composition of our clients interacting with one of the three media. For instance, group composition is much cheaper than individual composition per unit of a professional helper's time. Nonverbal approaches would be more effective with groups than with individuals, because their use with individuals would be as expensive per unit of a professional helper's time as the spoken medium. Of the three media, the written may be the cheapest yet, whereas the spoken, especially with individuals, may be the most expensive.

Face-to-face contact with an individual client is the norm in traditional psychotherapeutic practices. It is also the most expensive because it fills up the therapist's time. As soon as a therapist adds one more client in the office, the cost of the therapy hour is halved. By adding a third client in the same office, the cost is reduced by one third, and so on. Of course, our clients want the privacy and privilege of being seen individually, because they see themselves as losing face, or other characteristics, by being in a group. Yet group therapy is certainly more cost effective than individual psychotherapy. Insurance providers, therefore, will have to insist, and even demand, that clients will be reimbursed for group therapy, and only in exceptional cases for individual sessions. Standard insurance practices still reinforce the use of individual sessions; only under special conditions do they reimburse marital and family therapy. In fact, many insurance companies do not reimburse either marital or family therapy.

Not only are group sessions cheaper than individual sessions, but the use of written homework assignments in parallel with face-to-face sessions may also decrease the number of sessions needed to achieve the desired outcome. Once we introduce these two factors into cost effectiveness, more people can be helped for each unit of a professional's time.

Evaluation as Standard Operating Procedure

The normative state of affairs in the mental health field consists of practitioners doing psychotherapy without evaluation and researchers doing evaluation without psychotherapy. There is a great deal of research on evaluative instruments (L'Abate & Bagarozzi, 1993). It is really not necessary to proffer evidence to support this conclusion—a perusal of the majority of mental health and clinical psychological journals will provide support. However, more often than not, research for evaluation instruments is performed without pairing it with psychotherapy process and outcome. As a result neither the field of evaluation nor the field of psychotherapy profit by the experience of the other. They are two completely separate fields of experience with little if any feedback from one to the other. Combinations of both into one process are few and far between. Usually, it takes a research grant to combine them. The use of writing can overcome this disadvantage, as discussed at length in Chapter 6 in this book and elsewhere (L'Abate, 1992, 1994; L'Abate & Baggett, 1997).

Briefly, no matter how much we may justify and rationalize the importance of evaluation, the technique has failed to become an integral part of psychotherapeutic practices. Most of us still rely on the interview and hence on the spoken medium to arrive at an understanding of what is going on with our clients. The reason for this failure lies in the inadequacy of the spoken medium to direct treatment. As long as evaluation is based on the spoken word, treatment planning and treatment in general will be based on a catch-as-you-can basis and not on rationally or even empirically based grounds. Only if part of treatment is based on written homework assignments can evaluation can be linked with treatment.

Furthermore, evaluation performed initially, before treatment, to meet external demands or routines is limited in its value unless it is performed again at the end of treatment. However, unless a contract to this effect is made at the very outset of therapy, may clients who quit prematurely will not be reexamined at the end. Is a rationale for reevaluation necessary? How can we assess whether we have been of help? How can we distinguish whether our clients have "improved" by feeling better or by negotiating a better life-style? How can we check on self-reported comfort when we cannot find out whether changes have taken place at different levels and parts of the context of change? Is the interview sufficient in suggesting treatment planning and predicting treatment progress? It is definitely necessary, but is it sufficient? Without some objective ways of verifying whether change has taken place, how can we document our competence? A solution to this problem would be to charge clients for both pre- and posttreatment evaluation from the very beginning of therapy. If clients drop out of treatment without re-evaluation, they are going to lose the amount prepaid. Pre- and posttreatment evaluation, of course, would not be the only means of evaluating a therapist's practice. The number of sessions, drop-out rates, and no-shows, as well as self-reports of client's satisfaction, could be used as other indicators of substantive professional practice

Sharing Results with Colleagues or External Evaluators

Most war stories from psychotherapists focus on extreme and exotic examples of deviancy, reliance on a newly found gimmick, and claimed successes indicating the undisputed competence of the therapist. Thus far, no objective method has been found to document therapeutic competence. I have not yet found one therapist who doubted in any way his or her clinical and therapeutic competence. They were licensed, were they not? Most practicing therapists need to bolster their self-esteem or sense of importance by their successes. Very few therapists seem to focus on their failures or to learn from failures as much as it would be necessary. We learn from our failures, not from our successes. Private practice, after all, is based on the marketplace. Supposedly competent therapists are sought after and those less competent have to make a living the best way they can by reducing their fees to accommodate a larger number of clients. Sharing our results with our peers? Who has heard of such a weird idea? It would require making our results available intersubjectively in a way that would violate all standards of accepted practice. Why should we?

If we were to evaluate our clients on a pre- and posttreatment basis as a standard operating procedure, perhaps this practice might obviate the need to make our procedures open to scrutiny and inspection from outsiders. Lacking this practice, however, we need to ask how we are credentialed by state agencies and how these credentials allow us to practice within existing legal and ethical guidelines. The credentials have been granted on the basis of paper examinations and not on the basis of visible, observed hands-on practice, as done, for instance, in advanced certification for board examinations. Certainly, opening our files to external scrutiny would raise a great many questions about issues of confidentiality. On the other hand, without such a scrutiny, we would leave open and unanswered the whole issue of professional competence.

CONCLUSION

The answer to the initial question of how does a whole profession change, is slowly, painfully, and, very likely, as a result of external pressure. It is no longer possible to use the monolithic term "psychotherapeutic community" to describe a homogeneous group. This community admittedly encompasses a variety of disciplines and organizations made up of professionals with very different value systems and practices even within the same organization or discipline. Some therapists may find it difficult to practice according to new, cost-effective ways of helping people. Some will strongly deny the need for any change and continue in their own merry, traditional ways. Some undoubtedly and inevitably will attack the validity of the present thesis and recommendations for change, but will buckle down to face reality. Therapists in the private sector, those who are doing well financially and who are not concerned about the public sector and about seemingly academic issues like costs, cost effectiveness, accountability, verifiability, and outcome in large scale preventive and therapeutic interventions, may well rebel against and reject vehemently what they perceive as a direct threat to their *status quo.*

Who will be ripe and ready for change? Very likely, therapists in the public sector may be ready to consider this proposal. Psychotherapists whose major professional identification is scientific/artistic, rather than the other way around, "pure" psychotherapists whose major identification is as artists, may well be concerned about some of the issues mentioned here, and welcome change.

REFERENCES

Anderson, C.M., Reiss, D.J., & Hogarty, G.E. (1986). *Schizophrenia and the family: A practitioner's guide to psychoeducation and management.* New York: Guilford.

Averill, J.R., & Nunley, E.P. (1992). *Voyages of the heart: Living an emotionally creative life.* New York: Free Press.

Bloom, B.L. (1992). Computer-assisted psychological intervention: A review and commentary. *Clinical Psychology Review, 12,* 169–192.

Cantor, N., & Kihlstrom, J.F. (1987). *Personality and social intelligence.* Englewood Cliffs, NJ: Prentice-Hall.

Deci, E.L., & Ryan, R.M. (1987). The support of autonomy and the control of behavior. *Journal of Personality and Social Psychology, 53,* 1024–1037.

Ehrenwald, J. (Ed.). (1991). *The history of psychotherapy.* Northvale, NJ: Aronson.

Foa, U.G., Converse, J., Jr., Tornblom, K.J., & Foa, E.B. (Eds.). (1993). *Resource theory: Explorations and applications.* San Diego, CA: Academic Press.

Foa, U., & Foa, E. (1974). *Societal structures of the mind.* Springfield, IL: C.C. Thomas.

Freedheim, D.K. (1992). *History of psychotherapy: A century of change.* Washington, D.C.: American Psychological Association.

Gibbs, J.P. (Ed.). (1982). *Social control: Views from the social sciences.* Beverly Hills, CA: Sage.

Gibbs, J.P. (1989). *Control: Sociology's central notion.* Urbana, IL: University of Illinois Press.

Giles, T.R. (1993). *Managed mental health care: A guide for practitioners, employers, and hospital administrators.* Boston, MA: Allyn & Bacon.

Goodman, M., Brown, J., & Deitz, P. (1992). *Managing managed care: A mental health practitioner's survival guide.* Washington, DC: American Psychiatric Association.

Gordon, R.E., & Gordon, K.K. (1981). *Systems of treatment for the mentally ill: Filling the gaps.* New York: Grune & Stratton.

Horwitz, A.V. (1990). *The logic of social control.* New York: Plenum.

Hunt, W.A. (Ed.). (1971). *Human behavior and its control.* Cambridge, MA: Schenkman.

L'Abate, L. (1986). *Systematic family therapy.* New York: Brunner/Mazel.

L'Abate, L. (1990). *Building family competence: Primary and secondary prevention strategies.* Newbury Park, CA: Sage.

L'Abate, L. (1992). *Programmed writing: A self-administered approach for interventions with individuals, couples, and families.* Pacific Grove, CA: Brooks/Cole.

L'Abate, L. (1994). *A theory of personality development.* New York: Wiley.

L'Abate, L., & Bagarozzi, D.A. (1993). *Sourcebook of marriage and the family.* New York: Brunner/Mazel.

L'Abate, L., & Baggett, M.S. (1997) *Distance writing and computer-assisted training in mental health.* Atlanta, GA: The Institute for Life Empowerment.

L'Abate, L., & Colondier, G. (1987). The emperor has no clothes! A critique of systems thinking and a proposal. *American Journal of Family Therapy, 15,* 19–33.

L'Abate, L., & Platzman, K. (1991). The practice of programmed writing (PW) in therapy and prevention with families. *American Journal of Family Therapy, 19,* 99–109.

Langer, E.J. (1983). *The psychology of control.* Beverly Hills, CA: Sage.

Liberman, R.P., DeRisi, W., & Mueser, K.T. (1989). *Social skills training for psychiatric patients.* Des Moines, IO: Allyn & Bacon.

Liddle, H.A. (1992). Family psychology: Progress and prospects of a maturing discipline. *Journal of Family Psychology, 5,* 249–263.

McFarlane, W.R. (1991). Family psychoeducational treatment. In A.S. Gurman & D.P. Kniskern (Eds.), *Handbook of family therapy: Volume II* (pp. 363–395). New York: Brunner/Mazel.

Merkel, W.T., & Searight, H.R. (1992). Why families are not like swamps, solar systems, or thermostats: Some limits of systems theory as applied to family therapy. *Contemporary Family Therapy: An International Journal, 14,* 33–50.

Pennebaker, J.W. (1990). *Opening up: The healing power of confiding in others.* New York: Morrow.

Prochaska, J.O., DiClemente, C.C., & Norcross, J.C. (1992). In search of how people change: Applications to addictive behaviors. *American Psychologist, 47,* 1102–1114.

Ridgewood Financial Institute, Inc. (1993). *Psychotherapy finances: Managed care handbook.* Jupiter, FL: Suite 407, 1016 Clemons Street, 33477.

Rodin, J., Schooler, C., & Schaie, K.W. (Eds.). (1990). *Self-directedness: Cause and effect throughout the life course.* Hillsdale, NJ: Earlbaum.

Rogers, C.R. (1957). The necessary and sufficient conditions of therapeutic personality change. *Journal of Consulting Psychology, 21,* 95–103.

Searight, H.R., & Merkel, W.T. (1991). Systems theory and its discontents: Clinical and ethical issues. *The American Journal of Family Therapy, 19,* 19–31.

Selvini-Palazzoli, M., Cirillo, S., Selvini, M., & Sorrentino, A.M. (1989). *Family games: General models of psychotic processes in the family.* New York: Norton.

Stolorow, R.D. (1991). The intersubjective context of intrapsychic experience, with special reference to therapeutic impasse. In R.C. Curtis (Ed.), *The relational self: Theoretical convergences in psychoanalysis & social psychology* (pp. 17–33). New York: Guilford.

Stricker, G. (1992). The relationship of research to clinical practice. *American Psychologist, 47,* 543–549.

Wegner, D.M., & Pennebaker, J.W. (Eds.). (1993). *Handbook of mental control.* Engle-
    wood Cliffs, NJ: Prentice-Hall.
Winegar, N. (1992). *A clinician's guide to managed mental health care.* New York:
    Haworth.
Yates, A. (1991). *Compulsive exercise and the eating disorders: Toward an integrated theory
    of activity.* New York: Brunner/Mazel.

3

Employee Assistance Programs and Managed Care: Merge and Converge

DARREN W. ADAMSON, Ph.D.

MICHAEL D. GARDNER, Ph.D.

EAPS: WHERE THEY BEGAN AND WHAT THEY ARE

History and Growth

Several definitions of employee assistance programs (EAPs) have emerged over the past 20 years. Roman and Blum (1987) broadly define EAPs as "mechanisms to increase the chances for continued employment of individuals whose job performance and personal functioning are adversely impacted by problems of substance abuse, psychiatric illness, family difficulties or other personal problems" (p. 221). Another, perhaps more specific definition is offered by Sonnestuhl and Trice (1986). They state that EAPs are: "job based programs operating within a work organization for the purpose of identifying 'troubled employees,' motivating them to resolve their troubles, and providing access to counseling or treatment for those employees who need these services"

(p. 176). While these and other definitions of EAPs differ, it is generally recognized that most EAPs are accessed after a problem or issue has occurred (Roman & Blum, 1988). However, it is important to note that employees can access their EAP on a voluntary basis (when no work performance problems are evident) if they have a desire or need to do so. In such cases EAPs can play a preventive role by assisting employees before the problem affects work performance.

Employee assistance programs trace their roots to industrial alcoholism and occupational mental health programs that began during World War II (Quick, Sonnenstuhl & Trice, 1987). In 1970, when the National Institute of Alcohol Abuse coined the term "employee assistance," there were approximately 450 programs in the workplace. In 1987 there were 18,000 (Quick et al., 1987). By 1991 the Association of Labor-Management Administrators and Consultants on Alcoholism (ALMACA) estimated that there were 19,000 to 20,000 EAPs in operation, with an annual growth rate of approximately 49% (ALMACA, 1991).

Philosophy and Structure

Since the emergence of EAPs in the early 1940s, many changes have occurred in their structure and the type of delivery they provide (Trice, Smithers & Neck, 1983). A movement that initially dealt only with alcoholism, it now offers a veritable smorgasbord of services ranging from alcohol and drug treatment to financial, emotional, and marital counseling to health promotion and disease prevention programs (Quick et al., 1987). One of the most recent changes in the evolution of EAPs is the role they play in the management of mental health benefits for cost-conscious corporations.

The settings in which these services are offered vary as greatly as the types of services offered. One structure, common among the national EAPs is a telephone or "800 number" service. In this type of EAP the client calls the number and a counselor either speaks with the client and helps resolve the issue or refers the client to services in the local area, based on zip code.

On the other end of the spectrum is the full-service or broad-brush EAP. This program offers a full range of services, including assessment and referral of "troubled employees" to appropriate services, short-term counseling, inservice training to work groups, management consultations, organizational development consultation to management, and so on.

One other distinction is whether the EAP is in-house or contracted. The in-house EAP usually is closely allied with the company's human resources department. Contracted EAPs are private companies that provide services to corporations on a fee-for-service basis or under a capitated (one yearly fee with assumption of financial risk) contractual arrangement.

Cost-Benefits of EAPs

One motivator to establish an EAP in a corporation is the strong positive message it sends employees, telling them that they are important to the corporation, that the corporation desires to meet their needs. This can engender loyalty and increase morale among employees.

However, even though morale and loyalty are important, the most powerful motivator for providing EAP services to employees is the cost-benefit realized by the corporation. Cost-conscious corporations have a particular interest in determining if the results of a specific program are really worth the costs of maintaining that program. The empirical data on the cost-effectiveness of EAPs are limited. Several articles discuss the need to conduct cost-effectiveness studies within the EAP industry, and provide advice on how to do so, but actual published studies are virtually nonexistent (Decker, Starrett, & Redhorse, 1986; Masi & Goff, 1987; North, 1992, Roman, Blum, & Bennett, 1987).

In one study reviewed by North (1992), the Campbell Soup Company used its EAP to incorporate managed behavioral health care services. This pilot program covered three sites and affected 10,000 people. Campbell set out to meet three objectives: (a) reduce psychiatric and substance abuse costs by 20%; (b) provide the most effective and efficient treatment; and (c) improve or maintain employee satisfaction with health care service delivery. After its first year the company exceeded its expectations. Health costs were reduced by 36%, and behavioral health care costs were reduced from 11.5% to 6.7%. The company's objective to provide high quality treatment and maintain high employee satisfaction was also met (North, 1992).

A cost-benefit study of the McDonnell Douglas EAP, which included approximately 5,492 cases seen in the company's EAP between 1985 and 1988, showed similarly impressive results. Of the 5,492 cases in the sample, 1,032 had conditions that could be affected by services offered by the EAP. The results indicate that the EAP saved the corporation $5.1 million over the four-year period. Savings were realized by reducing absenteeism by 6,121 days ($.8 million), reducing employee medical claims ($2 million), and reducing dependent medical claims ($2.3 million) (McDonnell Douglas Corporation and Alexander Consulting Group, 1989).

A cost-benefit study of the Intermountain Health Care EAP demonstrated similar results. The employees who utilized EAP services used leave time 20% less often than employees who did not utilize the EAP. It is apparent what a 20% reduction in use of leave means to a company's bottom line. Even more impressive were the reported cost savings from decreased medical and psychological insurance claims. The group that did not utilize the EAP spent six times more on medical claims than the group serviced by the EAP. Savings in claims for psychological services were even more dramatic. The group that didn't utilize the EAP spent over fourteen times more on psychological claims than the group that did. The total cost savings for one year were nearly $600,000 (Gardner, Adamson, & Stahmann, 1993).

Ah ha! This is why EAPs are so attractive. These demonstrated cost savings have also strengthened the argument for the management of mental health care in general and for that management to be done by EAPs in particular.

EAPS AND MANAGED CARE: MERGE AND CONVERGE

The most current, and perhaps the most complicated, role played by the EAP is in managing mental health benefits. EAP professionals are now frequently asked to become involved in managed care. This has not been easy for many EAPs. The role of patient advocate is more complex under managed care and occasionally feels more like patient antagonist. As mental health care dollars shrink and the need for mental health services grows, EAP professionals are being required to do more with less.

Another, certainly less difficult, change involves the evolution of the familiar language of EAPs, which is coming to match that of third party payors. For example, the central role of assessment and referral is more often being called case management. In order to assist the practitioner in speaking the language of managed care we have included a list of some of the more commonly used terms.

Terminology of Convergence

This list is certainly not exhaustive but it does provide a notion of the language of managed care as it differs from some of the third party payor language we have become accustomed to.

ADMISSION REVIEW: The evaluation of a particular case by an external reviewer to determine medical necessity of treatment and appropriateness of an admission. This review usually occurs at the beginning or immediately following the beginning of treatment.

ANCHOR GROUP: A multidisciplinary group practice that receives preferential referral consideration because of the "full-service" nature of the practice.

BENEFIT INCENTIVE: A benefit plan designed to encourage appropriate, cost-effective use of the plan through little or no out-of-pocket expenses to the patient, with further cost savings to the employer (for example, through the use of outpatient rather than inpatient services).

BRIEF THERAPY: Therapy designed to provide resolution of specific patient complaints in a time-limited and goal-focused context.

CAPITATED CONTRACTS: An arrangement in which contracted health care sources provide as much care to patients as is needed for a predetermined and preset fee. Most health maintenance organizations use capitated contracts.

CASE MANAGEMENT: The process of tracking the treatment of a patient or family by a case manager. The goal is to identify and recommend the most appropriate treatment and then coordinate the treatment, and often with EAPs, its payment.

CLOSED PANEL: A health care product in which participants are required to receive services from approved providers or facilities. This term has also been used to refer to provider panels that do not accept applications from new providers.

CLOSED PANEL HMO: An HMO model wherein health services are provided by full-time salaried physicians and allied professionals and all correlated health services are owned by the organizations itself.

COBRA (CONSOLIDATED OMNIBUS RECONCILIATION ACT OF 1985): Federal legislation that requires employers to make available continued insurance coverage to employees whose employment is terminated for up to 18 months for employces and 36 months for dependents.

CONCURRENT REVIEW: Continued review of cases to determine medical necessity and appropriateness of treatment during the time treatment is being provided.

DEPENDENT: A member who is eligible for benefits under the subscribers health plan.

DSM-IV (DIAGNOSTIC AND STATISTICAL MANUAL, IV): Published by the American Psychiatric Association, this manual is the standard by which case managers determine medical necessity of treatment.

EXCLUSIONS: Services or procedures excluded from coverage under the health care plan (for example, evaluation of ADHD is covered but treatment is not).

GATEKEEPER: An entity or person that must be contacted prior to services being obtained. The role of the gate or gatekeeper is to evaluate the case and make appropriate referral for treatment. In some cases the gate serves both the role of case manager and preauthorization agent. Most health care products incentivize the subscriber to go through the gate by enriching the benefit for compliance.

HEALTH MAINTENANCE ORGANIZATION: An arrangement to organize and deliver comprehensive health care services to a defined population on a prepaid basis, emphasizing preventative health care. Normally, the patient is not required to pay additional costs beyond the prepaid premium. There are essentially two types of HMOs: (a) closed panel—services provided by staff clinicians at the HMO facility; (b) Direct contract—services are provided by individual or small group practitioners on a fee-for-service or capitated basis at their offices.

MANAGED CARE: A system wherein each case is managed typically through the use of a small managed care panel of providers. These providers have accountability to provide quality services in the most economically efficient manner. Managed care often utilizes a gatekeeping component or a process of preauthorization by a case manager.

MAXIMUM ALLOWABLE FEE: The maximum amount a third party payor will pay for a given procedure or service.

OPEN PANEL: A health care product that allows subscribers to use the provider of their choice

PEER REVIEW: The examination of patient cases to determine medical necessity and appropriateness of treatment typically performed by a clinician of the same specialty or by a team of clinicians.

PPO (PREFERRED PROVIDER ORGANIZATION): An arrangement whereby a third party payor contracts with a group of health care providers to furnish comprehensive health care services at negotiated rates in return for an expected increase in patient volume.

PREAUTHORIZATION: The requirement that any services provided be authorized in advance by a representative of the third party payor or managed care company. Services are authorized only if they are deemed medically necessary and appropriate given the diagnosis. Payment for services may be denied if preauthorization was not obtained.

TPA (THIRD PARTY ADMINISTRATOR): An organization that is not a third party payor but is structured to process insurance claims in behalf of a corporation. Their role is to oversee and control health care dollars.

UTILIZATION REVIEW/UTILIZATION MANAGEMENT: An independent or external company or department within an insurance company responsible for implementation of preauthorization and any review processes. Additionally, information gathered is used to determine health care product improvements or restrictions or, in some cases total elimination of certain features.

THE NEW ROLE OF THE EAP

Seemingly gone forever are the old EAP days, those days when EAP professionals were loved by all. They were loved by the supervisors because the "troubled employee" was taken care of; loved by employee, because this helped resolve problems with supervisors. The new role of the EAP puts them in the position of effectively managing the mental health services of an employee population, while still maintaining the traditional function of helping troubled employees. This role is more comprehensive and more complex than the old one had been.

A central role of the EAP in managed care (called EAP Care in this chapter) is choosing practitioners to be on the preferred provider panel. The following section will address getting on the panel.

Empowerment by Becoming Known to Those Who Determine Empanelment and Reimbursement

One of the indicators of success in the EAP Care environment is the ability to get paid for the services you provide. As recently as just a couple of years ago the service was provided, a bill was submitted, and fees were collected. Today this process is complicated by preauthorization, medical referrals, EAP Care referrals, paneled provider status versus non-paneled provider status, and so on. In today's managed care environment, therapists need not only the clinical skills to treat their clients, but also the business/insurance savvy to remain viable in this dynamic period in the mental health market. This section will teach providers how to become empaneled (sounds like the cure for a disease) and empowered as a player in EAP Care.

The Do's and Don't's of Applying for Preferred Provider Status

One of the first steps in becoming a preferred provider with an EAP Care manager is the application process. Before applying consider the following: Is there sufficient volume of clients in my geographical area to justify the time-consuming, lengthy, sometimes costly application process? (Some EAP Care companies charge an application fee, a portion of which is refunded if status is denied.) If there is not sufficient volume of potential clients, ask yourself if there is a possibility that there will be in the future. This is an important question for two reasons. The first reason involves the constant contract changes in the market from year to year. For example, a large manufacturing firm that employs 5,000 workers uses company X for its managed mental health plan. The following year company Y underbids company X by one dollar (or even 10 cents) per employee per month. When the manufacturing firm changes companies to save money, unless you are a preferred provider for both company X and company Y, you could lose clients. Situations like this one are occurring across the country on a regular basis. Reason number two is that panels that are open to new providers one day may not be open the next day. It is very common for providers to call a company to receive an application and information only to find that the panel is now closed. Closed panels mean that the EAP Care firm has enough preferred panel providers to meet the needs of the potential clients in that area, and therefore it is not accepting new applications. We strongly suggest, therefore, that if you have the opportunity to become empaneled, consider it seriously. The opportunity may be gone tomorrow.

Other questions to consider prior to the application process may include: What is the rate of reimbursement? How easy is it to collect fees from this company? What is their reputation among mental health professionals? What are the requirements for preferred panel status?

This question begs further comment. The application process for preferred panel status can take anywhere from ten minutes to several hours to complete and may require several pieces of documentation. Most EAP Care applications require things such as state licensure, malpractice insurance (usually in the amount of at least $1,000,000), two to five years (this is a recent change—it used to be one to two years) as a licensed provider of mental health services, willingness to submit records and provide treatment plans, and so on. Before you spend your valuable time applying, find out the specific requirements for provider status. You can do this in a couple of ways. Most applications come with a cover letter stating what the requirements for empanelment are. If this is not the case, call the company's provider relations department and ask for this information over the phone or have it sent to you. If you don't meet the requirements, talk to provider relations to see if they make any exceptions or have provisional status. If not, you may not want to take the time to apply as rejection seems assured.

Once you have considered those concerns and are ready to begin the application process, there are several things that will help you gain empanelment. One of the keys is being familiar with the "brief therapy" trend in the market. This is important because you will be asked about your therapeutic orientation, types of training, and philosophy about treatment. You must not appear to be a long-term therapist (15 sessions plus), but rather a short-term, solution-oriented therapist (15 sessions or less). If your average number of sessions is 32 the EAP Care manager may be leery of adding you to the panel.

Any seasoned therapist realizes that there are going to be a certain number of cases that require longer-term treatment. The EAP professional, too, is aware of these outliers. However, EAP Care companies want providers with a commitment to and philosophy of brief therapy. These questions usually will not be asked directly, so you are unlikely to be asked. "What is the average number of therapy sessions you provide your clients?" In a recent application filled out by one of the authors the following two questions were asked to get at this information: 1. Briefly describe your clinical orientation (please also describe your philosophy regarding the use of medications in treatment), and 2. Describe your understanding of the function of the insurance utilization management (UM) process. Most EAP Care applications include some version of questions like these. Keep in mind that the goal of EAP Care managers is to provide cost-effective treatment to their subscribers. You as a provider filling out the application want this to be reflected in your answers, so that the company's goals are congruent with yours. You may even consider answering the indirect questions with a direct answer, such as "My treatment philosophy allows me to treat the majority of my clients in fewer than 15 sessions." Data from your own outcome studies supporting your claims, if you have them (if you don't, consider beginning to collect them) can be very helpful.

The words you use on the application are very critical in showing that you are managed-care friendly. Avoid words that come from the more traditionally long-term therapy approaches. For example, terms or phrases such as insight-oriented, family of origin issues, supportive therapy, self-esteem, psychoanalytic, and so on, are red flags for application reviewers. Replace these terms with cognitive-behavioral, solution-focused, brief model, short-term, group approach, and similar constructions.

A few other general hints will help you gain preferred provider status. Always fill out the application in its entirety. Don't leave blank spots. They lead to assumptions—generally not favorable ones. Type the application whenever possible. Include any supporting documentation that you can attach directly to the application—a copy of your current license, proof of malpractice insurance, official transcripts, certificates of completion of brief therapy-related seminars, descriptions of or certificates from managed care conferences you have attended, and so on. Know the hospital affiliations of the company to which you are applying. Do not put in your application a strong affiliation with a competing hospital. It is also helpful if you can discover the makeup of the existing panel in your geographic area, along with the specialties of the paneled providers. With this knowledge you can try to fill in geographical or specialty gaps. Additionally, if you are unsure of what information is being requested, call the designated contact or the provider relations department and ask. If you are still unclear, try to find someone who has been empaneled by that particular company and ask to see a copy of his or her application and supporting documentation.

Inservicing and Information Brokering: Tools of Empanelment

Besides effectively filling out the application there are other ways to gain favor with EAP Care companies. One effective way is to communicate your willingness to provide *free* information and services that lie within your area of expertise to their employees or clients. An effective method of accomplishing this is to provide inservices and seminars on topics such as stress management, conflict resolution, drug and alcohol use and abuse, and so on. This accomplishes two objectives. First, it allows the company to know that you are willing to provide services for them without expecting to be paid directly. It indicates that you intend to develop a mutually beneficial relationship. This process also allows those EAP Care managers to assess your skills and abilities prior to any formal contract or preferred provider status being granted.

Secondly, through this process of providing pro bono services another vital message is communicated—the message that you are managed-care friendly. Your willingness to provide these services communicates that you understand the concept and philosophy of managed care and that you are willing to be a team player. EAP Care companies want providers who understand managed care and the changes associated with this new and evolving system of providing mental health care. By following the guidelines provided you will send the message to the EAP Care companies that you understand these changes and are willing to abide by them in order to remain viable in this dynamic period of health care reform.

YOU'RE ON THE PANEL!! SO NOW WHAT? MAINTAINING A SUPPLY OF REFERRALS

Staying Connected with your EAP Professional. How to Keep a Referral Source Happy and Active

Even though many EAP professionals are becoming managed care case managers they are still, for the most part, strong patient advocates. Therefore, they want an indication from you as the therapist that you too are a patient advocate as much as a professional who wants to get paid for services rendered.

A very basic way to do this is to discuss with the EAP your approach to aspects of practice that relate to patient advocacy. For example, whether it is hypothetical or real, talk about how you would handle a situation where a client's benefits are exhausted for a given year and he or she still needs additional sessions. Do you do any pro bono work?

Another indicator that is fairly specific to the EAP referral source is collaboration with the EAP in the client's work setting. Often the EAP needs assistance in advocating for the employee with a supervisor or at a worksite. Indicate to the EAP that you are willing, at either a reduced fee or no charge, to go to the workplace and advocate as necessary for the client, or that you are willing to provide information that would assist the EAP in doing the workplace intervention.

It is also important to include the EAP professional in the treatment team. Many EAP professionals are licensed mental health providers and can provide consultation and collaboration in the treatment of a client. The consultation can take the form of actual clinical suggestions, or you can function as an expert about workplace issues, how they may be affecting the client's well-being, and how they can be treated in therapy. Including the EAP, when appropriate, in the provision of therapy enhances the relationship and increases referrals.

Another indicator of a patient focus is to implement a tracking and reporting system in your practice. Send a brief note or call the EAP professional to inform him or her that the client did arrive for the initial visit and that you welcome any input from the EAP about the case. This is very reassuring, showing the EAP that he or she has succeeded in one of his or her most difficult tasks, assisting the client to have the confidence that the referral was appropriate. In making assessments and referrals, the EAP professional faces the task of creating client confidence in another therapist such that the client doesn't feel abandoned by the EAP and follows up with the therapist. Knowing that the transfer worked and the transition was smooth increases the EAP's confidence in continuing to refer clients to you. Additional followup information about how the client is doing during therapy and at discharge is also useful.

As mentioned earlier, any inservices that you would be willing to provide, free of charge, to assist the EAP in carrying out his or her other workplace-based responsibilities creates happiness and referring activity.

Whatever method you use to enhance the connection with an EAP referral source must have at its base the creation of a professional relationship with that person. An EAP wants to refer to people who are known and trusted. Get to know and become known by, in person or on the phone, the EAP professional.

Information Is Power: Supplying What Is Necessary

Since resistance tends to beget resistance, it is important that providers supply all requested information. Most EAP Care companies want very basic information about most cases. Cases that are outliers (for example, those that go beyond some set number of sessions, say 10) require more extensive information. Basic information includes: full name of client and subscriber; correctly spelled; subscriber SSN; diagnosis(es), preferably all five DSM-IV axes; brief social history; outpatient and inpatient treatment history, including use of psychoactive medications; brief summation of clinical issues to be worked on; treatment plan that is solution-focused including adjunctive therapies that will be employed—for example, groups, workbooks, and psychiatric consults; a statement of the number of sessions you are requesting (make sure this fits with the diagnosis); and so on. The key to providing this information is to be brief but thorough. EAP Care case managers are very busy, and if they are reassured of your intent they will learn to rely on you to do much of the case management for them. Provide them with information indicating that you have already looked at the costs of the care you are providing and have considered and implemented cost-conscious strategies.

Brief Therapy: Turn up the Volume of Referrals by Keeping the Numbers Down

To cost-conscious EAP Care firms the fewer the sessions the lower the cost. Therefore, it is vital that you as a practitioner utilize effective brief therapy strategies. A brief discussion of short-term treatment strategies follows.

One of the first things a practitioner can do is create client expectation of time-limited treatment. This can be accomplished simply by contracting with the client for a limited number of sessions. Client cooperation is enhanced if the practitioner clearly spells out the agenda or map of treatment so that the client can see how "doable" the plan is. The map includes a limited number of clearly identified problems.

Another strategy that needs to be implemented early in treatment is measurement of outcome. Obtain a baseline measurement of the various problems that have been identified for amelioration. As treatment proceeds and at the conclusion of treatment remeasure the same problem areas. As much as possible include the client in the interpretation of the data. Occasionally the client will interpret the data much more positively than the therapist.

To enhance the effect of short-term treatment, assess and intervene at the broadest system level possible. At a minimum, obtain data regarding the client's primary system, the family (or it's equivalent in the client's life). Where possible, include members of the primary system in treatment, either in person or through some other means. Working with an EAP can often include the work system as a target of intervention. This can be accomplished by coordinating with the EAP actually to include in treatment members of the client's work team or to simply include information obtained by the EAP about the client's work system.

For those diagnoses traditionally requiring longer-term treatment, it is useful to begin treatment by including adjunctive therapeutic resources. Create the expectation early on in treatment that the client will reach out for these additional resources. It helps if you or your support staff offer to act as case coordinator in obtaining and coordinating services offered by others. Adjunctive therapeutic resources include but are not limited to self-help groups, 12-step groups, support groups, massage therapy, biofeedback therapy, psychoeducational groups, community resources (county mental health services, battered women's shelters, welfare services, and so on), primary care physicians, psychiatrists, the EAP professional (this also encourages continued referrals), state rehabilitation services, community information services (lecture series, community education classes, and so on), spouses or other family members; neighbors, friends, and so on.

The use of adjunctive therapeutic resources also helps to support the power of a multidisciplinary approach. In working with other professionals to meet the needs of your client you enhance the effectiveness of therapy and reduce the number of sessions you are requesting of the case manager. Be sure to include the EAP case manager as an integral part of the treatment team.

As part of the assessment, include identification of precipitating events or triggers of the targeted problems. The client is assisted in identifying the people, places, situations, and circumstances that create or help to maintain the problem behavior. Next, carefully describe the thought processes in which the client engages that are associated with the precipitating events. By focusing on the thought processes, the therapist and client have more objective, measurable targets of change. This also helps to extend treatment beyond the active phase. Clients learn to identify these triggers and then learn compensatory behaviors to counteract them, thus becoming their own therapists.

From the inception of treatment and throughout its course, helping clients create a visualization of desired outcome enhances brief treatment success. As clients can visualize what their lives will be like with or without the targeted behaviors, two things are accomplished. One, therapist and client have a clear picture of when therapy is finished. The second benefit lies in the motivating power of mentally practicing the desired outcome. Many athletes perform better by visualizing their performance many times before the actual performance. With clients, very often the visualized performance becomes real.

Another very useful aid in brief therapy is the effective use of homework. Homework should be specific and clear, and it should also be goal-focused in two ways. One, link the homework to the content of the session in which it is assigned, and two, link it to the overall objectives of the treatment contract. The more effectively the therapist relates it to the symptoms and to the objectives the more useful it is. Homework has the obvious advantage of extending the power of the therapy session. Another advantage is the confidence that successful homework completion builds in the client. The more confidence the client has in him- or herself the less dependent he or she is on the therapist, thus leading to the necessity for fewer sessions.

Another effective strategy in brief therapy is to emphasize the contracted termination date throughout the treatment. This encourages the client to work hard to accomplish the specified goals of treatment. It is also helpful to communicate use of this strategy to the EAP Care case manager.

Obviously, this is not an exhaustive discussion of brief therapy concepts. To be effective in meeting your clients' needs and getting paid to do so, you are encouraged to become an expert in the provision of brief therapy.

SUMMARY

The changing third party payor market to a managed care market is anxiety-producing for most practitioners. To cope with these anxieties, a practitioner must learn to do what most of us recommend to our clients—we must enhance our support network by creating relationships with people who can be helpful to us. The suggestion of this chapter is that you as a practitioner expand your professional support network to include the EAP professional acting in the role of case manager. Create a working relationship with the case manager so that your clients benefit from being able to receive payment for your services and you benefit from the support received by adding another member to the client's treatment team.

It is hoped that the suggestions contained in this chapter will help in the relationship-creating effort advocated. Connecting with others facing the same struggle creates more hope and more influence to encourage a sane approach to this change.

REFERENCES

ALMACA. (Association of Labor-Management Administrators and Consultants on Alcoholism) (1991). Phone interview by Michael Gardner, August 1991.

Decker, J. T., Starrett, R., & Redhorse, J. (1986). Evaluating the cost effectiveness of employee assistance programs. *Social Work* (Sep.–Oct.) 391–393.

Gardner, M. D., Adamson, D. W., & Stahmann, R. F. (1993). *The Effects of Employee Assistance Program Services On Health Care Costs And Absenteeism.* Doctoral dissertation completed by Michael Gardner, Brigham Young University, Provo, Ut.

McDonnell Douglas Corporation and Alexander Consulting Group. (1989). Unpublished EAP Financial Offset Study.

Masi, D. A., & Goff, M. E. (1987). The evaluation of employee assistance programs. *Public Personnel Management, 16*(4), 323–327.

North, R. J. (1992). Striking the right balance with EAP based managed care. *EAP Digest* (Jan.–Feb.)

Quick, R. C., Sonnenstuhl, W., & Trice, H. M., (1987). Educating the employee assistance professional: Cornell University's employee assistance education and research program. *Public Personnel Management, 16*(4), 333–343.

Roman, P. M., & Blum, T. C. (1987). The relation of employee assistance programs to corporate and social responsibility attitudes: An empirical study. *In Research in Corporate Social Performance and Policy.* Greenwich, CT: JAI Press.

Roman, P. M., & Blum, T. C. (1988). Formal interventions in employee health: Comparison of the nature and structure of employee assistance programs and health promotion programs. *Social Science Medicine, 26*(5), 503–514.

Roman, P. M., Blum, T. C., & Bennett, N. (1987). Educating organizational consumers about employee assistance programs. *Public Personnel Management, 16*(4), 299–312.

Sonnenstuhl, W., & Trice, H. (1986). *Strategies for Employee Assistance Programs: The Crucial Balance.* Ithaca, NY: ILR Press.

Trice, H. M., Smithers, C. D., & Neck, M. (1983). EAPs: Where do we stand in 1983? *Journal of Psychiatric Treatment and Evaluation, 5*(6), 521–529.

4

Maximizing Psychotherapeutic and Psychopharmacological Outcomes: The Psychiatrist's Role in Managed Care

LEN SPERRY, M.D., Ph.D.

I can vividly recall my first week of college in 1957 and seeing a poster trumpeting the mental health care team in action. A male psychiatrist was in the forefront, with a nurse, a social worker, a psychologist, psychiatric aide, and a chaplain in the background. The identity and role of the psychiatrist was clearly that of expert healer as well as leader of the treatment team composed of other disciplines in supportive roles. Now, however, the identity and role of the psychiatrist is not quite so clear, particularly in managed care settings. A rather common, stereotypic view of the managed care psychiatrist is someone practicing second-rate medicine in a small back office, writing prescriptions, and signing off charts (Schneider-Braus, 1992). Today, a poster about managed care mental health might well show the psychiatrist in the background serving in a supportive role and function!

THE CHANGING ROLE AND IDENTITY OF PSYCHIATRISTS

That the identity and role of psychiatrists have changed considerably over the past 30 years is a given. How and why the psychiatrist's role has changed, the compatibility of this change with the values and ideals of psychiatry, and the needs of managed care is the focus of this chapter. As background for discussing the evolving role of the psychiatrist it will be useful to define terms and the context for these changes, including the evolving role of nonmedical therapists.

Professional identity refers to the image and self-concept attributed to members of a particular profession by those inside as well as those outside that profession. *Professional role* refers to specific expectations regarding appropriate behavior for members of a given profession. *Role function* refers to the characteristic patterns or ways of fulfilling expectations. While identity defines what a professional is, role and role function prescribes what the professional does or should do.

Giles (1993) has captured the essence of the traditional role of the psychiatrist in the following characterization: They were leaders in providing and administering mental health services, they prescribed and monitored medications and provided other medical services, they assumed primary responsibility for supervision of other therapists' work, and they provided policy input at both the local and the national level. Today, Giles notes that psychiatrists not only command higher fees for outpatient services but—perhaps incorrectly—they are perceived as willing to provide only longer-term, dynamically oriented psychotherapy. Therefore, managed care firms refer patients instead to nonmedical therapists who practice shorter-term, goal-oriented therapies. And when psychiatrists are retained, managed care administrators tend to limit their role and influence. Giles also notes that because of their mistrust of psychiatrists, these administrators typically deny them administrative positions. Not surprisingly, this distrust and delimiting of role and influence has been demoralizing for many psychiatrists (Siegler, Axelband, & Isikoff, 1993).

Understandably, psychiatrists have mixed feelings about managed care, and generally have been less than enthusiastic in embracing managed care practice. Undoubtedly, many psychiatrists can recount numerous horror stories involving experiences with prior authorization, unreasonable demands for the justification of continued care, denial of treatment, and premature discharge that have had various negative therapeutic consequences, including suicide (Westermeyer, 1991). Many are concerned about loss of autonomy in the way they chose to practice, loss of income, and the belief that managed care represents reduced quality of care. Unfortunately, organized psychiatry's response has been largely reactive and ambivalent. Because managed care has and no doubt will continue to shape the future of psychiatry, it is essential that psychiatrists become more proactive in articulating their unique identity and role. Failing this, psychiatry could further lose its leadership position—particularly its ability to influence policy—in regard to the future of mental health delivery (Siegler, Axelband, & Isikoff, 1993).

THE CHANGING ROLE AND IDENTITY OF THE NONMEDICAL THERAPIST

Thirty years ago the psychologist's function was primarily psychological assessment. Then, the social worker's function was taking a detailed social history and attending to the patient's social service needs. Similarly, the psychiatric nurse's function was administering medication and carrying out other medical orders. These role functions supported the psychiatrist's role as team leader and primary decision maker. Specific role functions of the psychiatrist included decisions about differential diagnosis and differential therapeutics, especially somatic therapies such as medication.

Outside the inpatient setting, this team concept has largely disappeared today. In place of the differentiated roles that supported the psychiatrist as team leader, today social workers, psychologists, and psychiatric nurses are more likely to function in relatively autonomous capacities in diagnosing, deciding, and providing psychosocial therapies in the roles of psychotherapists or nonmedical therapists.

In the past three decades the identity of *psychotherapist* has evolved out of the unsuccessful efforts of psychiatry to retain *medical psychotherapy* as an exclusive role for those with the identity of licensed physicians (Ludwig, 1987). Now psychotherapist is an inclusive identity and refers to social workers, psychologists, marital and family therapists, mental health counselors, pastoral counselors, and psychiatric nurses who practice various forms of psychotherapy or other psychosocial treatments. In the managed care literature it is commonplace for the term *nonmedical therapist* to refer collectively to mental health professionals and paraprofessionals who provide some form of psychotherapeutic service (Feldman, & Fitzpatrick, 1992; Giles, 1993).

It should not be surprising that managed mental health care firms have a preference for short-term, goal-oriented therapies, and thus seek out providers who not only value but are skilled in providing this kind of treatment (Giles, 1993). Budman (1992) has described several value differences between those who champion short-term therapy compared to those who advocate long-term treatment. For instance, long-term therapy emphasizes basic character change and sees a patient's being in therapy as the patient's most important priority. Short-term therapy prefers the least radical intervention, does not endorse the concept of care, and views being in the world as more important than being in therapy. While long-term therapy posits that changes take place in the course of treatment, brief therapy accepts that many changes will occur after therapy because ultimately change occurs as a result of the patient's efforts and responsibility for implementing change.

Formal training and the attainment of certification or licensure mark the evolution of the identity and role of nonmedical therapists in managed care practice. Whether their discipline is social work, psychology, mental health counseling, or chemical dependency, these individuals have forged an identity and role that managed care administrators understand and appreciate as compatible with managed care policy. Presently, the same cannot be said for the identity and role of psychiatry. Of course, admitting inpatients and prescribing and managing medication is still largely the province of psychiatrists, but whether and how long this will continue is uncertain. Efforts to gain or increase prescription privileges by nonmedical therapists are underway. In the meantime, others, including Kisch (1991) and Sovner (1991), advocate an expanded role for nonmedical therapists in what they call "collaborative psychopharmacology," an area where nonmedical therapists have increased input in decisions about medication and somatic treatments.

PROPOSED ROLES AND ROLE FUNCTIONS FOR PSYCHIATRISTS

Relatively little has been written about the developing identity and proposed alternative roles for psychiatrists. This section summarizes that literature. It also proposes and articulates an integrative role and role functions for psychiatrists in managed care.

The psychiatric community recognizes that changes in identity and role are necessary. Sabin and Borus (1992) contrast traditional fee-for-service psychiatric practice with managed care psychiatric practice with regard to role. They indicate that there is a major change in role involved, from independent professional in traditional practice to independent professional *and* employee partner in managed care practice. This implies a shift in role from an authorative to a collaborative relationship with other mental health personnel. Others (Blackwell & Schmidt, 1992; McNutt, Severion & Schomer, 1987) also advocate the collaborative role for the psychiatrist. To effect this role change, Blackwell and Schmidt (1992) conclude that psychiatrists need to be educated in four content areas: short-term therapy skills, ethical concerns, cost-efficient care, and professional role development. They believe that professional role development is learned through appropriate role modeling and supervised experiences in collaborative relationships with multiple providers from other disciplines. Sabin (1991) and Sabin and Borus (1992) suggest that six new skills are required for this role change: collaborative program development, individual practice management, ethical analysis, advocacy beneficence, a developmental model, and a broad repertoire of treatment methodologies. Sabshin (1987) describes the changed role of the psychiatrist in the 1990s as a generalist who can integrate a mixture of combined techniques and will be able to titrate each, or move from one to the other with a diverse patient population.

These characterizations—collaboration, advocacy, short-term therapy, and integrative and combined interventions—stand in stark contrast to both the traditional image of the psychiatrist as an expert, authoritative team leader, and the current stereotype of the managed care psychiatrist as a passive prescription-writing functionary.

An evolution of the psychiatrist's role and role functions is underway that will have a profound implication not only for managed care but also for psychiatric practice outside managed care settings. This chapter proposes a specific integrative, collaborative role and three role functions for psychiatrists in managed care. The role is *maximizing psychotherapeutic and psychopharmacological outcomes*. The role functions are evaluator, provider, and consultor.

Let's start by defining and articulating this role. Begin with the word outcomes. The managed care psychiatrist would conceptualize all treatment endeavors—from diagnosis to monitoring results of interventions—in terms of outcomes. This contrasts with traditional psychiatry's focus on process. Being outcome-oriented means paying attention to quality, efficacy, cost-effectiveness and accountability.

The managed care psychiatrist's focus on outcomes involves both psychotherapeutic and psychopharmacological interventions. I agree with Hyland (1991) that because medication has demonstrated effectiveness for a number of psychiatric conditions the question of psychopharmacology needs to be addressed in each patient evaluation. Similarly, the question of psychotherapy needs to be considered at the onset of every psychiatric treatment. Combined treatment, particularly integrating pharmacotherapy with psychotherapy, is the cutting edge of mental health today (Beitman, 1993a; Beitman & Klerman, 1991) and reflects psychiatry's biopsychosocial perspective.

Psychiatrists continue to maintain their primary role in psychopharmacology. However, there is considerable discussion about the involvement of psychiatrists in psychotherapy. Should they be primary providers of psychotherapy? Or psychotherapy supervisors? Or principal decision makers about psychotherapeutic management?

Ludwig (1987) reviews the psychiatrist's role in the practice of psychiatry from the mid-1800s through the present. He notes that psychiatry has played a dominant role in psychotherapy until recently, when non-medical therapists have challenged that role. Medical psychotherapy has been defined as "a series of medical procedures carried out by a physician trained to treat mental, emotional, and psychosomatic illness through relationships with the patient in an individual, group or family setting, utilizing verbal or nonverbal communication with the patient" (Katz, 1986). Ludwig (1987) believes that there is a difference between psychiatrists and nonmedical therapists when it comes to conceptualizing, approaching, and managing clinical problems with psychotherapeutic methods. He claims that psychiatrists are trained to conceptualize problems from a medical and biopsychosocial perspective and tend to think in terms of diagnosis, differential diagnosis, differential therapeutics, and prognosis more than nonmedical therapists. Regarding their approach and management of clinical problems, Ludwig says that "inculcated with a sense of medical responsibility and Aesculapian authority, psychiatrists have been trained to take authoritative stands when necessary and make life-and-death decisions, intervening when the potential of suicide or violence exists and resorting to hospitalization or restraint under certain circumstances" (Ludwig, 1987, p. 365).

In short, he believes that because of their medical training and experience, and because they can administer a wider variety of medical and psychosocial interventions than nonpsychiatrists, psychiatrists are able to conduct psychotherapy in its broadest sense. Munoz (1994) agrees but extends the psychiatrist's role beyond provider and supervisor of psychotherapy. Munoz agrees that the psychiatrists should be the principal strategist in psychotherapeutic management, and decide on matters of differential psychotherapeutics (Francis, Clarkin, & Perry, 1984). Presumably, this would include deciding on the setting, duration, and focus, and the specific interventions to be utilized by the assigned therapist.

An important word is "maximize", and it is my contention that psychiatrists are the most qualified among the mental health disciplines to exercise leadership and accountability for ensuring that quality mental treatment that is both efficacious and cost-effective is provided. According to Jaques and Clement (1991), "in order to discharge accountability, a person in a role must have appropriate authority" (p. 8). Medical license and board eligibility or certification in psychiatry provides such authority. Speaking about managerial role, Jaques and Clement note that "every manager must be held accountable for the work of subordinates, but also for adding value to their work . . . second, he or she must be held accountable for sustaining a team of subordinates who are capable of doing their work; and third, he or she must set direction for subordinates and get them willing to work alone, with him or her in that duration, that is to say, he or she must carry leadership accountability" (p. 111). It is my belief that psychiatrists, like managers, can and should carry leadership accountability by ensuring that treatment outcomes are maximized.

Unlike the leadership style of the traditional psychiatrist, which tended to be authoritative—or even authoritarian—the leadership style of the managed care psychiatrist would be consultative and collaborative. Such a leader seeks input on decision and expects others to be accountable for their work tasks, but ultimately makes and takes responsibility for certain treatment decisions and outcomes. And given current malpractice and liability statutes (Woodward, Duckworth, & Guthiel, 1993), the psychiatrist necessarily would have an oversight function.

I propose that the psychiatrist in a managed care setting be accountable for maximizing psychotherapeutic and psychopharmacological outcomes. Essentially, this means ensuring that quality, cost effectiveness, and efficacious care. This does not mean that the psychiatrist provides all services, but rather that the psychiatrist has sufficient involvement and decision-making authority for treatment offered by all providers involved with a given patient. And, because the psychiatrist is legally accountable for treatment outcomes, he or she must exercise an oversight function. Specifically, this means that all mental health personnel will be held accountable for their particular role functions. For instance, each provider would be accountable for maximizing his or her particular treatment outcome, the case manager would be accountable for maximizing the coordination of various providers, and the managed care administrator would be accountable for maximizing cost effectiveness. In short, the psychiatrist's accountability would be to ensure that all psychosocial and somatic treatment outcomes were maximized.

Supporting this proposed role change are three interrelated role functions: evaluator, provider, and consultor. These role functions simultaneously promote collaboration with patients (evaluator and provider) and other managed care personnel (consultor), reflect the realities of managed care policies, and respect and enhance the psychiatrist's medical training and the unique biopsychosocial perspective of psychiatry. Table 4-1 summarizes this change and evolution of role and role functions.

THE EVALUATOR ROLE FUNCTION

Bennett (1993) describes contemporary managed care as atheoretical and highly pragmatic. He believes that the essence of managed care can be reduced to three questions: What does the patient need? How

TABLE 4-1

Change and Evolution of the Scope of Roles for Mental Health Professionals

Time Frame / Professional	Yesterday	Typical Managed Care Setting	Proposed
psychiatrists/ medical therapists/ prescribing clinicians	differentiated and wide	delimited and differentiated	focused (evaluator, provider, consultor)
	authoritative/ leadership	subordinate/ supportive	collaborative leadership
nonmedical therapists	differentiated and narrow (social worker, nurse, psychologists, etc.)	undifferentiated and broad (nonmedical therapists)	focused
	subordinate/ supportive	independent (quasi)	interdependent/ collaborative

can the need be met? And how do we know when this outcome is achieved? It is my conviction that these three questions essentially reflect the psychiatrist's evaluator role function. Answering these questions goes beyond the traditional discipline boundaries, psychology, social work, nursing, and psychiatry and is based on demonstrated efficacy rather than on ideology.

In a number of respects, the evaluator role function described here is distinct from the traditional psychiatric evaluation. Traditionally, a psychiatrist performs a psychiatric evaluation consisting of a description of the present illness, past psychiatric history, a social and developmental history, and a mental status exam that led to a diagnostic formulation—usually in DSM-IV categories—and a treatment plan. While such an evaluation addresses the first and second questions to some extent, it seldom addresses the third managed care question. This is because the standard psychiatric evaluation process is largely a symptom narrative and insufficiently focuses on the patient's level of functioning, coping resources, readiness, and capacity for treatment. Furthermore, while a diagnostic formulation summarizes the patient's symptomatic presentation with a diagnostic label (question 1), and while the treatment plan may focus on symptomatic relief, it may not reflect how the patient's need can be best met (question 2). And, of course, the traditional psychiatric evaluation was not designed to address issues of accountability or the monitoring of outcomes (question 3).

The proposed evaluator role function is then both broader and more focused than the traditional diagnostic-oriented evaluation process and role. While the traditional evaluation emphasizes data and content, the treatment-oriented evaluation emphasizes function and prognosis or treatability—the extent to which a patient expects and is willing and capable of modifying or changing behavior, as well as the patient's level of functioning, deficits, and coping resources. The evaluator engages in focused listening, picking out of the patient's story and symptom narrative the prognostic indicators and clues regarding potential therapeutic leverage. Therapeutic leverage refers to the change potential that accrues from prognostic factors and treatment interventions that unbalance the patient's dysfunctional pattern of functioning, thereby increasing treatability and therapeutic outcome.

Such an evaluation would consist of seven dimensions—seven Ps—presentation, predisposition, precipitant, pattern, perpetuants, prognosis, and (treatment) plan (Sperry, Gudeman, Blackwell, & Faulkner, 1992). Of these the dimensions of presentation, pattern, perpetuants, and prognosis are most critical and central to all three of the psychiatrist's role functions (see Figure 4-1).

Presentation refers to the patient's symptoms, mental status, diagnosis, and perception of need. Pattern refers to the patient's consistent

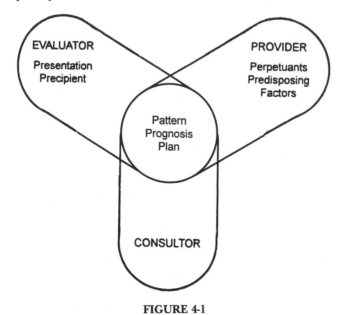

FIGURE 4-1

The Interrelationship of the Evaluator, Provider, and Consultor Roles and the Centrality of Pattern, Prognosis, and Plan

and predictable behavioral and emotional response and functioning in the face of specific triggers and stressors. Perpetuants refer to intrapersonal, interpersonal, and environmental factors that serve to reinforce and confirm the patient's pattern of functioning. Prognosis refers to the patient's treatability and expected response to treatment.

Completing a treatment-focused evaluation requires somewhat different information from the patient—and corroborators—because the emphasis is on treatability; that is, on readiness and functional capacity. Readiness is a function of the patient's expectation for treatment, and his or her willingness and capability to engage in change. Patients with higher expectations of improvement respond better to medications and psychosocial interventions than those with lower expectations of improvement (Sotsky et al, 1991). Similarly, patients who have accepted their diagnoses, decided to cooperate with treatment, and made efforts to change are more likely to have positive treatment outcomes than patients who have not (Beitman, 1993). Furthermore, patients who can modulate their affects, cognitions, and behaviors are more capable of collaborating in treatment than those who remain parasuicidal or engage in treatment sabotage or escape behaviors (Linehan, 1987). Functioning can be estimated by the Global Assessment of Functioning (GAF) Scale of Axis V of DSM-IV, or more specifically by five subscales for Axis V: psychological impairment, social skills, dangerousness, occupational skills, and substance abuse (Kennedy, 1992).

To gather such focused information quickly and accurately requires considerable cooperation and collaboration by the patient and corroborators. Thus, efforts to establish rapport and engage the patient in the evaluation process are as important for the psychiatrist functioning in the evaluator role as in the provider role. The following case illustrates this type of evaluation.

The Case of C.W.

C.W. is a moderately obese, never-married, 38-year-old white female clerk-stenographer who presented with a two-week onset of spontaneous crying, sad mood, decreased sleep with early morning awakening, and increasing social isolation. She had not showed up for work for four days, prompting the psychiatric referral. Her history and mental status exam are consistent with a diagnosis of major depressive episode, as well as meeting the criteria for avoidant personality disorder *(Presentation)*. Cutbacks at her office led to her transfer out of a close-knit typing pool, where she had been for 16 years, to a receptionist-typist position for a new sales manager in another location. This transfer was viewed by her as a significant loss and appears to have triggered her depressive symptoms and social isolation *(Precipitant)*. No personal, family psychiatric, alcohol, or substance abuse history was reported. However, C.W. described intense feelings of humiliation and rejection following the birth of a younger brother after early nurturing by her parents. She came to believe that the opinions of others were all that counted. However, she was teased and ridiculed by her peers for her personal appearance, especially her obesity. There were also strong parental injunctions against discussing important matters with "outsiders" *(Predisposition)*. It appears that she distances and isolates herself from others, anticipating and fearing their disapproval and criticism. She views others as critical and harsh and is convinced she is viewed by others as inadequate. Therefore, she is slow to warm up and trust others, and tests others' trustability by being late, cancelling, or missing agreed-upon engagements *(Pattern)*. Lack of social skills in relating to new or less known individuals, and a limited social network—she is a homebody who spends much of her time reading romance novels, watching soap operas, or knitting—further contributes to an isolative life-style and reinforces her beliefs about self, the world, and others. *(Perpetuants)*. With the exception of social relations she has functioned above average in all life tasks. She agrees that she is severely depressed and wants to cooperate with combined treatment involving medication and monitoring on an outpatient basis along with time-limited psychotherapy. She does not appear to be particularly psychologically minded and has moderate skill deficits in assertive communication, trust, and friendship skills, and it can be anticipated that she will have difficulty discussing personal matters with health providers, that she'll test and provoke providers into criticizing her for changing or cancelling appointments at the last minute, being late, and the like. Nevertheless, she continues to be nicotine-abstinent some three and half years after completing a smoking cessation program. Her support system includes some contact with an older female cousin and a pet dog. *(Prognosis)*. Combined treatment with an antidepressant and psychotherapy focused on ameliorating symptoms, returning to work and establishing a supportive social network there, and increasing interpersonal skills were the initial treatment outcome goals established *(Plan)*.

PROVIDER ROLE FUNCTION

The evaluator role function, then, emphasizes conceptualization and planning intervention based on treatability and patient functional capacity. The provider role function, on the other hand, emphasizes

tailoring and combining treatment based largely on pattern, perpetuants, and prognosis.

Currently, medication management is the main provider role function for psychiatrists in outpatient managed care settings. Typically, the
psychiatrist evaluates the appropriateness of medication for a patient
referred from a nonmedical therapist. If a medical trail begins, the
psychiatrist monitors the individual weekly or biweekly until a maintenance dose is achieved. Thereafter, medication checks are scheduled
monthly, bimonthly, and quarterly.

These brief sessions (usually 15 or 20 minutes each) provide an
extraordinarily opportunity to maximize treatment outcomes. Unfortunately, many psychiatrists skilled in managing the psychological issues
of psychotherapy do not routinely utilize these skills when they provide
medical treatment. Ward notes: "Too often, they neglect invaluable
psychotherapeutic approaches and use only explanation and admon-
ishment to get patients to take medication" (1991, p. 69). It is not
only possible but highly probable that patients can achieve maximal
pharmacological benefits within the context of an optimal patient–
psychiatrist relationship.

Skilled medication management (Eckuren, Liberman, Phipps, &
Blair, 1990) requires awareness of the patient's pattern, prognostic
factor, and overall treatment plan, particularly if the patient is concurrently involved in psychotherapy with a nonmedical therapist. An understanding of the psychology of medication compliance or adherence
(Blackwell, 1976; Doherty, 1988) and the placebo effect (Beitman,
1993b; Spiro, 1986) are important. The involvement of family members
in ensuring medication compliance (Doherty, 1988; Doherty & Baird,
1983) is also crucial.

The psychiatrist must consider what type of relationship—that is,
how much dependency to allow the patient and how much authority
to exert—he or she will strive to develop. In addition, the psychiatrist
must negotiate a treatment agreement that maximizes medication compliance and the placebo effect, as well as considering psychological
reactions to dosage, side effects, main effects, and the influence of
the patient's social network on compliance. Furthermore, transference
reaction must be anticipated and recognized, as they may either facilitate or sabotage treatment outcomes, as well as countertransference
reactions that may distort proper management (Busch & Gould, 1993).

Ward (1991) describes specific strategies for effectively dealing with
narcissistic, obsessive, histrionic, borderline, avoidant, schizophrenic,
and paranoid patients in medication management contexts. Ward also
provides a number of useful guidelines for structuring and tailoring

management sessions based on the patient's treatment expectations and other prognostic factors.

The other psychiatric provider role function involves combined treatment, which has been heralded as the basis of clinical psychiatry practice in the 21st century (Beitman, 1993a). In this context the psychiatrist sees the patient and provides combined treatment—medication and psychotherapy. The sessions may be scheduled for 30, 45, or 50 minutes, depending on the managed care policy and the psychiatrist's training and cost of the session. The nature of the psychotherapy may be supportive, interpersonal, cognitive, dynamic, or strategic in focus. In addition to utilizing the same kind of strategies noted above for medication management, the psychiatrist also works to maximize psychotherapeutic outcomes.

Most psychiatrists are familiar with the early results of the NIMH Treatment of Depression Collaboration Research Project (Elkin, et al. 1989) wherein cognitive or interpersonal therapy was combined with antidepressant treatment. However, fewer psychiatrists are aware of numerous other efforts to combine psychosocial modalities with medications for specific Axis I and II disorders.

Beitman and Klerman (1991) offer cogent guidelines and protocols for combining and tailoring medication and psychotherapy for various anxiety, mood, psychotic, and personality disorders. There are other forms of combined treatment, such as medication and family therapy, medication and group therapy, and individual with family and marital therapy (see Beitman, 1993a; Glick, Clarkin & Goldsmith, 1993). These and other combined biopsychosocial interventions will further help the psychiatrist in maximizing psychopharmacology and psychotherapy.

The Case of C.W., Continued

The treatment plan for C.W. was developed based on her presentation as well as her pattern and prognostic factors. The treatment and strategic goals were developed to facilitate therapeutic outcomes by maximizing therapeutic leverage while minimizing the influence of previous perpetuants and other forms of resistance to change.

Treatment consisted of a trial of a serotenergic antidepressant that would be minimally stimulating. Twenty minute weekly outpatient sessions with the psychiatrist focused on symptom reduction and returning to work. This meant that some collaboration with C.W.'s supervisor about work and peer support was initiated. The supervisor agreed that C.W. needed a familiar, trusting social support, and was able to assign one of C.W.'s coworkers to the same office to which C.W. had been moved. An initial treatment agreement was established for six 45-minute sessions combining medication and interpersonal therapy. They also discussed that skill-oriented group therapy was probably the treatment of choice for C.W. to increase her trustability and decrease her social isolation. Aware that C.W.'s pattern of avoidance would make entry into and continuation with the group difficult, the plan was for the individual sessions to serve as a transition into the group, after which shorter individual sessions would focus on medication management, probably on a monthly and then a bimonthly basis.

Aware of her pattern, the psychiatrist anticipated that C.W. would test the psychiatrist and group therapist's trustability and criticalness. Throughout treatment both clinicians continued to be mindful of the therapeutic leverage (success with nicotine abstinence, relations with cousin and pet, closeknit typing pool) as well as the perpetuants that would likely hamper treatment.

THE CONSULTOR ROLE FUNCTION

There are various ways in which psychiatrists can interface with other professionals, organizations, and government bodies. They can advocate and advise on policy matters, as well as supervise, collaborate, or consult on health and mental health issues. Psychiatrists have made significant contributions to local and national health and mental health policies in the past, and need to become more proactive in this area now and in the future. This section focuses on the psychiatrist's role function as consultor in maximizing psychotherapeutic and psychopharmacological outcomes. It does not discuss advocacy or policy advising dimensions.

As noted earlier, the consultor role function shares commonalities (plan, pattern, and prognosis) with the evaluation and provider roles. However, there are notable differences as well. First, in the consultor role function the psychiatrist may have little or no face-to-face contact with the patient, and instead interfaces with a nonmedical therapist and occasionally with nonpsychiatric physicians. Second, relationships with nonmedical therapists take on different forms with varying degrees of legal liability (Applebaum, 1991).

The American Psychiatric Association (1980) outlines three kinds of relationships between psychiatrists and nonmedical psychotherapists: consultative, collaborative, and supervisory. In the consultative relationship, the psychiatrist has no ongoing relationship with the patient and the therapist is not obliged to follow the psychiatrist's counsel. In the collaborative relationship, responsibility for treatment is shared, and so the psychiatrist is responsible for the patient's medications and physical complaints. Finally, in the supervisory relationship, the psychiatrist actively directs all facets of the nonmedical therapist's work. Applebaum (1991) adds that in the supervisory as contrasted with the consultative relationship, the nonmedical therapist is obliged to follow the psychiatrist's counsel.

In this chapter the consultor role encompasses supervisory, consultative, and collaborative relationships and a specific oversight function. This contrasts with the traditional psychiatrist role function as supervisor and team leader. Unlike the authoritative, independent role of the past, it emphasizes an interdependent-collaborative relationship with nonmedical therapists, particularly regarding medication and combined treatments.

The advent of increasingly effective psychotropic medications with fewer side effects and better safety profiles has led to growing collaboration between nonmedical therapists and prescribing psychiatrists. This collaboration not only can lead to the amelioration of symptoms, but also can increase the patient's availability for and capacity to respond to psychotherapy. However, efforts to collaborate can confuse, complicate, and even sabotage both treatments. The addition of a second professional in the treatment matrix can engender negative transference as well as problematic countertransference (Busch & Gould, 1993).

This can occur because the collaborating clinicians tend to have a different treatment focus and goals, and relate to the patient differently in terms of duration and frequency of sessions. While the prescribing psychiatrist may be focused principally on managing relationships with the patient and psychotherapist to maximize medication compliance and, it is hoped, to increase a positive placebo response (Spiro, 1986), the nonmedical therapist is focused principally on enhancing the patient's self-management and interpersonal relationships functioning. Furthermore, the two collaborators usually differ in gender, age, interpersonal style, professional discipline, and attitudes toward somatic and psychosocial therapies. Not surprisingly, projective identification and splitting can be expected.

Projective identification refers to the patient disavowing unacceptable parts of the self and attributing them to one of the clinicians, who begins to behave as of the patient's attributions were true. In splitting, this projective process extends so that the clinician becomes idealized and feels compelled to nurture and protect the patient, while the other clinician is devalued and feels like attacking or rejecting the patient. If not carefully managed, splitting can sabotage the treatment process. Early signs of splitting include distorted perceptions such as idealization or devaluation of the other clinician. When splitting is present, coordination of treatment with the other clinicians becomes crucial. Both must be willing to step back and clarify the perception of each other that the patient has presented. Then, they must be able to present a unified front to the patient, supporting each other's treatment approach in interactions with the patient. And, if necessary, they should see the patient together until a resolution of the splitting is achieved (Woodward, Duckworth, & Guthiel, 1992).

It is for such reasons that some caution against overly close collaboration between psychiatrists and nonmedical therapist. For instance, Kelly (1992) insists that frequent communication between clinicians and sharing impressions about the patient's problems and progress toward treatment goals can be destructive to treatment. Kelly believes that it can engender unacknowledged and unchecked competition between the clinicians, and it can infantilize the patient as well. Instead, he proposes that the prescribing psychiatrist relate to the nonmedical therapist as a consultant rather than as a collaborator or supervisor, since he doesn't believe real collaboration is possible when individuals are trained in nonmedical disciplines.

On the other hand, many others (Beitman, 1991; Blackwell & Schmidt, 1991; Busch & Gould, 1993) advocate collaboration. When the roles of both clinicians are clearly distinguished, frequent discussions about the patient and treatment goals can facilitate treatment outcome. In fact, Busch and Gould (1993), a psychiatrist and a social worker who routinely collaborate, find that the quality of collaboration is crucial to treatment outcomes. They indicate that mutual respect, trust, and openness are necessary in developing an effective collaboration. They point out that collaborative communication can be quite useful to both clinicians if they sensitize each other to their concerns. For instance, because the therapist sees the patient more frequently, he or she should be able to recognize early signs of hypomania in a patient who is taking an antimanic medication. Or, the prescriber, concerned that a patient's inability might be a side effect of fluoxetine, can learn from the therapist that the patient is usually irritable.

Several authors (Applebaum, 1991; Beitman et al, 1992; Chiles, Carlin, Benjamin, & Beitman, 1991) have extended the discussion of collaboration between prescriber and therapist to include the patient. They recognize that a three-way therapeutic agreement must be reached covering the purpose of each treatment, the clinician's roles, the patient's roles with each clinician, frequency and duration of sessions, policies for communication between the clinicians, any supervision of one clinician by the other, arrangements for emergencies and coverage after hours, and exceptions to confidentiality of records. This agreement can be summarized in writing. The frequency of collaboration of a managed care setting is largely influenced by practice guidelines. At a minimum, it should occur at the beginning and end of treatment, when problems arise or major changes in medication or treatment modalities occur, or at times when either clinician is unavailable because of vacation or sick leave (Woodward, Duckworth, & Guthiel, 1993).

Training psychiatrists for these consultor role functions will facilitate the adoption of these role functions (Blackwell & Schmidt, 1991; Kay, 1991; Sabin, 1991; Sabin & Borus, 1992). Kay (1991) believes that future psychiatrists will receive training to teach and supervise other health care personnel as well as in leadership and administrative skills.

The Case of C.W., Continued

The initial treatment plan for C.W. involved the combined modalities of medication management and a short course in interpersonal psychotherapy for depression with gradual transition into a time-limited group therapy focused on interpersonal skill development. As C.W.'s depressive symptoms ameliorated and a maintenance medication schedule was established, the psychiatrist began preparing her for transition into the group. Because of C.W.'s fear and ambivalence about the group process, the psychiatrist suggested and C.W. agreed that it might be helpful to meet with the therapist who led the interpersonal skills group she was slated to join. During their fifth session the group therapist was briefly introduced to C.W. and there was some discussion of a three-way treatment agreement. The three agreed that C.W. would continue in individual weekly appointments concurrent with weekly group session. And assuming things were proceeding well enough, sessions with the prescribing psychiatrists would be reduced to monthly medication checks.

A subsequent two-way discussion between therapist and psychiatrist concluded that there was little likelihood that projective identification and splitting would be issues with C.W. Instead, difficulty in maintaining active group participation and follow-up on homework between group sessions was predicted. The psychiatrist agreed to encourage and support the patient's group involvement in his concurrent individual sessions with her. Furthermore, the therapist and the psychiatrist planned on conferring after the third group session regarding the transition from weekly to monthly sessions with the psychiatrist.

CONCLUDING COMMENTS

The identities and roles of mental health professionals will continue to evolve in the coming years. It has been my purpose to give an overview the nature of these changes, particularly as they affect the psychiatrist practicing in a managed care setting. I have proposed a specific role for the psychiatrist to match the psychiatrist's unique training, values, and biopsychosocial perspective, as well as the values and demands of

TABLE 4-2

Role Functions with Differing Role Definitions for the Psychiatrist

Authoritative/Independent Leadership	*Supportive/Subordinate Position*	*Collaborative Leadership*
expert diagnostician		principal evaluator
differential therapy prescriber		differential therapy evaluator/prescriber
psychosocial therapy provider		focused combined treatment provider
somatic therapy pre-scriber/provider	somatic therapy pre-scriber/provider/referrer	somatic therapy pre-scriber/provider
medical evaluator/ provider/referrer		medical evaluator/ provider/referrer
treatment team leader and supervisor	"sign off" supervision	treatment team consul-tor: (supervisor, consult-ant, oversight function)

managed care. The role involves a collaborative leadership relationship with other health and mental health personnel for the purpose of maximizing psychotherapeutic and psychopharmacological outcomes. Table 4-2 compares this role and role function with previous ones.

This role and the functions of evaluator, provider, and consultor require a somewhat different leadership style and focus on treatment outcomes rather than on treatment and service delivery per se. Nevertheless, I hope that psychiatrists can be trained to collaborate effectively with other mental health professionals to provide state-of-the-art combined treatments that are both cost effective and efficacious. For not to prepare, educate, and mentor psychiatrists and psychiatrists-in-training about roles in managed care "is to fail in our responsibility to the future of psychiatry" (Lewis & Blotcky, 1993, p. 192).

REFERENCES

American Psychiatric Association (1980). Guidelines for psychiatrists in consultation, supervisory, or collaborating relationships with nonmedical therapists. *American Journal of Psychiatry, 137:* 1489–1491.

Applebaum, P. (1991). General guidelines for psychiatrists who prescribe medication for patients treated by nonmedical psychotherapists. *Hospital and Community Psychiatry, 42:* 281–282.

Beitman, B. (1993a). Combined Treatments. In Oldman, J. Riba, M. and Tasmen, A. (Eds.) *American Psychiatric Press Review of Psychiatry, Volume 12.* Washington, DC: American Psychiatric Press, pp. 517–519.

Beitman, B. (1993b). Pharmacotherapy and the stages of psychotherapeutic change. In Oldman, J. Riba, M. and Tasmen, A. (Eds.) *American Psychiatric Press Review of Psychiatry, Volume 12.* Washigton, DC: American Psychiatric Press, pp. 521–540.

Beitman, B. & Klerman, G. (Eds.) (1991). *Integrating pharmacotherapy and psychotherapy.* Washington, DC: American Psychiatric Press.

Beitman, B. (1991). Medication during psychotherapy: Case studies of the reciprocal relationship between psychotherapy process and medication use. In Beitman, B. and Klerman, G. (Eds.) *Integrating Pharmacotherapy and Psychotherapy.* Washington, DC: American Psychiatric Press, pp. 21–44.

Bennett, M. (1993). View from the bridge: Reflections of a recovering staff model HMO psychiatrist. *Psychiatric Quarterly, 64:* 45–75.

Blackwell, B. (1976). Treatment adherence. *British Journal of Psychiatry, 129:* 513–531.

Blackwell, B. & Schmidt, G. (1992). The educational implications of managed mental health care. *Hospital and Community Psychiatry, 43:* 962–964.

Budman, S. (1992). Models of brief individual and group psychotherapy. In Feldman, J. and Fitzpatrick R. (Eds.). *Managed Mental Health Care.* Washington, DC: American Psychiatric Press, pp. 231–247.

Busch, F. & Gould, E. (1993). Treatment by a psychotherapist and psychopharmacologist: Transference and countertransference issues. *Hospital and Community Psychiatry, 44:* 772–774.

Chiles, J., Carlin, A., Benjamin, G., & Beitman, B. (1991). A physician, a nonmedical psychotherapist and a patient: The pharmacotherapy-psychotherapy triangle. In B. Beitman and G. Klerman (Eds.), *Integrating pharmacotherapy and psychotherapy.* Washington, DC: American Psychiatric Press, pp. 105–118.

Dekle, D., & Christensen, L. (1990). Medication management. *Hospital and Community Psychiatry, 41:* 96–97.

Doherty, J. (1988). Managing compliance problems in psychopharmacology. In F. Flach (Ed.), *Psychobiology and psychopharmacology.* New York: Norton, pp. 12–31.

Doherty, W., & Baird, M. (1983). *Family therapy and family medicine.* New York: Guilford.

Eckuren, T., Liberman, R., Phipps, C., & Blair, K. (1990). Teaching medication management skills to schizophrenic patients. *Journal of Clinical Psychopharmacology, 10:* 33–38.

Elkin, I., Shea, M., Watkins, J. *et al.* (1989). NIMH treatment of depression collaborative research program I: General effectiveness of treatments. *Archives of General Psychiatry, 46:* 971–982.

Feldman, J. & Fitzpatrick, R. (Eds). (1992). *Managed mental health care: Administraitve and clinical issues.* Washington, DC: American Psychiatric Press.

Frances, A., Clarkin, J., & Perry, S. (1984). *Differential therapeutics in psychiatry: The art and science of treatment selection.* New York: Brunner/Mazel.

Giles, T. (1993). *Managed mental health care: A guide for practioners, employers, and hospital administrators.* Boston: Allyn and Bacon.

Hyland, J. (1991). Integrating psychotherapy and pharmacotherapy. *Bulletin of the Menninger Clinic, 55:* 205–215.

Jaques, E., & Clement, S. (1991). *Executive leadership: A practical guide to managing complexity.* Cambridge, MA: Blackwell Business.

Katz, P. (1986). The role of the psychotherapies in the practice of psychiatry. *Canadian Journal of Psychiatry.*

Kay, J. (1991). The influence of the curriculum in psychiatry residency education. *Psychiatric Quarterly, 62:* 95–104.

Kennedy, J. (1992). *Fundamentals of psychiatric treatment planning.* Washington, DC: American Psychiatric Press.

Lewis, J., & Blotcky, M. (1993). Living and learning with managed care. *Journal of Psychiatry, 17:* 186–192.

Ludwig, A. (1987). The role of psychiatrists in the practice of psychotherapy. *Journal of Psychotherapy, 41:* 361–368.

Munoz, R. (1994). Commodity markets and the carving of psychiatry. *Clinical Psychiatry Quarterly.*

Sabin, J. (1991). Clinical skills for the 1990's: Six lessons from HMO practice. *Hospital and Community Psychiatry, 42:* 605–608.

Sabin, J. and Borus, J. (1992). Mental health teaching and research in managed care. In Feldman, J. and Fitzpatrick, R. (eds.) *Managed Mental Health Care: Administrative and Clinical Issues.* Washington, DC: American Psychiatric Press.

Sabshin, M. (1987). The Future Role of Psychiatrists. In Adelson, C. and Rabinowitz, C. (Eds.) *Training Psychiatrists for the 90's: Issues and Recommendations.* Washington, DC: American Psychiatric Press.

Schneider-Braus, K. (1992). Managing a mental health department in staff model HMO. In Feldman, J. and Fitzpatrick, R. (Eds.) *Managed Mental Health Care.* Washington, DC: American Psychiatric Press, 125–141.

Siegler, J., Axelband, M. and Isikoff, J. (1993). Psychiatry: Taking a leadership role in managed health care. *Psychiatric Times.*

Sovner, R. (1991). A Psychopharmacology service model. In Austad, C. and Berman, W. (Eds.) *Psychotherapy in Managed Care.* Washington, DC: American Psychological Association, pp. 86–97.

Sotsky, S., Galss, D., Shea, M. et al. (1991). Patient predictors of response to psychotherapy and pharmacotherapy: Findings in the NIMH treatment of depression collaborative research program. *American Journal of Psychiatry, 148:* 997–1008.

Sperry, L., Gudeman, J., Blackwell, B. & Faulkner, L. (1992). *Psychiatric case formulations.* Washington, DC: American Psychiatric Press.

Spiro, H. (1986). *Doctors, patients and placebos.* New Haven, CT: Yale University Press.

Ward, N. (1991). Psychosocial approaches to pharmacotherapy. In Beitman, B. and Klerman, G. (Eds.) *Integrating pharmacotherapy and psychotherapy.* Washington, DC: American Psychiatric Press, 69–104.

Woodward, B., Duckworth, K. & Guthiel, J. (1993). The pharmacotherapist-psychotherapist collaboration. In Hham, J., Riba, J., and Tasmen, A. (Eds.) *American Psychiatric Press Review of Psychiatry, Volume 12.* Washington, DC: American Psychiatric Press, 631–649.

Westermeyer, J. (1991). Problems with managed care without a psychiatrist-manager. *Hospital and Community Psychiatry, 42:* 1221–1224.

5

Brief Group Therapy

HENRY I. SPITZ, M.D.

INTRODUCTION

The challenge of providing excellent clinical care on a cost efficient basis to large groups of people has been a primary focus in the mental health field for decades. In recent years, the emergence of innovative and creative models of health care delivery have emerged and can be broadly subsumed under the rubric of *managed care*.

Although the language of managed care has found its way into common clinical parlance in the mental health field, the majority of practitioners do not feel a corresponding level of comfort with many of these new formats for the provision of treatment of emotional disorders. This trend is reminiscent of the prevailing clinical climate that followed the movement towards the deinstitutionalization of chronically mentally ill patients in the late 1960s and early 1970s. Mental health care providers were faced with serving the needs of enormous numbers of patients and found themselves understaffed and armed with inadequate funding and training.

It was then at this period in history when group techniques began to develop as a partial solution to this clinical dilemma. Groups were able to accommodate greater numbers of people, required less staff time, and cost about one third to one half as much as conventional long-term individual psychotherapy. The experimentation that took place within the group field led to the emergence of shorter-term, more eclectically based treatment modalities aimed at the resolution of troublesome psychiatric conditions.

The current crisis in the American health care system demands similar treatment efforts that are relatively brief, more targeted at specific symptoms (rather than at global and/or vague diagnostic entities), clearly defined, documentable, and lend themselves to the scientific study of treatment outcome and efficacy (Feldman & Fitzpatrick, 1992; Goodman, Brown, & Dietz, 1992).

The group milieu has much of value to offer to clinicians, administrators, employers, and most importantly to the patients or consumers of sorely needed psychological services.

The focus of this chapter will be on an overview of the ways in which conventional group treatment methods can be adapted to meet the needs and concerns of all who are interacting under the managed care system.

OVERVIEW OF SHORT-TERM GROUP PSYCHOTHERAPY

Brief group psychotherapy formats have followed the lead of their individual psychotherapeutic counterparts and subscribe to many of the same principles. Budman & Bennett (1983) originally characterized six factors that are found in all time-limited groups. They emphasized the necessity of "focality of treatment," which encompasses the notion of a realistic and thoughtful but circumscribed goal setting for group members. Secondly, they noted the centrality of active group leadership. Because time is limited in brief groups, the leader must be active from the outset. If properly done, appropriate leadership activity will result in theraputic group norms and the rapid emergence of a third essential factor, early group cohesion. Group cohesion is the interpersonal cement that bonds group members and allows for an accelerated first phase of group therapy. Cohesion provides an emotional cushion for members and protects them from avoidable problems such as interpersonal attack or scapegoating in the group.

A clear time limit on both the length of each session and the duration of the group experience over time is also considered to be essential to the conduct of a short-term group. This format creates a sense of theraputic urgency in the group and helps define what are attainable goals for participants within a fixed time span. In order to accomplish this task, the leader of the short-term therapy group strives to keep the group focus in the here and now, with only occasional forays into the past if historically relevant patterns or themes are being demonstrated in the current group process. This technique in the outpatient setting follows the guidelines for examination of intragroup interactions in the style suggested by Yalom (1985), who studied short-term groups in hospital settings. Yalom discussess groups whose leaders had to conduct groups for patients with short hospital stays.

Lastly, Budman, Bennett, and others familiar with the time-limited group model (such as MacKenzie, 1990) stress the issue of careful patient selection designed to maximize similarities among members, another element that leads to a rapid induction and cohesion stage in a new group.

Several other points about which there is consensus in the literature on short-term groups underscore the need not only for careful member selection but also for thorough attention to the pregroup phase. It is important for the therapist to obtain preauthorization for one or two evaluation/preparation sessions at the outset. The key elements to be accomplished prior to the first formal group session include individual and interpersonal diagnostic evaluations and an orientation session for prospective group members. Both of these factors are correlated with a lowering of the dropout rate from groups and a group membership that enters with realistic expectations of the group experience to come (Piper, Debanne, & Bienvenu, 1982).

The application and modification of these generally accepted criteria for short-term groups when the context in which the group is conducted is a managed care setting will form the bulk of the material to follow in this chapter. The orientation will be aimed at the group leader and will address many of the major pragmatic issues that affect both clinical decisions and matters related to the procedural and acountability aspects unique to group therapy in the managed mental health care system.

CONSTRUCTION OF THE GROUP

1. The Role of the Leader

The eventual success or failure of many psychotherapy groups often can be traced back to leadership decisions made prior to the start of the group experience. In managed care systems it is particularly important that the group leader review several key areas of group treatment prior to the initial contact with the prospective group member.

First, the therapist's theoretical orientation and personal belief system regarding psychotherapy can be a major help or hindrance to the theraputic endeavor. The group leader has to be flexible in adapting his or her preferred way of working in order to meet both the time limits and the needs of the patient populations found with the managed care system.

It is generally acepted in group circles that extremes of leadership styles usually result in trouble for the group. In Liberman, Yalom, and Miles (1973) study on psychological casualties resulting from encounter group experiences it was shown that extremes of leadership style, the charismatic on one end of the range and the passive on the other, represented the most high risk leadership postures. Because managed care groups are time-limited, the leader has to be active but not charismatic. Constructive leadership activity finds the therapist active in structuring the group experience, making sure that theraputic group norms emerge, maintaining the relevant group focus, and guarding against potential harmful trends in the group. Passive leaders do not provide enough direction, structure, and orientation for brief therapy group experiences and as such provide poor role models for members and make work with more seriously impaired psychiatric patients nearly impossible.

Leaders who subscribe to a predominantly psychoanalytic or psychodynamic orientation must give careful thought and planning to the modifications of traditional technique in order to accomplish more ambitious goals in the short-term setting. Many therapists mistakenly equate brief therapy with superficial therapy or see it as a quick fix. Short-term groups for higher functioning patients can be extremely effective both at symptom removal and in helping to change some aspects of personality structure.

A central function in all brief therapies is the leader's ability to formulate the work to be done and to be unrelenting in keeping the group focused on the group goals (Budman, 1992). There are many stages in groups where the group will avoid, resist, or drift away from the work focus. (These stages are discussed later in the chapter.) Alert leaders recognize these deleterious trends and plan therapeutic interventions to keep the group centered on its primary tasks.

In sum, the clinician's ability to attain his or her own sense of clarity referable to the understanding of the "managed care group" is critical to the process of making sensible determinations about the choice of "ingredients" and their proportions in the "recipe" for the creation and ongoing management of therapeutic group experiences aimed at addressing a range of problems for which managed care providers will be called upon for their expertise. Budman's (1992) term, *informed eclecticism,* captures the spirit of a sort of leadership that is most likely to maximize the inherent resources of the time-limited group.

The similarities and differences among three major representative group formats can be seen in Table 5-1.

2. Establishment of Group Goals

Goal specificity is a hallmark of managed mental health treatment. The more precise the clinician can be in both planning and describing a proposed treatment plan, the more likely it is that the plan will be approved for reimbursement under managed care.

Because groups are composed of not one but many members, the issue of goal setting takes on added significance insofar as plans must be made for each member and for the group as a whole. On the group level, the leader has clinical decisions to make that rely heavily upon determining whether the group alone will suffice or whether the group will serve as one important part of a more comprehensive treatment program for its members.

Two goals that apply to all members of short-term groups include the notion of increased patient responsibility for change and the transfer of learning of information gleaned in the group to life outside the group. In time-restricted formats, both of these factors are central to the attainment of theraputic goals. Adjunctive use of community support options, 12-step derived programs, and similar resources are frequently employed to enhance the accomplishment of goals for brief therapy groups.

Each individual member of the group should have a clear and well-thought-out reason for his or her placement in a specific group. All too often, people are inappropriately referred to groups for reasons that are destined to make the group experience a failure or defeat for the member, leader, and group. Common examples include the referral of someone to a group because other therapies have been unsuccessful, referrals made solely on the basis of economics (group therapy is cheaper than other therapies), or such misconceptions about time-limited groups as the myth that brief therapies are only suited to higher functioning patients.

In the section to follow, the pragmatics of evaluating a patient for short-term group therapy will be highlighted.

3. The Pregroup Phase

Careful attention to the issues of the pregroup phase both helps to ensure a reduced dropout rate and increases the likelihood of a successful

TABLE 5-1

Typology of Groups

	Self-Help Group
Size	Large (size often unlimited)
Leadership	1. Peer leader or recovered substance abuser 2. Leadership is earned status over time 3. Implicit hierarchical leadership structure
Membership Participation	Voluntary
Group Governed	Self-governing
Content	1. Environmental factors, no examination of group interaction 2. Emphasis on similarities among members 3. "Here and now" focus
Screening Interview	None
Group Processes	Universalization, empathy, affective sharing, education, public statement of problem (self-disclosure), mutual affirmation, morale building, catharsis, immediate positive feedback, high degrees of persuasiveness
Outside Socialization	1. Encouraged strongly 2. Construction of social network is actively sought
Goals	1. Positive goal setting, behaviorally oriented 2. Focus on the "group as a whole" and the similarities among members
Leader Activity	1. Educator/role model catalyst for learning 2. Less member-to-leader distance
Use of Interpretation or Psychodynamic Techniques	No
Confidentiality	Anonymity preserved
Sponsorship Program	Yes (usually same sex)
Deselection	1. Members may leave group at their own choosing 2. Members may avoid self-disclosure or discussion of any subject
Involvement in Other Groups/Programs	Yes
Time Factors	Unlimited group participation possible over years
Frequency of Meetings	Active encouragement of daily participation

---

*Adapted from Spitz & Rosecan (1987). *Cocaine abuse: New directions in treatment and research.* (pp. 162–163). New York: Brunner/Mazel.

Psychotherapy Group	Managed Care Group
Small (8–15 members)	Small (8–10 members)
1. Mental health professional 2. Self-appointed leadership 3. Formal hierarchical leadership structure	Professional mental health leadership
Voluntary and involuntary	Voluntary
Leader governed	Leader governed
1. Examination of intragroup behavior and extragroup factors 2. Emphasis on differentiation among members over time 3. "Here and now" plus historical focus	1. Examination of intragroup issues and transfer of learning to life outside group 2. "Here and now" focus
Always	Always and strong pre-group orientation
Cohesion, mutual identification confrontation, education, catharsis, use of group pressure re: abstinence and retention of group membership	Cohesion, peer support, homogeneous group factors
1. Cautious re: extragroup contact 2. Intermember networking is optional	1. Depending on nature of group 2. Usually is optional
1. Ambitious goals: immediate problems plus individual personality issues 2. Individual as well as group focus	1. Crisis resolution 2. Specific target symptoms or behavior 3. Life-cycle issues
1. Responsible for therapeutic group experience 2. More member-to-leader distance	Leader very active in structuring group experience
Yes	Usually not (exception-high functioning groups)
Strongly emphasized	Strongly emphasized
No	No
1. Predetermined minimal term of commitment to group membership 2. Avoidance of discussion seen as "resistance"	1. Members may be screened out during orientation phase or in first 1–2 sessions
Yes–eclectic models No–psychodynamic models	Yes
Often time-limited experiences	Strict time limitations
Meets less frequently (often once or twice weekly)	Usually once per week; cognitive/behavioral and in-patient groups meet more frequently

group experience for members. This phase consists of several components: individual diagnostic evaluation, assessment of group functioning, and the preparation and orientation of every incoming group member.

While this is good practice in any group, short or long-term, it takes on central significance when prepaid health care organizations are financing the treatment services. Time spent with a potential group member before the first actual group session is what constitutes the pregroup phase. The more specific the provider can be concerning the elements in this phase, the more likely it is that a reasonable time- and cost-efficient treatment plan will emerge.

The initial aspect of the pregroup stage begins with the first contact with a person being considered for group therapy and ends with a face-to-face orientation about the group and its key elements. Because this is such a critical phase of group treatment, it will be described in some detail. This will serve the dual purpose of delineating the essential features of pregroup preparation and detailing the process of implementing it in an actual managed care clinical setting.

The issue of diagnostic evaluation in managed care formats puts greater emphasis on functional impairment, medical necessity for treatment, and signs and symptoms that are consistent with some generally accepted diagnostic instrument such as the DSM III-R or DSM-IV. In this regard, the clinician can conduct a thorough diagnostic assessment and conceptualize it in standard diagnostic terms: however, it is preferable to present the Axis I and/or Axis II diagnoses in a form that stresses symptoms and behavioral problems. In so doing, the provider can more efficiently communicate the target treatment goals and subsequent rationale and plans for their management into treatment objectives and strategies.

The special concern for group therapists is that conventional individual methods of evaluation usually focus more on individual psychopathology, but group therapy is an interpersonal form of treatment. Consequently, any comprehensive initial assessment of an individual should include some measure of historical and current interpersonal strengths and weaknesses.

A simple way to get a rough gauge of this dimension of someone's life is to incorporate a group function history as part of the initial interview. To accomplish this, the evaluator looks at an individual's interpersonal patterns in natural groups. The simplest way to do this is by taking a chronological view of the patient's life, starting with family of origin, going on to peer group relationships in childhood and adolescence, through school history, work function, capacity for forming and sustaining friendships and romantic or sexual relationships, and any other large or small group experience (for example, military service or athletic team participation) that might identify functional or dysfunctional group capacity.

As a case in point, consider two prospective group members who both meet the criteria for Dysthymia (300.4 DSM-IV). If one has a pattern of interpersonal avoidance, anxiety in new situations, and a capacity for developing trusting relationships once he or she feels comfortable with people, and the other has a poor family history, difficulty with authority figures, a longstanding feeling of mistrust of others, and substance abuse, their theraputic fate will be easier to determine if conceptualized from a combined individual and interpersonal perspective. In the above example, Patient 1 might do very well in a short-term, supportive, social skills group with a cognitive/behavioral focus. Patient 2 would be less likely to do well in such a setting, and an observer might be led to wonder about the existence of other concurrent personality disorders.

In addition to initial interviewing methods there are instruments for evaluating interpersonal themes. When considering someone for group placement it may be helpful to administer one or more tests that emphasize an interpersonal focus. MacKenzie (1990) suggests the value of five measures that are useful in this regard. He cites the Core Conflict Relationship Theme (CCRT), the configurational analysis, the interpersonal content thematic evaluation, the life-stage developmental perspective, and the Structural Analysis of Social Behavior (SASB) as aids in the quest for relevant interpersonal information that will help in appropriate group composition and placement of patients in short-term groups.

In clinical setttings where the evaluator is someone other than the group leader and in many outpatient clinic settings, it is very important to have a systematized mechanism for referring patients to groups once the evaluation process is completed. Patients, therapists, and groups themselves should all be compatible in order to maximize the groups' theraputic power. Exhibits 5-1 and 5-2 illustrate a sample method of group referral and therapist response forms that ensure that optimum group matching takes place.

Once the diagnostic segment is complete, the group leader should have a complement of members ready to join a new group. The next major task prior to the first meeting is to thoroughly orient and prepare individuals for the group experience that lies ahead.

The group literature on patient pretraining (Piper, Debanne, & Bienvenue, 1982) clearly suggests that realistic pretreatment expectations for patients, eventual ease of group management for group leaders, and positive outcome for the total group are directly enhanced by effective pretraining efforts. Pretraining takes many forms, including

EXHIBIT 5-1

Group Therapy Referral Form

Patient's name: _____ Case number: _____

Home phone number: _____ Work phone number: _____

Age: _____ Sex: _____ Referral source: _____

Brief psychiatric history (include hospitalizations, type and extent of previous treatment, known stressors to symptom upsurge): _____
_____
_____

Current symptoms: _____
_____

Present social circumstances (include family situation, involvement with friends, family, and social/community networks): _____
_____
_____

Describe reason for referral to group therapy: _____
_____

What type of group do you recommend for this patient? _____
_____

What are the goals for this patient and how will group placement help implement them? _____
_____

Is group therapy to be primary modality or adjunctive? _____
Psychiatric diagnosis: _____
_____

Medical status: _____
_____

Current medications: _____
_____

Are there any scheduling problems (work, school, other therapies, etc.)?
_____

What is the patient's reaction to discussion of referral to group? _____
_____

Other information or considerations that might be important to patient's ability to participate or remain in group treatment. _____
_____
_____

EXHIBIT 5-2
Group Therapy Referral Follow-up Form

To: **Referral Source**
From: **Group Leader**
Re: **Patient 'X'**

____(A) We suggest your patient join the following group: (Name of group, leader's name, day, time, and place of meetings)

_____

_____

Please contact _____ (usually group leader's name and phone number) to arrange placement into group.

____(B) At this point in time we do not have an appropriate group for your patient but will place the patient on the waiting list and notify you as soon as a place is available.

____(C) We do not feel that this patient is suitable for our group at this time. (Please provide an explanation for this decision.)

_____

_____

_____

_____

_____

_____

_____

_____

_____

_____

_____

_____

_____

the distribution of written orientation manuals for members, actual waiting list or orientation groups, and others.

The author finds that the use of a pregroup checklist (see Table 5-2) facilitates the process of patient preparation for group leaders and members. Some of the salient items for short-term groups include clarity regarding group goals and time restrictions, confidentiality, coordination of other simultaneous therapies or medications, and whether the group will be open or closed to new members once it has begun.

When the pregroup phase is successfully completed, the patient should have a picture of what to expect in sessions, his or her anxiety about group entry should be diminished, and the motivation for therapy should be reenforced. The remaining work for the leader prior to the first session is to construct a group of well screened and properly oriented members who will function well together in a time-limited group. The section that follows addresses the factors to be taken into account in composing a group that will maximize its therapeutic potential when conducted in an atmosphere where time is of the essence.

4. Group Composition with Respect to Managed Care Settings

The traditional wisdom in composing therapy groups has been to try to achieve a sense of balance between homogeneous and heterogeneous

TABLE 5-2

Pregroup Preparation Checklist

1. General purpose and goals of the group
2. Group composition and size
3. Role and activity level of the leader
4. Observers, audiotaping, or videotaping of sessions
5. Physical arrangement of therapy room
6. Time period of each session; duration of the group (long-term versus time-limited)
7. Loss and addition of group members
8. Rules about attendance
9. Fees and billing procedures
10. Other coexisting treatment: drugs, hospitalization potential, other therapies (simultaneous individual therapy)
11. Contacts and/or socialization among members outside the group
12. Modifications of the group contract (e.g., individual scheduling problems)
13. Confidentiality
14. Questions and answers about group therapy (try to clarify myths, misconceptions about group and elicit early resistances to group participation)
15. Anything unique about the patient's life situation that might intrude on his/her ability to join, remain in, or participate in the group

Reprinted from Spitz & Rosecan (1987). *Cocaine abuse: New directions in treatment and research.* (p. 179). New York: Brunner/Mazel.

elements. Primarily due to the abbreviated or uncertain time frame of the managed care group, most practitioners have emphasized the critical nature of similarities among members as the cornerstone of this modality.

The obvious benefits of homogeneous factors shared by all members are evident in a quick induction into group, fewer feelings of isolation, a clearer immediate sense of group purpose, and the more rapid emergence of group cohesion. Cohesion, as originally defined by Yalom (1985), was described as the members' attraction to one another and to the idea of the group itself. Group cohesion is not necessarily synonymous with comfort, nor was it a change unto itself, but it is a necessary precondition for change without which the critical formative stages of the group would be adversely effected if not destroyed.

Consequently, advocates of the brief group therapy model have put a very high premium on the forces that promote cohesion, and they suggest composing groups wherein members share the same problem set. Homogeneous factors can be related to psychological symptoms, age, gender, history of prior psychiatric treatment or group treatment, occupation, and the like. The leader of the group in the managed care context is well advised to look for similarities to obtain those benefits. However, what is sometimes overlooked or underemphasized in short-term groups are the positive influences of heterogeneous factors.

Whether a group functions homogeneously or heterogeneously is largely related to leadership style. Leaders who emphasize sameness and "groupness," and who tend to intervene at the level of the group as a whole, promote a degree of homogeneous group function that they regard as essential to the therapeutic endeavor in managed care groups. The constructive use of the ways in which members differ also can be used to advantage, especially by the leader of a brief therapy group. Heterogeneous elements favor the creation of a manageable baseline intragroup tension and form the building blocks for group interaction, both of which can accelerate the pace of a group.

In time-limited groups one can see many of the elements of longer-term groups in miniature. The same blend of homogeneous and heterogeneous factors found in open-ended groups can be very helpful in striking a sense of balance in the group and affording the leader more therapeutic leverage and options. Certain themes related to individuality, separateness, and autonomy can be utilized in short-term managed care groups and derive directly from the differences rather than the similarities among group participants.

STAGES OF SHORT-TERM GROUP DEVELOPMENT

All psychotherapy groups, like all human beings, go through natural developmental stages over the course of their lives. It is essential that the leader of a brief therapy group has some idea of phases of group development because they emerge very rapidly in shorter therapeutic experiences and can be a source of confusion for leaders and members alike. On the other hand, a clear knowledge of where a group is in its life cycle helps immeasurably in plotting a therapeutic course and in timing the sequencing of group interventions.

Numerous authors have described and labeled stages of group development as a therapeutic roadmap for the group leader. For practical purposes, the stages in a short-term managed care group can be conceptualized as follows: (a) pregroup phase, (b) induction into group, (c) establishment of group cohesion, (d) the working group phase, (e) individuation and differentiation phase, and (f) transition out of group/ termination phase.

As a matter of convenience, these group phases are presented separately. However, in actual practice there is considerable overlap among the various stages, and it is helpful for the leader to have a general idea of where the group is developmentally as a guide for planning treatment events.

For example, the induction phase of the group can be used as an extension of the screening process by seeing the members in action in a real therapy group. In the first one or two sessions, the leader may discover that a particular member is experiencing undue difficulty and perhaps group placement was premature. This makes it possible to remove a member early in the life of the group so that the group will not be adversely affected by an excessive focus on this member. Similarly, members for whom short-term groups are experienced as overwhelming or too emotionally intense can be spared a negative therapeutic outcome or failure and may be protected by leaving the group at a very early stage.

Building cohesion occupies much of the initial group focus. Cohesion must precede confrontation so that strong peer support can build a safety buffer against ill-advised interventions by the leader and/or potentially damaging encounters with other group members.

The working group phase is the longest and most difficult to describe. In long-term groups, this stage occupies the bulk of the group experience and is the stage during which most learning takes place. Some group therapists liken the working phase of short-term groups to a condensed version of the application of insight and experiential learning that is characteristic of this phase in open-ended, psychodynamically oriented groups.

As the work of the group progresses and members come closer to reaching their individual goals, the stage of individuation and differentiation usually is reached. Members are not afraid to express themselves and risk real or imagined challenges from the therapist or other group members.

The transition out of group consists of a review of each member's initial problems and how far each has come in reaching or falling short of these goals. A group review with a positive and supportive emphasis takes place during this stage. Significant shared experiences are revisited in an effort to consolidate and reenforce gains made in the group.

For many, group is only one aspect of what their psychological conditions require and for these members plans for further therapy, aftercare, relapse prevention, and other options are discussed in the group. In the managed mental health model, group therapists must be aware of the overall needs of the people they see in group and be clear about the role of group treatment in the broader treatment plan for a given individual.

It is essential that the group leader keep notes throughout all the stages of the group, both for his or her own understanding of the stage and state of the group and its members and to facilitate the process of reporting central treatment issues verbally or in writing to managed care case reviewers. This author discourages the taking of in-session process notes because it distances the therapist from the group interaction. Recording significant group events and individual changes (patient placed on antidepressant medication, patient has become progressively more appropriately assertive in sessions, patient described having a successful job interview, etc.) following each meeting gives the therapist accurate observational data to substantiate reports given about group members at various stages of group development.

CONDUCT OF THE FIRST SESSION IN THE MANAGED CARE MODALITY

Many of the theoretical and clinical issues described earlier come to life in the group's first meeting. The task of the leader in the managed care group is to facilitate a rapid start and get the group launched in the first session. Although this may sound like a daunting task, much of the work done in the pregroup phase is enormously helpful in simplifying the leader's job.

The first meeting calls for active leadership both in helping all members break the ice and simultaneously in attempting to program future group behavior that will be maximally conducive to the utilization of the inherent theraputic potential available in all sensibly designed psychotherapy groups.

The exact nature of a particular group determines the form and style of leadership used to conduct the first session. Therefore, it is easier to illustrate these principles using a clinical vignette. Consider the example of the initial meeting of a short-term outpatient group for substance abusing patients.

The leader begins by introducing herself and asks the members to do the same. Next, the therapist reviews the ground rules for the group. Despite the fact that all members have heard them in the pregroup orientation, they bear repetition for several reasons. First, by taking an active stance the therapist begins to take control of the group and models participation rather than withdrawal. Secondly, the content of the ground rules helps set a firm but fair set of boundaries on the group experience and a set of expectations that all members will adhere to theraputically designed group regulations.

In the substance abuse group a representative set of ground rules might be as follows:

1. The goal of the group is for each member to help him or herself and the others to abstain from drug and alcohol use.
2. Each member agrees to be totally honest about current or historical drug use.
3. An absolute commitment is made to refrain from using any mind or mood altering substances.
4. Regular attendance is mandatory and excessive absences are destructive to the group and its therapeutic mission.
5. No one may come to the group while actively under the influence of drugs and/or alcohol.
6. Slips—using drugs during the course of the group—will be treated initially as potential learning experiences. However, repeated slips are self-defeating and may require treatment other than short-term group therapy, such as hospitalization.
7. All group members agree to random urine testing for drugs at the discretion of the group leader.
8. Members are asked not to socialize with each other outside of group sessions throughout the course of the group experience.
9. Group therapists have each member's permission to be in contact with other family members and with any other therapists who may be involved in his or her care.
10. Absolute confidentiality is a nonnegotiable core element in the group. Anything said in the group must be respected and not used for gossip or other countertheraputic purposes outside the group. Breaches of confidentiality are considered to be very serious matters and are grounds for immediate dismissal from the group (Spitz, 1987).

Once again, because time is of the essence, it is advantageous to both the leader and the group members to have a clearly defined baseline from which the group begins. The themes of commonalities among members, the desire for inclusion in the group, advice giving, social chatter, premature self-disclosure (when a member inappropriately presents personal material before he or she knows who the group members are), testing the group leader, silences, and confusion about how help will come from peers are all recognizable first-session themes. These themes can dominate the group in a negative way if the leader is not active enough in a directorial sense.

Alternatively, the same behavioral phenomenology can be utilized in concert with the group goals by a leader who is alert to early anxieties in members, recognizes characteristics maladaptive coping mechanisms, rigid social roles, and extreme psychological defenses, and incorporates them into the group design in such a way as to be helpful to the membership in altering or resolving these behaviors.

The initial session has been a notorious source of anxiety for both therapists and patients in groups. The time limits of the managed care group motivate the group leader to have a therapeutic plan or agenda that helps minimize therapist apprehension concerning issues in the general category of "What shall I do if. . . ?" Brief group therapy encourages the therapist to anticipate potential pitfalls, resistances, and other problems that complicate group therapies by creating and sticking to a plan of therapy that helps the group successfully traverse therapeutic roadblocks.

THE MIDDLE PHASE OF BRIEF GROUP THERAPY

In a clinically oriented presentation it makes sense to focus briefly on the middle phase of therapy, where most of the work in the working stage takes place. Certainly, in long-term groups this is the longest phase and in many ways the most difficult to describe in the short-term milieu. One useful way to approach the topic is to view the phase as one that presents many opportunities for change and growth along with strong forces for sameness and inflexibility. The effective leader can demystify the potentially confusing events and actions that characterize the middle phase of brief group therapy by conceptualizing it along two cardinal dimensions: membership issues and leadership concerns.

One inevitable aspect of the middle phase of brief therapy is the growing awareness for therapist and patient alike that the group is moving closer to its endpoint. The denial of the ending of group and the sense of security that emanates from a firm sense of group cohesiveness that typify earlier stages in the group begin to compete with the contrasting emotions that stem from the knowledge that with each passing session the group is nearing its time limit. This frequently creates a sense of urgency and anxiety among group members that time is running out and that there are still issues to be resolved.

The group often feels frustrated, frightened, and angry. Any or all of these feelings can be directed towards the leader who the group feels may have disappointed them. At times, this amalgamation of emotions can reach crisis proportions that pose a threat to the viability of the group. Ambivalent attitudes complicate the work of the group and call for astute leadership and therapeutic skill in order to avert a potential group disaster.

The leader can capitalize on the peer support elements to help members learn to reach out to contemporaries, rather than to the parental figure personified by the therapist, in order to cope with trying emotional times. This is also a time where it is the leader's responsibility to keep the group focused on its original task and not get detoured into other topics that were not part of the original group contract.

A favorable byproduct of the highly charged group atmosphere is the opportunity for experiential learning that can transpire. If the leader utilizes the affective elements and helps the group couple them with a realistic cognitive structure, then profound theraputic gains can be made in a short time. The technique of keeping the group theme oriented at these times usually helps members coalesce and reconstitute more rapidly.

The working phase allows the therapist to employ educational elements, experiences in the constructive expression of affect, and the acquisition of insight, as well as cognitive skills, to underscore the sense of universality among members as a force that counters hopelessness and demoralization, to demonstrate the use of confrontation in a caring and sensitive way, and to identify deleterious tendencies such as subgroup formation, and ultimately decode its meaning in terms of both individual and group processes.

The net effect of sensible management of the multitude of issues that emerge during the middle phase of group is the strengthening of group members and a logical transition into the termination stage of the group.

TERMINATION PHASE: ISSUES AND MANAGEMENT

While certain aspects of brief group therapy are indeed unique, there are some generic themes that are common to all psychotherapies. Termination of treatment is a case in point. The feelings of anticipated loss and separation are commonplace in most therapies. Similarly, the reactivation of historical experiences with death nearly always accompany the end of a psychotherapeutic relationship.

While there may be common problems associated with termination, the options available for handling them are increased in therapy groups. The issue of time limitations often has been viewed as a troublesome problem for therapists who are used to working in open-ended psychotherapy models. The brevity of the work in the short-term group makes for an intense but short-lived experience. When it comes to terminating a brief therapy group the task is facilitated by the fact that members have not known each other over a period of years, as is the case in most psychdynamically oriented groups. Furthermore, the intensity of the relationship of member to therapist is diluted in groups, as contrasted with dyadic therapies, because all members must share the leader. Because successful group experiences teach group members to rely on peers as well as authority figures, members who are leaving groups are doing so with enhanced interpersonal skills and a greater ability to find rewarding relationships in their personal and professional lives.

Termination in brief groups is different from other group therapies in that all members terminate at the same time. This phenomenon does not single out any particular group member and so helps to avoid the undue feelings of competition and failure that sometimes arise in long-term groups when one member reaches his or her goals and departs while others remain.

A final caveat for the leader of the brief therapy group is to stick to the original time frame no matter what pressure the group exerts to extend the sessions. While this may be patently obvious, the group leader is far from immune to the forces at play in groups and may be tempted to depart from the agreed-upon therapeutic plan.

There appear to be at least two ways of understanding how this could become a problem for the therapist during the temination stage of the group. The articulation of aspects of the therapist's personality with a particular group or group members, more traditionally described as a "countertransferential blind spot," can often form the basis of the leader's temptation to agree to extend the group's life. Secondly, from a social systems vantage point, the concept of group pressure or "system suction" is a powerful influence on even the most seasoned group therapist, and it may seem quite reasonable to go along with the group's wish for more time.

In either case, the leader is wise to consider and discuss the time issue openly for its value to the group in helping the members comprehend the power of terminations, but he or she should not make a policy change at this late juncture in the group's life. Not only will the therapist's credibility suffer but the group itself is not given a vote of confidence for its positive accomplishments, which have prepared them for coping with life's transitions, separations, and losses.

Brief groups conducted under the auspices of managed care also provide members with a reevaluation of their target goals and how close they have come to reaching them. While the review is ideally cast in positive terms, it should not be at the expense of the truth. Group members who need further therapy have their cases reviewed by the leader, who then confers with the managed care reviewer in discussing further treatment options, including family and community resources that may be considered helpful as an extension of the work done in the short-term group.

The specificity of goals and their ongoing monitoring, as required by managed care organizations, is tailor-made for brief group psychotherapy for patients with a broad range of psychological impairments.

EVALUATING THE GROUP EXPERIENCE

The group psychotherapy profession historically has been weak in evaluating treatment outcomes. In the past decade, a major thrust in the field has been towards putting group therapy on firmer footing with respect to scientific standards. (Hamilton, Courville, et al., 1993) The group therapy literature reflects this trend and is moving away from a largely anecdotal and narrative form to one that attempts to answer the questions of what actually transpires in group, which factors are deemed most helpful for which patient populations, and how standardized instruments that measure results can be developed. Are there techniques or protocols for therapy that are clearly delineated so that they can be replicated elsewhere and the issue of outcome in group therapy can be clarified?

The results of these efforts will have special significance to all those involved with group therapy in the managed care arena. Towards this end, Dies and MacKenzie (1983) began a systematic process of evaluating outcomes in group psychotherapy. Outcome research has been approached in two ways—measures of individual progress within the group and observations about the characteristics of groups themselves have been gathered and studied.

Some of the individual assessment tools used to evaluate patients prior to group entry are often readministered at the close of the group. Representative examples of this type include the Symptom Checklist

90 (SCL-90R), the Global Assessment of Function Scale (GAF or GAS), the Social Adjustment Scale (SAS), and the MMPI.

Groups can be evaluated from the dimensions of group content, group process, and the prevailing group climate. The most familiar tests for assessing these elements of psychotherapy groups are the Harvard Community Health Plan Group Cohesiveness Scale (HCHP-GCS), the Hill Interaction Matrix, the Group Environment Scale, and the Group Climate Questionnaire. For a more detailed description and discussion of these measures of outcome in group psychotherapy, the reader is referred to Garfield and Bergin (1986), Fuhriman and Packard (1986) and MacKenzie (1990).

Although the outcome research on brief group psychotherapy is still in its infancy, several general observations on the efficacy of group psychotherapy emerging from the literature cited above suggest the following trends: groups appear to be the treatment of choice when interpersonal problems are the chief complaint; proper preparation of patients and positive attitudes by therapists about the therapeutic value of groups appears to be correlated with both a reduced drop-out rate from treatment and more successful outcomes in terms of symptomatic improvement in group participants; in several studies group therapy compared favorably with individual therapy and was found to offer extra benefits not found in dyadic therapies; and groups offer greater opportunity for modeling and teaching in the therapeutic milieu.

The extra benefits alluded to above derive largely from the presence of many participants in the same therapeutic experience. Groups more closely approximate a microcosm of the outside world and allow people to be in actual relationships in a safe and controlled setting. Feedback in groups is direct and the possibilities for participants to obtain information about themselves is multiplied. This enhanced stimulation is one contributing factor in accelerating the therapeutic process and provides a large part of the rationale for creating time-limited groups.

The healing potential of groups, sometimes described as therapeutic or curative factors, are the natural resources available to group participants and have been well studied in long-term psychotherapy groups. As Yalom (1985) conceptualized them, the factors of realistic hope for change, universalization, the reactivation of family feelings, altruism, imitative behavior, and cohesion, among others, increase the options for constructive or corrective interventions and permit more therapeutic work to be done in a shorter time.

Currently, similar studies are underway that will help elucidate the inner workings of the brief therapy group and will support the clinical enthusiasm voiced by practitioners of these methods.

RECORDING AND REPORTING THE GROUP EXPERIENCE

Responsible group therapists keep good records of the significant elements in their groups regardless of the context in which they are working. In the context of managed care, regular record-keeping simplifies the process of reporting patient information to reviewing sources.

The recording process starts during the evaluation phase and includes a working diagnosis and a set of initial, intermediate, and long-term goals for the patient. There should also be a statement describing the role of this particular group at this particular time, and its relationship to each patient's overall treatment plan.

When the sessions begin, notes taken immediately afterward focus on two areas in the individual patient's course in the pursuit of his or her goals (see Exhibit 5-3) and the critical events in the transactions of the group itself (see Exhibit 5-4). A member referred to group for issues related to his or her excessive anxiety about speaking in groups should have the reduction of this anxiety as the target goal. Notes about this member should reflect changes in his or her behavior with specific reference to performance anxiety—for example, Fred opened the group today by discussing a presentation he will have to make at his job in a few weeks. This was the first time that Fred initiated conversation in the group. Similar notes, once again focused more on behavioral change and less on diagnostic language, helps track a patient's progress and will be appreciated by case reviewers for the help it affords them in understanding the course of therapy.

From a practical point of view, the author finds it useful to make an individual note in each member's chart following the group session and to also keep a set of group notes that highlights the course of the whole group and serves as an aid in plotting a therapeutic path for future meetings.

Recording group phenomenology provides a data bank to which the therapist can refer for a variety of purposes. Group notes should include a record of attendance, the major group theme or themes discussed in each session, any crisis situations, unexpected or unusual behaviors that arise, which members were active and which were withdrawn, and a plan for the next group session.

When the time comes to communicate with the managed care organization, the information contained in the group record and the individual charts forms the basis for a successful dialogue. Because it is likely that the group leader will be asked by the reviewer to describe a member's clinical course, it is useful to have a conceptual framework in mind for thinking about therapeutic issues so that these ideas can be expressed in terms that make sense to both parties.

EXHIBIT 5-3
Individual Progress Note Form

Patient	Group	Date of session

Working Diagnosis: *309.24-Adjustment Disorder with anxious mood*

Major Symptoms: *Social isolation, somatic complaints—sweating, "rapid" heart rate, stomach pains; avoidant behavior in fearful situations.*

In-Group Behavior (level of participation, prevailing mood, main interpersonal posture adopted in sessions, attitude and behavior toward the therapist): *John remains on the periphery of the group and contributes infrequently. When confronted directly by members or the leader, he tends to give monosyllabic responses and says he is afraid to "expose" himself to others.*

Individual Treatment Goals: *Work on interpersonal anxiety utilizing the support elements present in group. Gently encourage more active participation and self-disclosure by modeling this with other group members and by judicious use of therapist self-disclosure in selected areas.*

Progress Towards Goal Attainment: *John still remains aloof but seems to have developed the beginnings of a bond with the other male group members. He described taking the same bus home from group with Felix after last week's session.*

Treatment Plan: *Therapist will sit next to John to concretize issues of support. Next group meeting will be theme-focused in order to take the pressure off John and to help him participate in group discussions around a shared group issue. Possibility of antianxiety medication will be considered if his progress continues to be slow or if he shows signs of regressing to earlier withdrawn behavior.*

Prognosis (some informal estimate of patient's capacity for change based on group participation to date): *John appears to be "coming out of his shell" and if this trend continues it appears that the group will be of great value to him.*

EXHIBIT 5-4
Group Note Form

Group Leader	Date
Members Present	Session #

Group Goals (eg., Social skills training) _____

_____

Focus of Current Session (eg., Group discussed anxieties connected with meeting new people or being in unfamiliar situations) _____

_____

Any Specific Problems Impeding Group Progress (eg., Mr. L. mentioned that he was thinking of dropping out of the group) _____

_____

Major Interventions/Techniques (eg., Utilized group support and universalization to reassure Mr. L. and encouraged him to remain in group. Also did brief role-playing exercise addressed at learning techniques for how to manage when meeting new people) _____

_____

Plans for Next Session (eg., Try to get Mr. L. to begin the group discussion; discuss his reaction and those of the other group members to today's session. Assign "homework" outside of group in which each member has to introduce themselves to a new person or "stranger" and report the experience back to the group) _____

_____

Therapist Factors (eg., Co-therapy issues; practical matters such as leader vacation schedule; need for consultation/supervision about a specific leadership or membership problem) _____

_____

Any Changes in Group Composition (eg., Dropouts from group; addition of new members) _____

_____

Other Comments (eg., Notify the group about upcoming holiday and discuss the possibilities for changing the meeting to another day of the week in order not to lose the continuity of the sessions) _____

_____

If this is a first review, the provider should explain, verbally or in a written report, his or her view as to why treatment is medically necessary at this time. What are the patient's functional deficits and current level of functioning? In addition, a formal Axis I and/or Axis II diagnosis should be included in the initial report.

When the case review takes place on the telephone, it is advisable to discuss it in everyday language and in an organized fashion. One way to do that is to follow the diagnosis with a description of the presenting problem, the relevant past history, and the current symptoms and behavior. Next, the clinician is usually asked to discuss the treatment goals and objectives and the plan for their implementation. When group therapy is indicated, the therapist should outline several reasons why this choice has been made.

Consider the following case example: Ms. K is a 45-year-old unmarried elementary school teacher who had been living with her aging mother until the mother's death three months ago. Since that time she describes feeling "all alone," sleeping excessively, and having a sense of hopelessness about the future. In addition, she has taken time off from work and feels "too depressed" to return to her job. She denies suicidal ideation but has frequent crying spells, about which she feels embarrassed and "weird." Her only sibling, a younger brother, lives far away, and they have a distant relationship. She feels as though she "has no family anymore" and her friendship network is small and does not consist of anyone with whom she would feel comfortable discussing her current emotional state. She has no prior history of psychiatric illness.

Initial diagnosis: Dysthymia (Depressive neurosis—300.4)
Presenting symptoms and behavior: Sleep disturbance, social isolation, feelings of sadness, indecisiveness, diminished ability to concentrate.
Treatment objectives: Immediate goals—1. Provide for patient's safety and monitor any evidence of self-destructive or suicidal thought or actions. 2. Establish a collaborative relationship with the patient and encourage her to follow through with a therapeutic plan. 3. Evaluate the appropriateness of antidepressant medication.

Initial treatment strategies: 1. Conduct a thorough evaluation with particular emphasis on the risk of suicidality. Order psychological testing if the interview suggests areas of doubt or concern. Consider whether the patient can care for herself or might have to be considered for hospitalization. 2. Try to establish a therapeutic alliance with the patient until an external support system can be established. Encourage her to talk about her feelings of sadness and other areas that are giving her trouble at present. Assess patient's strengths currently and historically. Look for instances where she might try to avoid or defer the decision to seek treatment at this time. 3. Evaluate the patient to see if neurovegetative symptoms are present that would have a favorable response to antidepressant therapy. Look for appetite change, sleep disturbance, diminished libido, impaired concentration, mood fluctuations, and other indicators of a drug-responsive affective disorder.

In this hypothetical case, assume that all the above has been completed and the results suggest that the patient is not a suicidal risk, her condition is neither better nor worse than before, and she would prefer not to take medication. She experiences great relief from "getting it off my chest" and would be interested in a "talking therapy" although she is not sure she would feel comfortable discussing her problems openly in a group of "strangers".

The next phase would naturally be one in which the decision regarding choice of therapy would take priority. Using the same format mentioned above, the therapist would reconfirm the initial diagnostic impression, reevaluate the prevailing problematic symptoms and behaviors, and plan for some short- to intermediate-term interventions aimed at stabilizing the patient and eventually getting her back to her premorbid level of function.

In this case, a decision was made to suggest that the patient join an eight-session bereavement group composed of adults, all of whom had experienced the loss of a significant family member. The basis for the choice of a homogeneous, brief group was severalfold. First, it was felt that the isolated position she found herself in would be countered immediately by group placement that could serve as an interpersonal anchor for her during this difficult time. Secondly, being in a group where all members have experienced the same life circumstances was thought to be useful in destigmatizing her embarrassment and feelings of "weirdness" for reacting to her mother's death in the way she did. Group was also considered likely to be helpful in addressing her tendency to keep things to herself and to allow her not only to experience the safety of opening up but to benefit as well from the empathic and supportive elements resulting from the identifications among members. The hope was that she would apply the skills gained in the group to her life outside the group and be better equipped to broaden her social network.

Although she was hesitant at first, Ms. K. began to self-disclose around the third session. Members quickly rallied to her side and helped quell her fears of humiliation or criticism from others. The homogeneous elements in the group bolstered her initially and helped normalize her intense feelings during the state of bereavement.

The group also supplied a large educational component in which the leader and members discussed normal versus pathological grief reactions, techniques for coping with loss, and ways to rebuild self-esteem. The patient's ability to stay in the group gave her a sense of strength and mastery because she had not run away from things she feared. There was a noticeable lessening of her symptoms related to depression as she grew better at regulating her sleep and she regained a normal appetite and a greater general interest in life. By the time the group was near termination, she felt "a bit shaky" but had returned to the classroom on a regular basis.

While she clearly missed her mother, she was no longer obsessively preoccupied with thoughts only of her. She described feeling "unstuck," which to her meant that she was no longer "paralyzed by fear and depression."

The very end of the group focused on planning for the future. Her plan included an assessment of the need for further therapy and to develop self-monitoring skills to recognize the warning signs of any subsequent depression along with a decision to join a local book club in order to expand her social and intellectual pursuits and to move into an apartment of her own. In this particular group extramural socialization among members was encouraged, and Ms. K left the group feeling that she had already begun to make new friends.

In this case the decision to pursue therapy was deferred pending a scheduled follow-up visit with Ms. K. in three months time. When she was seen at that point she was much improved. Her work function was back to normal, she had increased her friendship circle somewhat, and she described herself as becoming more "philosophical" in her attitude towards her mother's death.

This is an instance where short-term group psychotherapy centered around a common theme proved to be sufficient treatment for the particular member under discussion and for most of the members of the group as well. One or two others required some brief individual psychotherapy focused on life cycle developmental issues triggered by the loss of a significant other.

The bereavement group is but one of many short-term group models that attest to the broad applicability of utilizing a group format to address either a specific problem or a unique patient population. Broadly speaking, shorter-term groups of six to twelve sessions are more targeted at symptom removal and skills acquisition. These groups tend to be homogeneous in their makeup and have clearly defined goals and protocols for reaching those goals. A representative cross-section of groups in this category include a weekly communication skills training group for couples with mild to moderate marital problems, a twice-weekly behavior therapy group for smoking cessation, and a ten-session weekly cognitive/behavioral stress management group for people with anxiety disorders.

There is hardly a condition or person for which or for whom a sensible group cannot be devised (Spitz, 1984). Some groups begin with a short-term agenda but may require reassessment in the course of treatment. An example is found in an H.I.V. support group, which, like many other groups composed exclusively of patients with serious medical illnesses, is always influenced by the physical health of its members. Periodic rehospitaliztion, the death of a group member, or the deterioration in a member's mental or medical status are unfortunate but familiar examples of states that the leader must evaluate and that may cause modifications, time extensions, addition of new members, and other clinical decisions that extend the group beyond its strict short-term mandate or original design.

Generally, groups that require a longer-term format often are those that are heterogeneous in composition and have ambitious or global goals as their primary purpose. The most common instance is outpatient psychodynamically or psychoanalytically oriented groups that try to change basic aspects of personality structure and firmly entrenched maladaptive behavioral patterns in group members.

SUMMARY

Group therapy has always enjoyed a reputation for the flexibility it affords clinicians working with patients in nearly every diagnostic category or life circumstance. Groups also fit well as part of an overall approach to certain problems, such as those found in most psychiatric inpatient services. The group milieu is one that works very well in combining techniques that broaden its scope.

Leadership variations such as coleadership have found a place of favor in group circles in areas as seemingly diverse as the treatment of adolescents, substance abusers, and couples having relationship difficulties. Successful cotherapy pairs model constructive collaborative interaction between adults and usually mobilize feelings related to parents in the family of origin of group members. This, too, can speed up the group process when family issues are the reason someone seeks psychological assistance.

The focus of this chapter has been less on leadership or membership variables than on time factors. The burgeoning interest in time-limited therapies has brought with it a welcome spirit of further experimentation with the model of brief group psychotherapy. Preliminary results show that this group modality has much to offer in the resolution of some longstanding clinical dilemmas.

Economic factors have been the other force that has helped set the stage for expanded use of the short-term group. The skyrocketing cost of health care has given rise to the quest for new and imaginative forms of therapy that make both economic and emotional sense. Brief group therapies clearly offer a solution to many of these concerns.

Managed mental health care represents an effort at cost containment without sacrificing the quality of service. What form this will take in the coming years remains to be seen but it is clear that whatever incarnation the system presents, group therapies will play an ever-increasing role in it. Some estimates suggest that if the current trends in the mental health field continue, during the next five years approximately 70% of psychiatric patients will experience some form of group psychotherapy.

Even if these estimates are imprecise, what is apparent is that shorter-term, less expensive forms of psychiatric treatment appear to be the wave of the future. With this in mind, most people in the mental health field who actually work directly with patients would be well advised not only to become conversant with the concepts embodied by managed mental health care but also to develop a fluency in the theory and practice of short-term group psychotherapy.

REFERENCES

Budman, S. H. (1992). Models of brief individual and group psychotherapy. In J.L. Feldman & R. J. Fitzpatrick (Eds.), *Managed mental health care* (pp. 231–248). Washington, DC: American Psychiatric Press.

Budman, S. H., & Bennett, M. J. (1983). Short-term groups psychotherapy. In H.I. Kaplan & B. J. Sadock (Eds.), *Comprehensive group psychotherapy* (pp. 138–144). Baltimore, MD: Williams & Wilkins.

Dies, R. R., & MacKenzie, K. R. (Eds.) (1983). Advances in group psychotherapy: Integrating research and practice (A.G.P.A. Monograph #1). New York: International Universities Press.

Feldman, J. L., & Fitzpatrick, R. L. (Eds.). (1992). *Managed mental health care: Administrative and clinical issues.*

Goodman, M., Brown, J., & Dietz, P. (1992). *Managing managed care: A mental health practitioner's survival guide.* Washington, DC: American Psychiatric Press.

Hamilton, J. D., Courville, T. J., et al. (1993). Quality assessment and improvement in group psychotherapy. *American Journal of Psychiatry 150:* 315–320.

Lieberman, M. A., Yalom, I. D., & Miles, M. (1973). *Encounter groups: First facts.* New York: Basic Books.

MacKenzie, K. R. (1990). *Introduction to time-limited group psychotherapy.* Washington, DC: American Psychiatric Press.

Piper, W. E., Debanne, E. G., & Bienvenu, J. P. (1982). A study of group pre-training for group psychotherapy. *International Journal of Group Psychotherapy, 32:* 309–325.

Spitz, H. I. (1984). Contemporary trends in groups psychotherapy: A literature survey. *Hospital and Community Psychiatry, 35:* 132–142.

Spitz, H. I. (1987). Cocaine abuse: Therapeutic group approaches. In H. I. Spitz and J. R. Rosecan (Eds.), *Cocaine abuse: New directions in treatment and research* (pp. 156–201). New York: Brunner/Mazel.

Yalom, I. D. (1985). *The theory and practice of group psychotherapy* (3rd ed.). New York: Basic Books.

6

Distance Writing and Computer-Assisted Training

LUCIANO L'ABATE, Ph.D.

The purpose of this chapter is to introduce the reader to the many uses of writing for therapeutic, paratherapeutic, preventive, and parapreventive purposes. The term *therapeutic writing* means that this is the only form of treatment taking place. *Paratherapeutic writing* is used in conjunction with face-to-face psychotherapy. *Preventive writing* is any approach that attempts to avoid the occurrence of a breakdown by improving the resistance to breakdown. It takes place in group rather than in individual therapy. *Parapreventive writing* takes place in conjunction with a preventive program (L'Abate, 1990). When writing is used as an additional, complementary, or supplementary medium to face-to-face, spoken therapy, it should be established as a condition for treatment from the very outset. Even when writing is used as the sole medium of intervention, a clearly worded contract would help (L'Abate, 1986, 1992). Otherwise, a therapist will meet a great deal of resistance if he or she suddenly assigns a writing project to unsuspecting clients who have not agreed to it beforehand. An Informed Consent Form to be administered to all clients who agree to work through either Distance Writing (DW) or Computer Assisted Training (CAT) is available from the author upon request. This document is quite lengthy and complex to cover all possible ethical and professional bases but it can be shortened and compressed to suit the needs of therapists and clients alike.

It is useful to have a written contract *from the very first session* to cover this practice.

Writing, in its various applications (which are reviewed below), is but a skip and a jump from computer-assisted training (CAT) and psychoeducational skill training programs (L'Abate, 1990). Before a program is loaded into a computer, it has to be written (Brown & L'Abate, 1969). As Bloom (1992) concluded in his review on this subject: "even those who are quite disturbed interact very successfully with computers, including many patients who are unable to interact with mental health personnel" (p. 169). Therefore, writing can be used as a paratherapeutic or preventive medium in its own right or it can be seen as precursor or preliminary to its use in CAT.

The use of writing and CAT enlarges the therapeutic and preventive armamentarium manyfold, allowing a therapist to help many more clients, per unit of his or her time, than is possible using individual face-to-face verbal interactions. Even in group psychotherapy, writing and CAT can be administered and individualized before, during, or after face-to-face interaction. In preventive programs that treat less disturbed individuals, writing and CAT could be administered without face-to-face contact, through the mail (L'Abate, 1990, 1992). Thus, writing and CAT have the potential to decrease costs and increase efficiency in current mental health practices. Whether these approaches are as effective as spoken ones remains to be seen. Consequently, writing will be used as part of CAT. The reader who wants to learn more about recent developments in CAT should consult Bloom's (1992) excellent review. For what is now an historical introduction to the same area, the reader may want to consult Brown and L'Abate (1969).

TOWARD A CLASSIFICATION OF WRITING FOR PREVENTIVE, PARATHERAPEUTIC, AND THERAPEUTIC PURPOSES

Categories in which to classify writing include:

1. **Structure,** increasing from
   (a) least structured or *open-ended writing* (OW) ("Write anything that comes into your mind," as practiced in diaries or journals) to
   (b) *focused writing* (FW) ("Write about your past hurts for twenty minutes a day for four days") to
   (c) *guided writing* (GW) ("I have read what you wrote and I want you to answer the following written questions in writing during the next week") and, finally, to

(d) the most structured extreme, *programmed writing* (PW) ("I want you to work on this program for depression. This workbook consists of eight lessons. I am giving you the first lesson to work on for next week. Make sure you make an appointment with yourself to work on this lesson, and bring the completed lesson to the next session. I am looking forward to seeing what you wrote.")

2. **Content**—from *traumatic to trivial* as discussed in Pennebaker's (1990) work.

3. **Goal,** ranging from *cathartic to prescriptive.* At the cathartic end of the range, the respondent is to get in touch with sad or painful feelings, without having to do anything else. At the other extreme, the prescriptive, the respondent is to follow a step or a sequence of steps requiring doing or not doing something according to specified instructions. Of course, other minor dimensions could be added to this model, including the *level of abstraction* required of the respondent, ranging from very abstract to very concrete. However, this dimension would be a part of programmed writing. It would be difficult to control the level of abstraction in open, focused, or guided writing, unless specific instructions were given, making the format a programmed one.

A summary of this model is shown in Figure 6-1, where overlap between extremes on each of the three dimensions is shown in the three corners of the triangle. For instance, writing about past traumas would have a cathartic effect (Pennebaker, 1990). Some writing programs have a prescriptive component, suggesting that certain behaviors must be programmed to be repeated in specific ways in the coming week, between lessons or therapy sessions. A prescription usually needs to be programmed to achieve the desired effect. Among the four levels of structure, open writing runs the risk of being the most trivial. A respondent, unless told otherwise, could detail whatever has happened in a daily diary without getting down to innermost feelings and thoughts.

Consequently, the purpose of this chapter is to illustrate various applications of focused writing (FW) in either preventive or therapeutic interventions and programmed writing (PW) in psychotherapy research and applications. Open-ended (OW) and guided writing (GW) will not be considered here because their application is secondary to the purposes of this chapter.

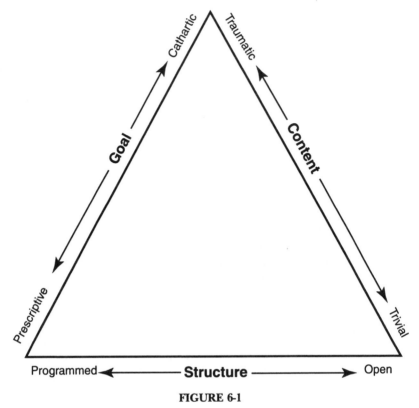

FIGURE 6-1

Toward a Classification of Preventive and Paratherapeutic Writing

EVALUATION AND WRITING

Elsewhere (L'Abate, 1990, 1992; L'Abate & Platzman, 1991), I have argued that the verbal, face-to-face relationship may be critical in dealing with clients as people, establishing rapport, trust, and communication with them through the use of warmth, regard, and empathy. The written medium, on the other hand, should be used to deal with referring symptoms or problems. The treatment of symptoms, *if it is to become an intersubjective method,* needs to be established through written-out plans. These plans or scripts should have been already tested on nonclinical populations. Consequently, as long as a part of treatment occurs in writing, it can be evaluated by more than one therapist in more than one clinical setting. For instance, workbooks for various clinical conditions, including depression and anxiety, have been created. Some of them were tried out with a nonclinical population of undergraduates who scored high on tests for depression and anxiety. It was found that indeed these workbooks significantly reduced high levels of depression and anxiety to normal levels, suggesting that they can be used with a clinical population (Bird, 1992). In addition, it was possible to administer a well-known personality test (Minnesota Multiphasic Personality Inventory-2, MMPI-2) and prescribe those programs that matched high peaks (highest deviance) on any of the 15 Content Scales (L'Abate, Boyce, Fraizer, & Russ, 1992).

There are now programs for various family dysfunctionalities, including negativity, lying, stealing, temper tantrums, sibling rivalry, and abuse, and they are used as homework assignments (L'Abate, 1990, 1991). Of course, homework assignments beg the question: "If these assignments are administered on the basis of the presenting symptom, what do we need an evaluation for?" This is an important issue that needs highlighting. Prescription of a written program or workbook should be based on both a test profile and the specific nature of a symptom. I argue here and elsewhere (L'Abate, 1990, 1992) that part—and in some cases all—psychological treatment can and should take place through the written modality. Once the written medium becomes an additional or alternative way to intervene, the linkage between evaluation and treatment will become feasible, practical, straightforward, and cheap! Linking evaluation with treatment has been a crucial problem since the historical beginnings of the testing movement (Weiner, 1976). Supposedly, tests are to be used to understand the extent and type of dysfunctionality. They are also to provide relevant recommendations for a specific match with the most appropriate form of treatment. This ideal, however, although desired and desirable, has never been reached, as far as I know (Howard, Nance, & Myers, 1987; Hurt, Reznikoff, & Clarkin, 1991; Kennedy, 1992; Moncher & Prinz, 1991; Okun, 1990; Perry, Frances, & Clarkin, 1985; Seligman, 1990).

Evaluation in Current Clinical Practices: Critical Remarks

Evaluation is not as valued by the mental health establishment as it should be. This situation should not distract us from stressing the importance of evaluation in spite of its consistent devaluation by the mental health and psychotherapy professions (L'Abate, 1990). Most evaluative practices in the mental health and psychotherapy fields consist, at best, of an interview and a history. Why should we waste our time and energy and a client's time, energy, and money to evaluate above and beyond an interview? Why not accept as a given existing evaluative practices, no matter how inadequate, and go with the flow instead, accepting things as they are? Were we willing to conform to accepted practices, no matter how inadequate or irresponsible, it would be tantamount to giving up, accepting the status quo without questioning it.

The status of evaluation in the mental health field, whether with individuals, couples, and families, is unacceptable, especially in trying to link and connect evaluation with therapy, rendering it practically irrelevant to the whole enterprise. This is one of the major failings of evaluation as traditionally practiced in mental health. If we cannot link evaluation with treatment, why should evaluation be performed? Evaluation is not part of standard operating procedures in the mental health field. Almost everybody who enters the any of the various mental health professions wants to become a therapist. Most mental health trainees do practice evaluation, seeing it as being part and parcel of being a therapist. Often, evaluation is seen as an unnecessary requirement and an irrelevant, time-consuming chore rather than a necessary and crucial part of therapy. As shown later in this chapter, as long as the spoken medium is used, specific links between evaluation and treatment planning will be difficult and expensive if not impossible. With the written medium it is possible, easy, and inexpensive to successfully achieve such a link. However, before dealing with this issue we need to compare the three media for psychological interventions.

COMPARING THE THREE MEDIA

It is important to compare the pros and cons of each medium with the other two, continuing a process already started in Chapter 2.

Advantages of Nonverbal over Spoken Medium

Because the nonverbal medium is based directly on the body, it is the most primitive or earliest medium of communication, and children are able to develop their nonverbal communication skills medium earlier than the other two. Hence, this medium could become a depository of stored memories—witness the admittedly impressionistic reports from clients who are undergoing "body work" such as Rolfing or massage (L'Abate, 1994; L'Abate & Baggett, 1997).

The many different expressions of nonverbal behavior allows therapists to enlarge their practices as much it it would allow them to widen the range of problems they may be able to deal with. The use of art, dance, play, movement, and other awareness-directed activities would allow them to see more clients per unit of time than when they rely solely on the spoken word. Many nonverbal techniques lend themselves to group activities than would not be feasible through the spoken word (except, of course, group psychotherapy). Many people with character or personality disorders, who typically are resistant to verbal therapy may benefit by nonverbal approaches *before* any other medium of intervention is attempted.

Advantages of Nonverbal over Written Medium

The written word is not as immediately available as the body is. The body may allow access to stores of painful memories imprinted in it that may not be as immediately accessible through spoken face-to-face spoken contact. Many nonverbal awareness exercises may open up a flood of past experiences that may need to be followed up through the written medium. The media, of course, may complement each other, even though nonverbal activities lend themselves to group interventions, while written experiences, as shown below, may lend themselves to a more individualized approach.

Advantages of Written over Spoken Medium

The written medium is determinably explicit while the spoken medium is indeterminably liable to distortions, deletions, and misinterpretations. The written medium is explicitly specific, making it controllable, while the spoken medium is not. We can neither predict nor control what clients and therapists are going to say. The use of training manuals for therapists may limit the therapist's variability but they do not limit the clients', because the spoken word is essentially infinite, while the written word, especially when programmed, is finite. Depending on its structure, content, and focus, writing can be controlled, while the spoken word cannot be (see Table 6-1).

When they are written, treatment plans become intersubjective and amenable to verification by colleagues. The written medium allows us to work at a distance from clients while the spoken word does not (unless we use the phone). Working at a distance from people means enlarging and expanding the written medium to the following populations: (a) existing clients, who can and do use written homework assignments, on a pre-, during-, or posttherapy basis; (b) clients who are no longer available, who have completed spoken, face-to-face psychotherapy but who could benefit by written booster shots; (c) clients who cannot afford therapists' fees but who could profit from a limited number of visits, perhaps once a month or once every few months, combined

TABLE 6-1

Differences between Traditional Psychotherapy, Focused and Programmed Writing

Traditional Psychotherapy	Focused and Programmed Writing
Style more important than method	Method more important than sytle
Reliance on style more than method	Reliance on method more than style
Style varies from one therapist to another	Little variance in method, style is either secondary or irrelevant
Process is idiographic	Process may be idiographic for FW and nomothetic for PW
Content varies	Content can be varied or fixed
Free-wheeling	
Flexible	
Very specific	Very specific in FW and general/ specific in PW depending on the nature of the problem
Costs: High	Costs: Minimal

with the administration of prearranged weekly written homework assignments; (d) incarcerated clients, whom we would have logistic and economical difficulties in reaching to talk face-to-face; (e) handicapped individuals or shut-ins who do not want or who are unable to leave their homes; (f) people in foreign lands who cannot relate to therapists in another language, including missionaries and military individuals and families. Finally, homework writing assignments can be administered while the therapist is on vacation, keeping clients in control of themselves.

Furthermore, the written word allows for comparative testing or theoretical and therapeutic approaches that would not be possible or would be very expensive through the spoken word. Such intersubjective testing can take place when treatment plans are detailed and put in writing (L'Abate, 1992). When writing is programmed, it can link evaluation with treatment in a way that is difficult if not impossible to do with the spoken word. For instance, once a set of programmed workbooks based on each of the fifteen content scales of MMPI-2 is complete, therapists will be able to choose the workbook that matches the scale with the highest elevation (L'Abate, Boyce, Fraizer, & Russ, 1992). By the same token, given specific symptoms, such as sibling rivalry, it is possible to administer a program that was specifically written for that symptom and not any others (L'Abate, 1992; L'Abate & Platzman, 1991).

A written program or workbook can be debugged and improved. However, it is very difficult to improve therapists because we still do not even have minimal standards to define what a competent therapist is. The process of granting licenses and degrees is based on paper credentials that do not take into account the proven therapeutic effectiveness of any therapist. How can we improve therapists if we do not know how they should be improved?

Advantages of Spoken over Written Medium

Admittedly, the spoken word may be necessary for rapport-building and motivation-imparting. However, this generalization needs to be qualified. There are externalizing, borderline, character disordered, acting out, and criminal individuals who use the spoken word for conning and manipulating by saying what they think the therapist will want to hear. Language is used to make a good impression, not to think or to introspect. If there seems to be a rapport, this quality is used to manipulate rather than to change. Hence, these individuals may benefit from nonverbal and written interventions rather than from interventions based on the spoken word. From all the evidence we have available, the spoken word is wasteful and highly inefficient with these individuals. By the same token, affective and depressive conditions, which are characterized by internalization and ruminative introspection, seem to benefit the most from talking. However, the comparative efficiency of spoken versus written media with depressed and anxious conditions has never been tested. It could be argued that affective conditions make for willing clients who might benefit from any kind of help, spoken, nonverbal, or written. Schizophrenic individuals and their families, on the other hand, may benefit from skill training, structured psychoeducational programs (the paratherapies) rather than psychotherapy, no matter what form that psychotherapy may take (Anderson, Reiss, & Hogarty, 1986; Gordon & Gordon, 1981; L'Abate, 1990; Liberman, DeRisi, & Mueser, 1989; Siani, Siciliani, & Burti, 1990).

Only comparative testing of the therapeutic effectiveness of the three media will tell us which clinical group will benefit from which medium and which sequence of media. For instance, as suggested earlier, depressed individuals may benefit from a sequence of verbal, nonverbal, and written interventions, while criminal and character disorders may benefit from a sequence based first on nonverbal, then written, and, if both media take, eventually the verbal.

THE CLINICAL USE OF FOCUSED WRITING

Focused writing suggests one specific topic that should be the major focus of concern of the writer—for instance, a client's autobiography or a narrative of depression or past hurts. After reading the written outcome of this assignment, the therapist has at least three choices available: (a) discussing the assignment, using it as grist for the therapeutic mill; (b) progressing to the next step of guided writing by assigning specific questions to be answered in writing—for instance, asking for elaboration of unclear passages in the earlier assignment; or (c) depending on what transpired during the face-to-face session, progressing to PW—that is, to a planned, already prepared approach based on previously designed series of lessons designed around a specific topic, forming a program or workbook (L'Abate, 1986, 1991, 1992; L'Abate & Platzman, 1991). These choices would not be available if the therapist relied solely on the spoken word.

Focused writing is usually ad hoc: that is, directed toward a specific issue or topic for which there is no program and for which the therapist may need to give specific instructions in writing on how the client needs to deal with that particular problem (in addition, of course, to face-to-face sessions). A basic issue concerning differentiation of applications between FW and PW relates to the comparative effectiveness of the two approaches. Is FW just as effective as PW? Perhaps in the future we shall be able to specify under what conditions each type of writing should be used, as suggested below.

Focused Writing At the Beginning of Therapy

By definition, FW takes place when a definite topic or assignment has been prescribed between therapy sessions. For instance, for theoretical, practical, and therapeutic reasons, I now routinely ask clients, whether individuals, couples, or families, to start writing about their "hurts" by listing them as they occur to them during preset times devoted to such assignments (for instance, twenty minutes a day for four days). These hurts include all of the possible traumas, rejections, failures, and painful o' troublesome experiences that may come to their minds in the weeks following the second therapy appointment.

In my practice, the first three sessions are framed as "evaluation." ("You are going to evaluate us, to see whether we can be of help to you or not.") The MMPI-2 and a marital questionnaire, the Problems in Relationships Scale (PIRS) described later in this chapter, are administered to the adults during the first and second sessions, with feedback given in the third session. At this point clients need simply to list their hurts. After this list is accomplished between the second and third sessions, if there is agreement over a therapeutic contract, clients are to rank these hurts in order of intensity, selecting those that were the most traumatic, expanding and elaborating on them in the following week(s).

In one instance, a client, who for many on-and-off years of therapy had avoided emotional confrontation, was able to remember the pain of moving into a house, a move his family had made when he was just two years old. The hurt of the experience, the coldness and emptiness of the house, brought tears to his eyes, as he recounted the many other times he had felt abandoned as he and his family of origin moved from one place to another without firm foundations. He repeated this experience with his family of procreation, which was now protesting and resisting yet another move. In another instance, a verbally resistant truck driver was able to write and to get in touch with the verbal and physical abuse he had received during his childhood from his alcoholic father, something he had not been able to reveal for years either to his wife or to himself.

The rationale for this initial step can be found in the position that hurt and the fear of being hurt is at the bottom of our human existence. The sharing of past hurt and fear of future hurt stands at the bottom of intimacy (L'Abate, 1986, 1994; L'Abate & Baggett, 1997). In addition to this theoretical rationale, there is another practical if not scientific reason to use this focused assignment at the outset of therapy. Pennebaker (1990), in his research on the use of writing about traumatic (hurtful) incidents, found that undergraduates writing about past traumatic experiences showed a significant improvement in physiological and immune system measures in comparison to undergraduates who wrote about trivial topics.

In my practice, I have given FW assignments to clients that asked them to concentrate on their defeats, on who defeated whom in their families of origin and/or procreation. They were to list which defeats they produced and which defeats they received. Couples and families were then to combine the individual lists into one grand list that would allow them to know who defeated whom. Sometimes, writing about these defeats was prescribed to achieve control over them. At this point, it seems more therapeutic to concentrate on hurts first, and only later, if necessary and relevant, on defeats. This practice covers the receptive, experienced aspects (hurts) of functioning: defeats, which are on the expressive side of an experiencing–expressing continuum, can be considered later.

Focused Writing during Therapy: Polarizations in Self-Definition

After dealing with the list of hurts, stressing most traumatic ones and achieving catharsis, there are a variety of directions that can be followed in the use of FW, depending on clients' immediate needs and the therapist's theoretical and therapeutic predilections. One direction that can be taken is to concentrate on self-definition. At the base of our existence is a basic definition of how we want to see ourselves—our self-concept. It undergirds the ways in which we think about ourselves and dictates how we act, even though often we are not aware of the connection between our internal self-definition and our external behavior (L'Abate, 1986, 1994; Quattrone, 1985). In dysfunctional relationships this definition is usually: (a) *dichotomous* (either-or); (b) *defensive* (to make up for perceived inadequacies); (c) *incomplete* (based on a one-sided and limited view of the self that includes just one or two attributes—it takes more than one attribute to make up a self); (d) therefore, *negative* ("bad" rather than "good"), and (e) *reactive* (to the individual's past and present experiences). This type of self-definition is bound to isolate the individual and produce a great deal of conflict in intimate relationships.

Because most dysfunctional partners meet, match, and marry on a complementary basis to fit into and satisfy their perceived definitions, they eventually are bound to clash about how they perceive themselves and each other, deteriorating into conflict and all of its possible negative outcomes. These partial self-definitions, of course, represent the outcome of generational and developmental deficits in past parenting and socialization experiences that left the individual with a partial and incomplete sense of self or no sense of self at all. As a result of this partial self-definition, the individual has to develop a self-image that will allow survival and perhaps even enjoyment of life. These definitions are at the bottom of the selfish–selfless polarities in marital relationships, characterized by repetitive, manipulative, and coercive patterns, and of the no-self polarity in many abusive–apathetic or neglectful family relationships, as found in many addictions and psychiatric conditions (L'Abate, 1990, 1992). Once the marital relationship is polarized, the same kind of polarization is likely to take place repetitively between parent and child, because the child will have to contend and react to a caretaker whose self-definition is lacking and who, most likely, may use the child to achieve what is perceived as an adequate sense of self.

Consequently, by concentrating on the partners' or caretakers' self-concept it is possible to undercut a variety of projections and externalizations. For instance, two of the most frequent self-definitions that lie at the bottom of a great many destructive conflicts in intimate relationships (between partners and between parent and child) are the good–bad and right–wrong dichotomies. Usually partners or parent and (adolescent) child are polarized around one of these two dichotomies, or there is a crossover between the individual who wants to be thought as right married (or parenting) to the individual who wants to be thought as "good." Either way, individuals with these self-definitions cannot win with each other. There is either "I win, you lose" outcome in the selfish position, or a "You win, I lose" in the selfless position. In the no-self position, both partners or parent and child lose and no one in the family wins. Of course, one could argue that if one partner or parent wins at the expense of the other, both partners or parent and child will lose. However, these defeats may not be perceived as such from the viewpoint of the partners or parents themselves. The one who wants to be right or correct finds the other (partner or child) always (or most of the time!) wrong, while the one whose self-conception is of being good finds the other bad. The worst outcome takes place when one partner or parent is both right and good, because there is no room left for the other partner or the child to be him- or herself.

The choice for clients is to stay the same or to find more acceptable and less destructive self-definitions, whether to retain the same, destructive labels (right vs. wrong and good vs. bad) or to consider more positive labels (helpful, effective, competent) for self-definition. The therapist should not accept any spur-of-the-moment decision, instead encouraging thinking and reflection on whether to retain or discard the old definition ("Why don't you think about it and let me know your decision next time we meet?"). Once the decision is made in favor of a more helpful and effective self-definition ("I would have found it hard to help you in retaining the old label . . . you could have kept it without my help"), the therapist can assign relevant focused homework assignments for anyone who is involved. Often, this confrontation brings a change in clients' self-image. However, if this initial assignment is insufficient to bring about any change in self-definition, additional assignments may be necessary. In this case, instructions can be given as follows, from one week to the next towards the end of the therapy session:

Week 1

"I want you to write down as many situations as you can remember about how often you were either "right' (or "good") in the past. Write down what happened and especially what happened to the person you were right with or good to. List as many people as you can remember. Keep this list open throughout next week and even later by adding to it as you think of others who were involved with you in being wrong and bad in the past. You are free to discuss this list with each other if it makes you happy. Make an appointment with each other at least 24 hours in advance. Whether you meet or not, bring a copy of this list to our next session."

After discussing the homework, with whatever implications and repercussions it may have brought about, congratulating whoever has done the homework, the therapist must consider whatever else may have happened that should be brought into the therapy session. At the end of this session, the therapist may give the second assignment.

Week 2

"I want you to write as many letters of apology as necessary to as many people who were judged by you to be wrong or bad. You may chose not to mail these letters, but their writing is necessary for forgiveness to take place (DiBlasio & Proctor, 1993; L'Abate, 1986). Your writing these letters is one way of showing that you may have forgiven yourself but you may need the forgiveness of those you love and who love you. If we cannot forgive ourselves for our mistakes, how can we forgive others? Discuss these letters with one another if you are comfortable at a meeting prearranged 24 hours in advance. If you do not find it comfortable to meet, just bring copies of these letters to the next session."

At the next session, after a discussion of the process of letter-writing, including the issue of whether or not to mail these letters, confront whatever issues ensue afterwards. At the end of the session give the third set of instructions.

Week 3

"Between today and next time we meet, I want you to monitor and write down all the situations where you were either right or good. What provoked you into being like that? What led into it and what followed from it? How did you feel afterwards? If you cannot find it in yourself to be right or good, pretend to be right or good and see what happens. In other instances, write down situations where you felt that you were right or good but chose to avoid being either but to be helpful and effective instead. Write all of these experiences down and discuss them among each other if you are comfortable. If you have given up being right or good, write what would have happened in the future if you had continued to define yourself that way. Either way, bring a list of your notes about these situations to our next session."

Once these homework assignments are completed, clients may be ready for completing as homework the first two written assignments of a Depression Workbook concerning the Drama Triangle and Distance Regulation (L'Abate, 1986).

Progressing from Experiencing to Expressing

Another application of FW, which is common in my clinical practice, relates to the experiencing–expressing continuum. This continuum is basic to personality and interpersonal functioning (L'Abate, 1994). Many dysfunctional individuals jump immediately from experiencing to expressing, without an intermediate step that would allow them to experience and process an emotional event before expressing it. In these individuals, experiencing painful feelings is equated and fused with expressing them, usually in a destructive fashion, through externalizations, accusations, and recriminations, or even worse, acting out, as in criminal behavior. Once the emotional experience is short-circuited, then there may be an enlarging of cognitive processing, ultimately resulting in obsessions and ruminations. Where cognition as well as emotionality are bypassed, then there is an enlarging of activity through impulsive, hyperactive, driven, or acting-out behavior (L'Abate, 1986; L'Abate & Baggett, 1997). In the latter case, the individual cannot stand the pressure of withstanding, much less experiencing, pain, discomfort, and unpleasant tension. Consequently, immediate discharge of painful or uncomfortable feelings is seen as the only way to get rid of those feelings, usually through anger, hostility, and acting out. These individuals are unable to process feelings rationally and to wait before saying or doing something that inevitably will be destructive, because no reflection or cognitive processing has taken place about how such feelings should be expressed in a helpful manner.

The therapist's task here is to help these individuals learn to differentiate experiencing from expressing feelings ("I am entitled to feel whatever I happen to feel. However, I am not entitled to hit you over the head with my feelings."). Once an awareness about the destructiveness of this pattern is reached, the decision of what to do about it has to be reached by the client(s) ("I need for you to think about this pattern between today and next time we meet. Then let me know whether you want me to help you with it or not."). After a decision in favor of abandoning this pattern is reached, the following lessons can be prescribed during the next three consecutive therapy sessions.

Week 1

"I want you to write down all the past instances when you jumped immediately from feeling something painful, unpleasant, or distasteful to expressing it by jumping into action or attacking an external target. Write down as many of these incidents as you can think of and add to this list as they come into your mind. Discuss this list with your family if you like, but only at prearranged appointment times (L'Abate, 1986). Bring this list to the next session." After a discussion of past instances when the client jumped from experiencing to expressing without using an intermediate, rational step, discuss whatever the client may bring to the session spontaneously. At the end of this session, say (or put it in writing):

Week 2

"During the next week, I want you to write letters of apology to whomever was the target of your attack. Do not mail these letters. Discuss them with your family if you like, but bring them to the next session so that we can go over them and improve them if necessary." During this session, the letters are gone over and editorial suggestions may be given by the therapist to ensure that their style and content are helpful and effective, following commonplace guidelines of helpful communication. After dealing with whatever else the clients may be bringing in to this session, say (or put it in writing):

Week 3

"During the next week, I want you to pay attention to when you jump from feeling something unpleasant or painful to expressing it immediately with anger. Write down what happened, what led into it, and what the outcome was for you and whomever was the target of your expression. I want you also to think of what would happen to you and those you love if you were to continue or persist in expressing immediately whatever you feel at the time. If possible, record instances where, instead of jumping into expressing the feeling, you processed and thought through ways and means of expressing feelings helpfully rather than hurtfully. Discuss your notes with your family if you like, but bring your records to the next session." This lesson could be broken up into two lessons, by dealing with the immediate present and the distant future, in terms of implications for the future if this pattern were to persist.

After this session is important to administer to clients lessons on how to express feelings nondestructively. An in-session exercise that I use quite often in my practice consists of the "Appreciation Game," in which we start by expressing "What I appreciate about me and what I do not appreciate about me." Clients begin by speaking about themselves and then they express feelings of appreciation to other family members. These feelings, however, have to be directed toward the performance or behavior of the self and others, but never to the person or personality. The same exercise can then be administered to families as an introduction to family conferences, or it could be used as an FW homework assignment.

Implications of Focused Writing for Help-Giving

A practical implication of this approach relates to how individuals want to assert their importance. We can do it by asserting our inherent righteousness and goodness and denying the existence of either of these qualities in those we love and who love us, or we can chose to assert our importance through relationally helpful and effective self-definitions. We may jump immediately into action or we may reflect on how we want to express what we feel. In FW, the overall process may be the same, even though the specific content may vary from one client to another. The sequence of instructions from one week to another can progress from dealing with and learning from the past (Week 1), to the process of asking for forgiveness from past targets (Week 2), to the present and the future (Week 3).

Focused writing is different from PW because it is constructed for the immediate and individualized needs of a specific client (individual, couples, or family). Responsibility for change lies in the client's hands, not in the therapist's head. If clients want change they can work for it by completing *in writing* assignments administered to them. In this approach FW assignments flow directly and idiographically from the problem at hand. In addition to the examples given here, there are many other conditions that could benefit by this approach.

Tentative differences between FW, PW, and traditional psychotherapy are summarized in Table 6-1. Here differentiation is needed between stylistic, relationship-oriented skills and structuring skills. Writing is one way of structuring therapy. Some therapists believe that style and the personal relationship between therapist and client is most responsible for change. Others believe that in addition to the personal relationship between therapist and client, there must be some structuring for change to take place. Furthermore, some would argue that relationship skills may be necessary for change to take place in individuals. However, these skills may be insufficient in helping couples and families—additional structuring skills, such as writing, may be necessary (L'Abate, 1986, 1991, 1992, L'Abate & Platzman, 1991).

The major issue with FW, and with writing in general, is no longer whether or not it helps. The evidence cited here and elsewhere (Esterling, L'Abate, Murray, & Pennebaker, in press; L'Abate, 1992; Pennebaker, 1990) supports its use as an ancillary or alternative medium of intervention instead of spoken therapy. The major issue is whether it will be used by the psychotherapeutic community, which must then find out what kind of writing will help whom, when, and where.

In conclusion, FW is an approach that requires the setting of personal, dyadic, or multirelational prearranged meetings where instructions for homework assignments are followed up, completed in writing, and then discussed with loved ones as well as with the therapist, producing three feedback loops: (a) from the questions asked in the lesson to the individual; (b) from the individual to the partner or other family members; and (c) from the individual, couple, or family to the therapist.

Once more information has been gathered, the therapist can switch from FW to PW. Neither approach is exclusive of the other. *Both can be administered in a sequentially flexible fashion. Which approach precedes the other depends very much on the particular needs of clients at the moment as perceived by the therapist and by the clients.* Both approaches, however, expect clients to work at these writing assignments, matching one hour of homework to each hour of therapy. With either approach, a major issue lies in finding evidence to support its responsible and responsive professional practice. Hence, this presentation will change from the clinical to the research applications of PW that are necessary to support its clinical practice.

THE USE OF PROGRAMMED WRITING IN PSYCHOTHERAPY RESEARCH

The purpose of this section is to argue that as long as the verbal modality is used as the major or only source of information about the process of psychotherapy, it will be difficult, if not impossible, to learn more about psychotherapy and answer the question about which method of treatment is better than others (Beutler, 1991). As long as treatment is verbal, the therapist must record and transcribe what is going on and then code it in order to reduce it to manageable units of research (Greenberg, 1991; Kolden, 1991). However, as long as we rely on the spoken word, the costs of studying therapist–client interactions, process, and outcome are going to be expensive if not prohibitive. Research will be limited to those few who are able to marshall grant support for this type of research. As Gottman (1979), among others, indicated, it takes at least 28 hours of clerical and technical time to reduce (score, classify) therapist–client interactions to manageable units of research. Using the written medium, either as an alternative or as an addition to the verbal medium, may allow us to learn more and faster about various methods of treatment than it would possible through an analysis of verbal interactions. The spoken modality is very expensive because it necessitates face-to-face interaction between a therapist and a client. Writing, if used properly, can be cost-effective because it does not necessitate a face-to-face interaction and puts more responsibility on the client for the conduct and progress of therapy.

Furthermore, as long as the spoken medium is used, it will be very difficult, if not impossible, to link evaluation with a specific form of treatment. This goal has been attempted conceptually in many instances but never substantiated empirically (Howard, Nance, & Myers, 1987; Hurt, Reznikoff, & Clarkin, 1991; Kennedy, 1992; Okun, 1990; Perry, Frances, & Clarkin, 1985; Seligman, 1990). It is possible to argue that as long as treatment relies mainly or solely on the spoken word such a link or match will remain virtually impossible for the large majority of psychotherapists, or certainly difficult and expensive to accomplish even for those few who can do it. The use of treatment manuals has been one way of decreasing therapist variability. However, thus far no one has won any prizes (Bleuter, 1991; Moncher & Prinz, 1991). Again, research will be limited to those few, very skilled, specialized researchers who are able to obtain research grants. However, the majority of psychotherapists will be unable to participate in research activities because of the time and energy required to find such a link through the verbal medium (Liddle, 1991). As Linden and Wen (1990) have found, publication trends in psychotherapy outcome research reflect a continuing lack of replication studies, plus a few other disadvantages that are peculiar to the nature of the spoken word. Writing, on the other hand, has the qualities of explicitness and specificity that cannot be found in the spoken word. Consequently, replication would take place at a much cheaper cost than would be possible with the spoken word. Writing can be replicated easily. The spoken word cannot be replicated. One advantage of PW, among others, lies in its potential to solve the long-standing problem of linking evaluation with treatment in a more specific way than can be accomplished through the spoken medium (L'Abate, 1992). Research advantages of PW will be illustrated through summaries of five research projects, three of which are still in progress.

Research in Progress on Programmed Writing

Programmed writing can help perform research functions at a cheaper and faster rate than the verbal medium (Bird, 1992; L'Abate, Boyce, Fraizer, & Russ, 1992). In the first study, undergraduates who scored on the upper third or half of the distribution on two paper-and-pencil tests for depression, the Center for Epidemiological Studies-Depression Scale (CES-D) and the Beck Depression Inventory (BDI) were selected as subjects. In a pilot study, *Ss* were divided into four groups. A control group (N = 16) received nothing and was retested at the same time as the other three groups. A second group (N = 13) received a workbook developed from this author's model of depression (L'Abate, 1986). A third group (N = 10) was administered a workbook developed from Beck's cognitive theory and treatment of depression (Beck, 1976). A fourth group (N = 11) received a workbook patterned after the MMPI-2 Content scale of depression (Butcher, Graham, Williams, & Ben-Porath, 1990). (This workbook, with others, is available in L'Abate, 1992). None of these *Ss* was ever seen face to face and the whole treatment was performed entirely through the mail. The average depression scores for all four groups before treatment were 25.83 (S.D. = 7.88) for the BDI and 34.95 (S.D. = 10.14) for the CES-D. On posttest after treatment (about 7 to 8 weeks), the control group means were 19.94 (S.D. = 7.54) on the BDI and 30.12 (S.D. = 8.91) on the CES-D. The means for the three treatment groups were 10.26 (S.D. = 11.34) on the BDI and 28.37 (S.D. = 13.09) for the CES-D. These results failed to reach statistical significance, but were suggestive and encouraging enough for the researchers to repeat and replicate the same procedure with another sample of undergraduates.

In this sample, the control group (N = 14) scored 22.79 (S.D. = 4.66) on the BDI and 34.21 (S.D. = 8.83) on the CES-D on pretest and 19.17 (S.D. = 8.82) on the BDI and 30.00 (S.D. = 8.55) on the CES-D on posttest. The three experimental groups scored means of 23.37 (S.D. = 7.42) on the BDI and of 33.28 (S.D. = 8.12) on the CES-D on pretest. On posttest these groups scored means of 12.52 (S.D. = 8.13) on the BDI and 19.68 (S.D. = 10.23) on the CES-D. An ANCOVA for repeated measures (4 × 2 × 2) yielded an F = 5.91 (df, 3,63), p < .001 for the BDI. The same level of significance resulted for the CES-D (F = 7.18, df 3,63), p < .001). A six month follow-up is now in progress and data collection and analysis is now taking place (L'Abate, Hamm, Russ, & Bird, in L'Abate & Baggett, 1997b).

A second study explored the effectiveness of using PW versus OW as treatment for generalized anxiety in undergraduates. They were selected on the basis of their T-scores above 65 on the Anxiety Content

Scale of the MMPI-2 (ACS). From a pool of volunteers, 35 males and 37 females were randomly assigned to one of three treatment groups. In the programmed writing group there were 13 males and 13 females. In the open-ended writing group there were 11 males and 12 females. In the comparison, control group there were 11 males and 12 females. From the original group of 72 Ss, 71.4% of the males and 81.1% of the females completed the study. They were administered Spielberger's State Trait Anxiety Inventory (STAI) as well as the ACS before and after completion of all written assignments. The PW group received six homework assignments designed to treat anxiety on the basis of the DSM-III definition of generalized anxiety disorder. The OW group was asked to write about anything that came to mind for about 30 minutes once a week for 6 weeks. The control group was tested before and after without any treatment. A factorial ANCOVA yielded significant treatment effects (p. < .05), that is, significant mean scores reduction, on the ACS and the State Anxiety scale of the STAI with no significant interactions or gender effects. Trait anxiety scores remained unchanged. There were no significant differences between PW and OW, a finding that substantiates Pennebaker's work (1990) as well as the replications of his work by Murray and his associates (Donnelly & Murray, 1991; Murray, Lamnin, & Carver, 1989). An examination of OW indicated that most were focused on anxiety-related topics, since this was the initial set for the study.

On the basis of these results from a nonclinical population, it seemed that PW could be now applied to a clinical sample, as in the study by Bird (1992). She evaluated the effectiveness of a stress-coping program with current and former clients to see which of four approaches improves self-esteem, self-disclosure, and coping skills. Half of her clients, randomly selected, received the coping program together with face-to-face counseling. The other half received only counseling. Former clients who accepted a letter of solicitation to participate in the study were assigned to either PW or to a no-treatment condition. The coping program consists of four lessons, and each lesson was assigned for four weeks. All clients were evaluated on a pre- and posttreatment basis with the Tennessee Self-Concept Scale, Rosenberg's Self-Esteem Scale, a Self-Profile Chart, and a Coping Resources Inventory. The 2 × 2 between Ss factorial design includes 15 Ss for each of the three experimental conditions and the comparison group for a total of 60 Ss. Bird's results supported the general use of PW on a posttreatment basis with former clients.

Another line of research, still in progress, deals with administering programs that are isomorphic with high peaks on the MMPI-2 Content Scales. On the basis of encouraging results in the pilot study described elsewhere (L'Abate, Boyce, Fraizer, & Russ, 1992), two more studies were conducted. In the first, results from undergraduates responding workbooks isomorphic with high peaks on the MMPI-2 Content Scales were compared with FW on trivial topics. Since this approach did not control well for the use of PW versus FW, in the second study PW lessons were compared with lessons dealing with trivial topics (L'Abate & Lambert, research in progress). Data analysis is now in progress.

Another line of research was suggested by the work of Blatt and his associates (Blatt, 1995) differentiating between self-concept and interpersonally derived depression. Two different programs, isomorphic with the two depressions described by Blatt, were administered to undergraduates on a random basis. Once the data are analyzed, we should be able to find out whether the matching or mismatching of the program with either type of depression is helpful. The overall practical outcome of this research for clinical practice is the existence of five depression workbooks, two already published (L'Abate, 1986, 1992), one (Beck, 1976) published in another work (L'Abate & Baggett, 1997a).

Toward Systematic Links between Evaluation and Treatment through Programmed Writing

The goal of linking evaluation with treatment can be accomplished through the creation of *prescriptive* rather than solely *descriptive* or, at best, *predictive* diagnostic instruments (L'Abate, 1990, 1992; L'Abate & Bagarozzi, 1993). In addition to the *descriptive–predictive–prescriptive* distinction, we need to consider two other distinctions of relevance to evaluation using a PW approach—the *nomothetic–idiographic* and the *direct–indirect*. Through PW we can use a nomothetic approach and apply it in an idiographic manner. Furthermore, evaluation can be direct, as, for instance, a semantic differential, or indirect, as in instruments to be described.

Evaluation and Programmed Writing with Individuals: Research in Progress

This approach, for example, can be accomplished with individuals using an objective like the Minnesota Multiphasic Personality Inventory-2 (MMPI-2). One study (L'Abate & Lambert, in L'Abate & Baggett, 1997b), for instance, evaluated whether programs specifically written for the 15 Content scales of the MMPI-2 (L'Abate, 1992b) could lower peak scores while a control group would write about trivial topics, as in the methodology developed originally by Pennebaker (1990). In a preliminary pilot study (L'Abate, Boyce, Fraizer, & Russ, 1992) peak and scale elevation scores on the MMPI-2 content scales could be lowered by administering matching written homework assignments. The sample of subjects and the type of controls used were too small to arrive at conclusive statements. The present study, consequently, is an example of how evaluation can be linked with treatment when programmed writing is used as a medium of treatment. It was designed to determine if a student's peak score and profile elevation from the Content Scales on the MMPI-2 could be lowered by completing programmed writing homework assignments (lessons) developed isomorphically to match each content scale (L'Abate, 1992).

A total of 266 undergraduates completed this study either for extra credit in an introductory psychology class or as part of the requirements for an abnormal psychology class. Out of this total number, 221 students completed all the assignments and both pre- and posttest administration of the MMPI-2. Forty-five subjects did not complete the posttest and 4 did not complete the testing in a way that could be used. Of the subjects who completed the study, 162 were females and 59 were males with a median age of 23 years.

All students who agreed to participate, after signing an informed consent form, were administered the MMPI-2 on a pretest–posttest basis approximately six weeks after completion of the written homework assignments. Subjects who returned test protocols initially were randomly assigned to one of three groups: (a) control focused trivia, (N = 48); (b) control programmed trivia, (N = 56); and (c) experimental (N = 117). The two control groups were combined after it was found that their performance on the before–after testing was not significantly different. Those who received assignments matching their MMPI-2 content scales were called "matched." Those who received general assignments directed toward supposedly trivial emotionally neutral topics were called "unmatched." All subjects completed four lessons from the workbook for the content scale based on their peak score or four assignments directed toward trivial topics, such as describing past cars, clothes, and places where they lived in the past.

Interventions consisted of programmed lessons developed (L'Abate, 1992) to match isomorphically the Content Scales of the MMPI-2. The structure of each lesson or homework assignment is generally the same. Respondents were asked to define in writing what their particular symptom or problem means to them and explain, in detail, how they experience the problem (e.g., social discomfort, depression, cynicism). Various dimensions of the symptom were identified and respondents were asked to "explain in detail" how each dimension applied to their experience.

They were asked to write about specific instances when they experienced the problem and how they felt about that experience. The next lesson involves evaluating or rating dimensions of the problems that were especially troublesome to them.

The peak or highest score on the content scales was considered the target score. In cases where there were two equal peak scores, a coin was flipped to determine which one became the target score. Once the peak score was determined for each participant, lessons specific for each scale were assigned. Students used their names when they volunteered as subjects, keeping contact with the experimenters through a mail box set up in the psychology department. There was no personal contact with the experimenters. Since students in the abnormal psychology class had personal contact with one of the experimenters, they used a five-digit identification number to remain anonymous. In both cases, all test protocols and lessons were received and sent via envelopes with either the participants name or code number on the front. In the first instance, all envelopes were passed through a box in the psychology office, and in the second instance, all envelopes were passed through a folder of envelopes on the instructor's desk.

Peak scores or spikes were obtained by subtracting the average on the other 14 content scales from the peak score. In other words, the overall scale elevation was removed by analyzing deviation scores only, regardless of scale elevation. Profile elevation was analyzed separately. Results showed that the interaction of matched versus nonmatched with time was significant, indicating that the nonmatched group improved more after treatment than the matched group. The main effect for time decrease due to treatment was significant. The main effect for treatment groups was significant, with the nonmatched subjects showing lower overall peak scores across time than the matched group. No other main effect or interaction was significant. When Hedges Unbiased Effect Sizes (UBS) were calculated as a function of matched and nonmatched treatment, the nonmatched group showed a larger UBS than the matched treatment group, which showed a medium UBS.

The above results are very surprising because of the unexpected changes in the behavior of the control group, which run counter to the original hypothesis. Writing about trivial topics, either focused or programmed, was more effective in lowering peak scores and scale elevations than matched programs with high content scales peaks. Impressionistically, the research assistants who conducted this study reported that students in the two control groups expressed very positive feelings about their homework assignments. Perhaps the pleasant quality of these assignments, which were less task-oriented and probably much less threatening than assignments directed toward lowering peak scores, may be somewhat responsible, paradoxically for these results. Furthermore, some of the so-called trivial assignments might have not been as trivial or neutral as it was thought initially, since some of them dealt with friends, for instance. There is also a possibility that because students were used as participants and earned school credit for their participation, those in the unmatched group may have felt they "got off easy" by not having to confront relatively threatening topics, which is what the matched group was asked to do. Another possibility could be that scores on post-test might decrease as a result of practice effects.

Another line of research has evaluated the effectiveness of programmed writing in dealing with depression in undergraduates. L'Abate and Lambert, in L'Abate and Baggett (1997b) evaluated two depression workbook programs based on either self-criticalness or overdependency. The call-sheet for this study specified that subjects had to admit being depressed, detailing many characteristics that are associated with this condition. The study was explained in detail through an informed consent form about the nature of the study, guaranteeing anonymity, and providing no consequences if participants were to drop out of the study. After the consent form was signed, subjects were mailed the test instruments, which they returned to a special box in the Psychology Department. No face-to-face contact between subjects and experimenters took place except by happenstance. Interactions between subjects and experimenters that were relevant to the administration of the study when necessary, took place by telephone.

Subjects were (N = 199) undergraduates who volunteered to participate in this study in exchange for course credits. One hundred and three subjects completed the study while 96 did not. Among completers, one subject did not complete one inventory but did complete the other two. Subjects were administered three paper-and-pencil, self-report instruments on a pre–postintervention basis. The two depression instruments administered were: (1) the Beck Depression Instrument (BDI); (2) the Center for Epidemiological Studies-Depression Scale (CES-D)— both instruments have received a great deal of research attention and are considered two of the most useful indicators of depression (L'Abate, Boyce, Fraizer, & Russ, 1992; L'Abate, Hamm, Russ, & Bird, in L'Abate & Baggett, 1997b); and (3) a self–other description inventory, the Self-Profile Chart (SPC). The SPC is a short rating scale designed to evaluate oneself on dimensions of personal (Self) and interpersonal roles (Others) on a 10-point range.

In a previous study with 52 former psychotherapy clients (L'Abate, Hamm, Russ, & Bird, in L'Abate & Baggett, 1997b), the SPC total self–other score was found to correlate positively and significantly with the Tennessee Self-Concept Scale and the total score of the Coping

Resources Inventory for Stress, suggesting that all three were measuring overlapping aspects of the self-concept. The SPC, however, takes only a few minutes to administer and less than a minute to score, while the other two scales take from 30 to 45 minutes to administer and at least five to ten minutes to score. The SPC, therefore, seems to fulfill some of the criteria set to select instruments for treatment outcome assessment. An item analysis of this instrument is in progress.

The interventions of this study consisted of two writing programs. One program focused on the nature of self-criticalness, while the other focused on overdependency. Forty-five subjects completed the overdependency workbook, 33 completed the self-criticalness workbook, and 25 students did not receive workbooks, serving as controls. Both programs were administered randomly through the mail, without the experimenters knowing anything about the nature of the subjects' depression, since all of the test instruments were scored after completion of these assignments. Both depression programs (or workbooks) consisted of four lessons administered once a week for four weeks, each lesson mailed on completion of the previous one.

Completers were not significantly different from noncompleters. Both groups combined were approximately 23 years old. The results indicated that both experimental groups (criticalness and overdependency) showed statistically significant lower depression scores on both the BDI and the CES-D than the control group. Hence, on the basis of previous and present evidence, it would seem that programmed writing for depression may be useful with at least nonclinical populations on a preventive basis. It will be important in the future to see how and whether the same approach can be used with clinical populations.

Symptom-Based Programmed Writing

Another, much more frequently used way to link treatment with evaluation can take place through the linkage of a specific treatment with a specific program. For instance, in dealing with individual symptoms, we have already shown how depression and anxiety can be linked through test scores and appropriate workbooks. This linkage, however, does not need to be limited to test scores. Scores may be necessary for experimental purposes in selecting *S*s from a nonclinical population, but they may not be needed (although they are desirable!) in dealing with a clinical population. Consequently, it is possible to take a symptom at face value and link the appropriate treatment with it. In dealing with acting-out juveniles and inmates, whose major characteristic is impulsivity, in addition to the MMPI-2 Content Scale for Antisocial Practices, which consists of only six lessons, a Social Training program consisting of 22 lessons, most of them designed to increasing thinking before acting, can be used. Two case studies were reported in conjunction with the appropriate workbook (L'Abate, 1992).

With couples, a different way of linking treatment with evaluation was accomplished by selecting two of the major symptoms of dysfunctionality, arguing and fighting, and linking them with the appropriate workbook. During the first lesson couples (or parents and adolescent) are asked to describe the frequency, duration, intensity, and content of their arguments. During the second lesson, they are asked to rank, in order of relevance to their personal (individual) experience, ten different (all positively framed) explanations of their arguments. During the third lesson they are asked to have an argument according to a structure that tells them how and when to have such an argument (prescription). They are to tape the argument and use at least six suicidal patterns they have used in the past, such as blaming, bringing up the past, mind reading, using threats, ultimatums, bribery, blackmail, and excuses. After they bring the tape to the therapist they are given written instructions on how to perform a content analysis of their individual patterns from the tape. After they complete this analysis they are given lessons that match those individual patterns that show up most frequently. Thus, therapists are able to give very specific lessons that are isomorphic with the patterns clients discover in their arguments (L'Abate, 1992).

With families the match between evaluation and treatment is even easier because symptoms are usually quite specific. Thus far programs dealing with the following symptoms have been published: negativity, verbal abuse, temper tantrums, shyness, stealing, sibling rivalry, domestic violence and child abuse, lying, and binge eating (L'Abate, 1992). All of these programs follow the same three-lesson format in which the first lesson deals with a description of the symptom in terms of frequency, duration, and intensity, the second lesson deals with positive reframings (explanations) of the symptom, and the third lesson deals with a specific prescription of the symptom according to a paradoxical strategy (Weeks & L'Abate, 1982). Our clinical evidence about the direct effectiveness of these programs at this moment is still admittedly anecdotal, even though, indirectly, paradoxical therapies may have shown a certain degree of effectiveness over more straightforward therapeutic strategies. The written format, however, would allow others besides the author and his associates to test the validity of this approach.

DISCUSSION

Among the many advantages of the written over the spoken word, in addition to cost, its potential to reach masses of individuals for both preventive and paratherapeutic purposes needs to be stressed (L'Abate, 1990). The studies mentioned above were conducted with a minimum of cost—payment went only to part-time research assistants, mailings, and data analyses provided by the institution, a large urban university. Thus, writing could be used in epidemiological and preventive interventions in ways that would be difficult and expensive to achieve through the spoken word.

The combination of the spoken with the written word—that is, the influence of the therapist's own style, which is mainly verbal and nonverbal, with the application of a replicable method of treatment through writing—should result in synergistic effects between the three modalities. This synergism, which thus far is only personally impressionistic in the writer's clinical practice, could accelerate the process of research about therapeutic change. This approach could enlarge the number of professionals who could become involved in research activities and the number of people who could be helped per unit of a therapist's time.

How much evidence will be necessary to change traditional therapeutic practices, which are now based mainly on the verbal medium, to include also both nonverbal and written modalities? No matter how much research evidence may be mustered, it is very doubtful whether any amount of evidence will hold sway on current verbally mediated psychotherapeutic practices. Ultimately, the decision to change and to incorporate new or even more cost-effective practices may need to be mandated by third parties, because change in current therapeutic practices will not take place otherwise. Resistance to the use of writing in psychotherapy practice and research, either by itself or in conjunction with the verbal modality, is inevitable. We psychotherapists are at least as resistant to change as are some of the very clients we want to help. However, if the process of therapeutic change consists of at least three components: (a) the existence of new responses—emotive, cognitive, or verbal—that were not repertoire *(novelty)*; (b) this new response needs to be of a positive nature, defined as being self-enhancing rewarding behavior that does not damage anyone else *(positivity)*; and (c) frequent repetition, practice, and rehearsal should increase the habitual preeminence of this new behavior in the repertoire of an individual *(strength)*, then the process of change for psychotherapists should possess the same characteristics. Professional change will take place if and when—and only if and when—we psychotherapists start practicing new, positive practices with sufficient intensity and strength to make a difference for ourselves and for our clients in terms of cost-effectiveness (that is, we become more effective in our procedures and pass along smaller costs to our clients). This change, of course, implies frequently using new, positive practices that we have not used in the past, such as writing in its different forms.

CONCLUSION

As long as psychotherapy is based mainly on the verbal medium, progress in psychotherapy will be slow and difficult, limited mostly to those few researchers who can receive research grants. Research in progress shows how it is possible to: (a) study comparatively different therapeutic models in the treatment of depression and reduce state anxiety through the use of programmed workbooks in student populations; (b) possibly increase coping skills in former clients, and (c) link and match evaluation with treatment through test scores or link specific symptomatologies with specific programs of treatment.

REFERENCES

Anderson, C. M., Reiss, D. J., & Hogarty, G. E. (1986). *Schizophrenia and the family: A practitioner's guide to psychoeducation and management.* New York: Guilford.

Beck, A. (1976). *Cognitive therapy and the emotional disorders.* New York: Meridian Press.

Beutler, L. E. (1991). Have all won and must all have prizes? Revisiting Luborsky et al.'s verdict. *Journal of Consulting and Clinical Psychology, 59,* 1–7.

Bird, G. (1992). *Programmed writing as a method for increasing self-esteem, self-disclosure, and coping skills.* Atlanta, GA: Department of Counseling and Psychological Services, Georgia State University.

Blatt, S. J. (1995). The destructiveness of perfectionism: Implications for the treatment of depression. *American Psychologist, 50,* 1003–1028.

Bloom, B. L. (1992). Computer-assisted psychological intervention: A review and commentary. *Clinical Psychology Review, 12,* 169–197.

Brown, E. C., & L'Abate, L. (1969). An appraisal of teaching machines and programmed instruction: With special relevance to the modification of deviant behavior. In C.M. Franks (ed.), *Behavior therapy: Appraisal and status* (pp. 396–414). New York: McGraw-Hill.

Butcher, J. M., Graham, J. R., Williams, C. L., & Ben-Porath, Y. S. (1990). *Development and use of the MMPI-2 content scales.* Minneapolis: University of Minnesota Press.

DiBlasio, F. A., & Proctor, J. H. (1993). Therapists and the clinical use of forgiveness. *American Journal of Family Therapy, 21,* 175–184.

Donnelly, D. A., & Murray, E. J. (1991). Cognitive and emotional changes in written essays and therapy interviews. *Journal of Social and Clinical Psychology, 10,* 334–350.

Esterling, B. A., L'Abate, L., Murray, E. J., & Pennebaker, J. W. (in press). Empirical foundations for writing in prevention and psychotherapy: Mental health outcomes. *Clinical Psychology Review.*

Gordon, R. E., & Gordon, K. K. (1981). *Systems of treatment for the mentally ill: Filling the gaps*. New York: Grune & Stratton.

Gottman, J. M. (1979). *Marital interaction*. New York: Academic Press.

Greenberg, L. S. (1991). Research on the process of change. *Psychotherapy Research, 1*, 3–16.

Howard, G. S., Nance, D. W., & Myers, P. (1987). *Adaptive counseling and therapy: A systematic approach to selecting effective treatments*. San Francisco, CA: Jossey-Bass.

Hurt, S. W., Reznikoff, M., & Clarkin, J. F. (1991). *Psychological assessment, psychiatric diagnosis, treatment planning*. New York: Brunner/Mazel.

Kennedy, J. A. (1992). *Fundamentals of psychiatric treatment planning*. Washington, DC: American Psychiatric Association.

Kolden, G. G. (1991). The generic model of psychotherapy: An empirical investigation of patterns of process and outcome relationships. *Psychotherapy Research, 1*, 62–73.

L'Abate, L. (1986). *Systematic family therapy*. New York: Brunner/Mazel.

L'Abate, L. (1990). *Building family competence: Primary and secondary prevention strategies*. Newbury Park, CA: Sage.

L'Abate, L. (1991). The use of writing in psychotherapy. *American Journal of Psychotherapy, 45*, 87–98.

L'Abate, L. (1992). *Programmed writing: A self-administered approach for interventions with individuals, couples, and families*. Pacific Grove, CA: Brooks/Cole.

L'Abate, L. (1994). *A theory of personality development*. New York: John Wiley.

L'Abate, L., & Baggett, M. S. (1997a). *The self in the family: A classification of personality, criminality, and psychopathology*. New York: Wiley.

L'Abate, L., & Baggett, M. S. (1997b). *Distance writing and computer-assisted training in mental health*. Atlanta, GA: The Institute for Life Empowerment.

L'Abate, L., Boyce, J., Fraizer, L., & Russ, D. (1992). Programmed writing: Research in progress. *Comprehensive Mental Health Care, 2*, 45–62.

L'Abate, L., & Bagarozzi, D. A. (1993). *Sourcebook of marriage and family evaluation*. New York: Brunner/Mazel.

L'Abate, L., Hamm, J., Russ, D., & Bird, G. (1997). Programmed writing: Two follow-ups and one application with clinical outpatients. in L'Abate, L., & Baggett, M. S., *Distance writing and computer-assisted training in mental health*. Atlanta, GA: The Institute for Life Empowerment.

L'Abate, L., & Kunkel, D. (research in progress). The problems-in-relationships scale (PIRS) and workbook program. Department of Psychology, Georgia State University, Atlanta, GA.

L'Abate, L., Lambert, R. G., Vardaman, P., Lewy, L., DaLee, D. & Hunter, L. (research in progress). Selfhood and depression: A test of a selfhood model of relational personality propensities.

L'Abate, L., & Lambert, R. G. (1997). Testing a model of psychopathology with the MMPI-2. In L'Abate, L., & Baggett, M. S. *Distance writing and computer-assisted training in mental health*. Atlanta, GA: The Institute for Life Empowerment.

L'Abate, L., & Platzman, K. (1991). Programmed writing (PW) in therapy and prevention with families. *American Journal of Family Therapy, 19*, 1–10.

Liberman, R. P., DeRisi, W., & Mueser, K. T. (1989). *Social skills training for psychiatric patients.* Des Moines, IO.: Allyn & Bacon.

Linden, W., & Wen, F. K. (1990). Therapy outcome research, health care policy, and the continuing lack of accumulated knowledge. *Professional Psychology: Research and Practice, 21,* 482–488.

Little, H. A. (1991). Empirical values and the culture of family therapy. *Journal of Marital and Family Therapy, 17,* 327–348.

Moncher, F. J., & Prinz, R. J. (1991). Treatment fidelity in outcome studies. *Clinical Psychology Review, 11,* 247–266.

Murray, E. J., Lamnin, A. D., & Carver, S. C. (1989). Emotional expression in written essays and psychotherapy. *Journal of Social and Clinical Psychology, 8,* 414–429.

Okun, B. F. (1990). *Seeking connections in psychotherapy.* San Francisco, CA: Jossey-Bass.

Pennebaker, J. W. (1990). *Opening up: The healing power of confiding in others.* New York: William Morrow.

Perry, S., Frances, A., & Clarkin, J. (1985). *A DSM-III casebook of differential therapeutics: A clinical guide to treatment selection.* New York: Brunner/Mazel.

Quattrone, G. A. (1985). On the congruity between internal states and action. *Psychological Bulletin, 98,* 3–40.

Seligman, L. (1990). *Selecting effective treatments.* San Francisco, CA: Jossey-Bass.

Siani, R., Siciliani, O., & Burti, L. (1990). *Strategie di psicoterapia e riabilitazione: Gli psicotici e il servizio psichiatrico.* Milano, Italy: Feltrinelli.

Weeks, G. R., & L'Abate, L. (1982). *Paradoxical therapy: Theory and practice with individuals, couples, and families.* New York: Brunner/Mazel.

Weiner, I. B. (Ed.). (1976). *Clinical methods in psychology.* New York: Wiley-Interscience.

7

Marital and Family Approaches

DENNIS A. BAGAROZZI, Ph.D.

INTRODUCTION

The future and viability of managed mental health care companies in the United States will depend, to a large degree, upon managed mental health care corporations' ability to demonstrate that their clinical practitioners are competent to provide high quality yet cost effective short-term mental health and psychological services to beneficiaries. Subjective anecdotal treatment reports and clinical summaries that claim psychotherapeutic success, no matter how skillfully written, will not be sufficient to satisfy beneficiaries and such independent evaluators, consumer protection groups, members of the major mental health professions, and officials from the various federal and state agencies that will be created once national health insurance is fully implemented. For accountability to be demonstrated satisfactorily, managed mental health care providers and the therapists they employ will have to document their effectiveness by using universally accepted scientific research methods and evaluation procedures. Reliable and valid tests, instruments, and other such tools that are behaviorally focused and sensitive to clinically produced changes must be used if claims of success are to be taken seriously.

In addition, clinicians who are members of service provider panels will be expected to demonstrate that the treatments they provide are equally as effective, if not more successful, in achieving positive therapeutic outcome, maintaining therapeutic gain, and causing less client deterioration than their fee-for-service counterparts (Rogers et al., 1993). Furthermore, managed mental health care practitioners will also be expected to show that their interventions are more effective (if not superior) in producing positive therapeutic outcome and reducing client deterioration than one routinely finds in untreated control group patients (Lambert, Shapiro, & Bergin, 1986).

With the full implementation of national health insurance, accountability will become increasingly more important. Practitioners who know how to select and use reliable, valid, easily administered, and time efficient behaviorally focused assessment instruments and procedures will be of immense value to managed mental health care organizations. It is possible that therapists who have been trained to be scientific practitioners will be more likely to secure places on service provider panels than those whose clinical training did not prepare them to conduct objective outcome evaluations of their practice.

MANAGED MENTAL HEALTH CARE AND MARRIAGE AND FAMILY THERAPY

Diagnosis

At the present time, most managed mental health care groups do not cover V-Code conditions listed in the DSM-IV as part of their benefit packages. V-Code conditions include marital problems, family problems, parent–child difficulties, academic problems, normal bereavement and grief reactions, life stage transitional problems, and other life circumstance difficulties. However, some managed mental health care organizations will permit a therapist to treat the identified client's spouse or other family members under certain circumstances for a limited number of sessions. These collateral contacts (as they are called) may also be approved for the treatment of some interpersonal sexual problems that cannot be treated adequately without the full participation of the client's spouse. In all cases where collateral contacts are deemed necessary by the therapist, prior approval must be received from a peer adviser, case manager, or review specialist. Although such exclusions may not be permitted under national health insurance, the current reality is that treating V-Code conditions and some types of sexual dysfunctions usually will require prior approval for a specific number of collateral contacts.

When collateral treatments are approved, assessment and outcome evaluations at both the individual and marital/family systems levels are warranted. How to conduct pretreatment and posttreatment evaluations under such conditions is the subject of this chapter.

PRETREATMENT ASSESSMENT AND PRETREATMENT

Decision Making in Terms of Individual Diagnosis and Marital/Family Systems Intervention

It is important to keep in mind as you read this chapter that within the managed mental health care models (as they now stand) marriage and/or family intervention is viewed as an adjunct to individually focused treatments, and the collateral involvement of other family members is only permitted for a limited number of sessions. This should not be disheartening to the marriage/family therapist, however, because marriage and family therapy, as originally conceived, was seen as a treatment of short duration whose major goal was the modification of dysfunctional interaction patterns and faulty communication-relationship structural arrangements (Haley, 1963; Jackson, 1959; Watzlawick, Beavin, & Jackson, 1967). The collateral inclusion of a spouse or other family member in treatment for a limited number of sessions, therefore, is in keeping with traditional marital/family systems treatment philosophy.

The selection of instruments and assessment procedures for both individual and marital/family assessment should follow logically from the therapist's theoretical/clinical orientation and should be relevant to the nature of the presenting problem. Evaluating the functioning of one or more individuals within a family does not mean that the therapist must abandon a systems orientation, because individual measures can be extremely helpful in determining how couples and family members function as interrelated components of a larger system (Bagarozzi, 1985; Bagarozzi & Anderson, 1989; L'Abate & Bagarozzi, 1993). When the therapist chooses an individually focused instrument to assess the client's presenting problem, that instrument should validly and reliably operationalize the concept (symptom) that is being assessed (for example, depression, anxiety, anger, guilt, shame, or self-esteem) in a way that makes short-term behaviorally focused treatment possible. In addition, the therapist must be sure that the instrument, test, or procedure chosen is one that is cost effective in terms of the time required for administration, scoring, and interpretation. Similarly, the therapist must be certain that he or she has had the proper training and relevant clinical experiences required for interpreting test scores and translating these scores and findings into concrete and achievable treatment goals.

For example, let us suppose that a 35-year-old man is referred for treatment because he is depressed. In addition to taking a routine personal history and a history of the presenting problem or symptom, there are a few brief self-report instruments that assess the severity of depression that a therapist might use. Examples include *The Depression Adjective Check List* (Liebin, 1965), *The Carroll Rating Scale for Depression* (Carroll, Feinberg, Smouse, Rawson, & Greden, 1981), *The Beck Depression Inventory* (Beck, 1979), *The Depressive Behavior Survey Schedule* (Cautela, 1977) and *The IPAT Depression Scale* (Krug & Laughlin, 1976).

In my work with individuals, couples, and family systems, I frequently use the Beck Depression Inventory (Beck, 1979). This scale is based upon its author's cognitive model of depression, and each of the 21 scale items is designed to operationalize a major aspect of depression (for example, depressed mood, pessimism, guilt, self-hate, self-accusation, irritability, loss of appetite, suicidal ideation, loss of sexual drive). The Beck scale items can be easily translated into concrete treatment goals and lend themselves very well to the cognitive behavioral intervention strategies that we have developed over the years (e.g., Anderson & Bagarozzi, 1983, 1988a, 1988b; Bagarozzi, 1981, 1982, 1983, 1985, 1986, 1988, 1990, 1992; Bagarozzi & Anderson, 1982, 1988, 1989; Bagarozzi & Giddings, 1983a, 1983b; Bagarozzi & Wodarski, 1977, 1978; Wodarski & Bagarozzi, 1979).

Defining and Conceptualizing the Presenting Problem or Symptom in a Manner that Allows for Objective Assessment and Brief Behaviorally Focused Intervention

In addition to using a standardized behaviorally focused assessment instrument, a situational analysis is also necessary for formulating an appropriate treatment plan and for determining whether collateral involvement would be appropriate. A brief outline of what should be contained in a situational analysis is presented below:

Situational Analysis

1. In what situations and environments does the symptom or problem behavior occur?
2. In what situations and environments does the symptom or problem behavior never occur?
3. In what situations and environments is the symptom or problem behavior most severe?

4. In what situations and environments is the symptom or problem least severe?

5. What situations, people, thoughts, feelings, and so on act as cues that set off the symptom or problem behavior?

6. How do the people who are present at the time behave once the symptom or problem behavior is exhibited and becomes evident to them?

7. How do you (the client, identified patient, etc.) feel when you are exhibiting the symptom or problem behavior?

8. What do you (the client, identified patient, etc.) say to yourself when you have these feelings and notice that you have become symptomatic?

9. How do the people who are present at the time feel and behave once the symptom or problem behavior has subsided or is no longer being exhibited?

10. What happens later on, after you and the people who were present when you were symptomatic have had a chance to think about what has transpired? How is your relationship with them affected?

11. What are the conditions and circumstances in your environment that you believe contribute to maintaining the symptom or problem behavior?

12. What are the conditions and circumstances in your environment that you believe contribute to reducing the symptom or problem behavior?

13. What have you done in the past to alleviate this symptom or to correct this problem behavior (e.g., psychotherapy, medication, use of drugs or alcohol, talking to a friend or member of the clergy, and so on)?

14. What have you found to be the most helpful?

15. What have you found to be the least helpful?

In addition to the situational analysis, an incentive analysis is also conducted. The major components of this analysis are as follows:

16. What positive behavioral self-control methods, procedures, techniques, and so on have you used in order to reduce the symptoms or to correct the problem behavior (e.g., self-reinforcement, tokens, positive self-statements)?

17. What negative behavioral self-control methods, procedures, techniques, and so on have you used in order to reduce the symptom or to correct the problem behavior (e.g., self-punishment, negative self-statements)?

18. Which of these self-control methods has been helpful?
19. What benefits would derive for you and significant others in your life if the symptom or problem behavior continued in its present form or intensity?
20. What benefits would derive for you and significant others in your life if the symptom or problem behavior got worse?
21. What benefits would derive for you and significant others in your life if the symptom or problem behavior were removed totally?
22. What are the disadvantages for you and significant others in your life if the symptom or problem behavior were to continue in its present form or intensity?
23. What are the disadvantages for you and significant others in your life if the symptom or problem behavior were to get worse?
24. What are the disadvantages for you and significant others in your life if the symptom or problem behavior were removed totally?
25. Is there anything else about the symptom or problem behavior that you think is important for me to know in order to help you?

Determining Who Should Be Included in the Assessment and Treatment Process: Abandoning Preconceived Notions Concerning the Identified Patient and the Nature of Treatment According to Managed Mental Health Care Philosophy

If, after the situational analysis is completed, the therapist determines that the client's symptom (for example, depression) is being reinforced by significant others in his or her life or that the client's depression serves a systemic function, it would be appropriate to request approval for collateral contacts with all family members who are actively involved on a day-to-day basis with the client.

Early systems theorists were behavioral and pragmatic (Bateson, 1935, 1936, 1972; Haley, 1963; Watzlawick, Beavin, & Jackson, 1967). They postulated that all behavior is communication and that all communication-behavioral exchanges were either symmetrical (based upon equality in power and status between and among interactants who reciprocate *identical* behaviors) or complementary (based upon inequality in power and status between and among interactants who reciprocate behaviors that are logically *opposite,* thereby maximizing the differences between and among them). If a therapist accepts this behavioral systems approach, then assessment of the identified patient's symptom of depression is only meaningful if all other family members are also evaluated along the same dimension. Only by having all significant family members complete the Beck Depression Inventory, or some other reliable and valid measure of depression, will the therapist be able to determine how complementary and/or symmetrical behavioral exchanges and role relationships serve to reinforce and maintain the identified patient's depression. For example, this man's depressed behavior—his self-recriminations, overeating, and lethargy—may be getting enough periodic reinforcement from his wife's and son's complementary upbeat behavior—their attempts to raise his self-esteem, to cheer him up, and to prepare him special meals that would temporarily relieve his sadness—so that he remains chronically depressed. Conversely, by administering the Beck Depression Inventory to all family members, the therapist may find a symmetrical pattern where all family members are depressed to some degree. In this case, depression may represent an affect that accompanies a systemic family theme, for example, unresolved mourning for a dead family member.

Choosing Appropriate Marital and Family Assessment Instruments and Procedures for Payment Under Managed Mental Health Care Authorization

The rationale for having all family members complete the same individual measures that are given to the identified patient has been discussed in the previous section. However, when it comes to choosing marital and family assessment devices and procedures for use in managed care settings, the choice may not be as clear cut as when choosing an individually focused instrument. The selection of appropriate tests, questionnaires, instruments, and other tools for the purpose of accurate marital and family assessment is an essential part of the therapeutic process. In previous writings (Bagarozzi, 1989, 1990), several criteria were identified as important when considering which instruments the family psychologist should choose. First, the therapist can select those instruments and procedures that have been shown to be reliable and valid measures of some important theoretical construct or group of related constructs that are consistent with the practitioner's theoretical/clinical orientation. For example, a therapist who subscribes to an intergenerational model of family dysfunctioning and family therapy might use the lengthy Personal Authority in the Family Systems Questionnaire (Williams, Bray, & Malone, 1984) to assess eight interrelated theoretical constructs (spousal intimacy, spousal fusion/individuation, nuclear family triangulation, intergenerational intimacy, intergenerational fusion/individuation, intergenerational triangulation, intergenerational intimidation, and personal authority). Essentially, theory determines which instrument is used. Translating test scores for each of these eight subscales into concrete intervention strategies requires sophisticated theoretical understanding, considerable training, and supervised practice, as well as a fairly high leve. of clinical expertise. For these reasons—the length of the PAFS-Q, the time required to complete it, and the clinical training and theoretical sophistication required to interpret PAFS-Q subscale scores and translate them into identifiable treatment goals and strategies—the Personal Authority in the Family Systems Questionnaire would be inappropriate for use in a managed mental health care setting. A more behaviorally focused and brief instrument such as the Spousal Inventory of Desired Changes and Relationship Barriers: SIDCARB (Bagarozzi, 1983), which takes each spouse approximately 3 to 5 minutes to complete, can be used to alert the therapist to the presence of intergenerational difficulties if they exist.

The second criterion identified by Bagarozzi (1989, 1990) has less to do with theoretical purity or theoretical orientation and is concerned primarily with the pragmatics of treatment. In such cases, the instrument is chosen because it makes it possible to identify particular presenting problems, problem constellations, or problem categories of marital or family dysfunctioning, disagreement, and conflict.

The Family Environment Scale (Moos & Moos, 1981) is a good example of such an instrument. The FES has ten subscales that are said to assess three underlying dimensions of family life—relationships, personal growth, and systems maintenance. The first dimension includes the following critical areas: cohesion, expressiveness, and conflict. The personal growth dimension is made up of five subscales: independence, achievement orientation, intellectual–cultural orientation, active-recreational orientation, and moral–religious emphasis. The final dimension has two components: organization and control.

The Family Environment Scale, although not grounded in a recognizable theory of family development, process, and change, is an early attempt to identify some areas where conflicts might develop in marriages and family systems. However, the comprehensiveness of the domains of marital and family life is far from complete and some of the areas that are included in the Family Environment Scale are of questionable relevance for clinical purposes. However, items that make up those areas of the FES that might be considered clinically important (for example, relationships, systems maintenance, independence, cohesion, expressiveness, and conflict) are not worded in ways that makes translation into specific behavioral interventions possible.

A third criterion that must be considered when selecting an instrument for use within a managed mental health care framework is time.

How long it takes the client to read and complete the instrument and how long it takes the therapist to score and interpret findings must be taken into account. As was mentioned earlier in this discussion, the Personal Authority in the Family Systems Questionnaire requires a considerable amount of time for family members to complete and for the therapist to score and interpret (it takes 20 to 30 minutes to complete and 10 to 15 minutes to score each family member's individual form). The Family Environment Scale, on the other hand, takes only about 10 minutes to complete and approximately 2 to 5 minutes to score. Plotting family scores on a graph takes the therapist an additional 10 to 15 minutes for a family of four.

While time is an extremely important consideration for managed mental health care practitioners, probably the most important criterion to take into account when selecting an assessment instrument is whether the information gleaned from the instrument can be translated easily into concrete treatment goals. It is essential, therefore, that the items and questions that make up instruments used in managed mental health care work are worded in ways that make problem identification specific and desired changes behaviorally explicit. Clinicians from behavioral schools of marriage and family therapy have led the way in this endeavor. For example, comprehensive and behaviorally specific instruments such as the 16-page Couple's Precounseling Inventory (Stuart & Jacobson, 1991), with its 12 separate subscales containing 341 bits of information, and the Spouse Observation Checklist (Patterson, 1976; Weiss, Hops, & Patterson, 1973; Weiss & Margolin, 1977) are excellent in terms of behavioral specificity and comprehensiveness but are impractical for use in managed care settings. There are, however, a number of brief behaviorally focused instruments that would be ideal for managed mental health care use. Examples include the 34-item Areas of Change Questionnaire (Weiss & Birchler, 1983), the 24-item Spousal Inventory of Desired Changes and Relationship Barriers (SIDCARB) (Bagarozzi, 1983; Bagarozzi & Atilano, 1982; Bagarozzi & Pollane, 1983) mentioned earlier, and the Marriage Inventory (Knox, 1971).

Unfortunately, behavioral specificity is not characteristic of the most commonly used family assessment instruments, such as the Family Adaptability and Cohesion Scales III (Olson, Portner, & Lavee, 1985), the Family Assessment Device (Epstein, Baldwin, & Bishop, 1983), the Structural Family Interaction Scale (Perosa, Hansen, & Perosa, 1981), the Family Process Scale (Berberin, 1982), the Family of Origin Scale (Hovestadt, Anderson, Piercy, Cochran, & Fine, 1985) and the Family Functioning Scale (Tavitran, Lubiner, Green, Grebstgein, & Velicer, 1987). However, the absence of brief and behaviorally specific family-focused instruments should not be interpreted as meaning that behaviorally specific treatment goals cannot be formulated for entire family systems. It simply means that a problem-focused assessment and treatment orientation is required. A problem-focused approach is very much in keeping with a managed mental health care philosophy of short-term intervention. The problem-focused approach to dealing with family difficulties has a long history (e.g., Epstein & Bishop, 1981), and there are a number of schools of family therapy that can be considered problem focused (for example, the structural, strategic, and functional). Unfortunately, none of these schools of family therapy has developed reliable and valid brief paper-and-pencil assessment measures that can be used by frontline practitioners in a managed mental health care setting.

These three problem-focused therapies rely heavily upon structured interaction interviews, which are conducted by highly skilled therapists who have been trained to observe, track, and evaluate the faulty family processes and dysfunctional hierarchical arrangements that are believed to maintain the presenting problem/symptom. Such diagnostic procedures and outcome evaluations are of little value to managed mental health care organizations, because the reliability and validity of such pretreatment assessments and posttreatment evaluations have yet to be demonstrated. Essentially, they are highly subjective and interpretive. We must, therefore, turn to assessment instruments that target specific family problems, dynamics, structural arrangements, issues, and so on if we wish to function successfully within a managed mental health care setting. In order to select the appropriate instrument for diagnosing the presenting family problem, the therapist must have some familiarity with the types of instruments that are available for use. For an overall view of instruments developed by family research- ers, the reader should be familiar with the *Handbook of Family Measurement Techniques* (Touliatos, Perlmutter, & Straus, 1990). These authors catalogue and abstract 976 instruments, which are grouped according to five general categories of marital and family life. Another volume that managed mental health care therapists might find helpful is the *Sourcebook of Marriage and Family Evaluation* (L'Abate & Bagarozzi, 1992), which was written specifically for clinicians. In this work, the authors offer critical analyses and in-depth discussions of the most common clinical tools and assessment procedures used by marital and family therapists.

BRIEF SHORT-TERM INTERVENTION IN MANAGED MENTAL HEALTH CARE: BASIC CONSIDERATIONS

Therapist Expertise and Training

The brief, short-term, time-limited, problem-focused model of intervention that is preferred by most managed mental health care organizations is more characteristic of behavioral therapies than more traditional forms of psychotherapy and counseling. Therapists trained in behavioral marital/family therapies and structural/strategic approaches to marital/family problem solving, therefore, probably will have less difficulty making the transition to managed mental health care models of intervention than therapists who were schooled in individual, relationship-interpretive, nondirective, existential, and experiential forms of psychotherapy, because these approaches usually place little emphasis upon objective and quantifiable behavioral outcomes.

In some instances, the retraining of therapists might be appropriate. Continuing education courses designed for this purpose should include training in:

1. Problem focused and behavioral approaches to marital/family intervention.
2. Behavioral diagnosis and assessment.
3. The selection, administration, interpretation, and clinical use of brief empirically developed and behaviorally focused tests and rating scales that can be used to help couples and family members identify desired goals and evaluate the progress each person has made toward achieving these goals.
4. Objective and empirical outcome evaluation.

This final skill, empirical evaluation, requires further discussion, because outcome evaluation is a complex and multifaceted phenomenon. Several clinical researchers (Bagarozzi & Anderson, 1989; Cromwell, Olson, & Fournier, 1976; Gurman & Kniskern, 1981; Kniskern & Gurman, 1983; L'Abate & Bagarozzi, 1992) have stressed the importance of gaining the perspectives of both insiders (spouse and all family members involved in the therapy) and outsiders (therapists, managed mental health care case managers, review specialists, and so on) when evaluating the effects of marital and family interventions. In addition to the insider–outsider dimension of evaluation, the degree of inference and subjectivity involved in outcome assessment also must be considered. These important issues are discussed in the following section.

Insider/Outsider—Subjective/Objective Considerations in Evaluating Treatment Outcomes, Successes, and Failures in Managed Mental Health Care

The most qualified person to judge the effectiveness, success, or failure of any psychotherapeutic intervention is the client (beneficiary) him-

or herself. This firsthand insider's view is indispensable. However, if such evaluations are simply open-ended, nonstandardized self-reports of satisfaction, an objective appraisal of therapeutic outcome cannot be obtained. The reliability and validity of such reports are suspect, because clients' feelings about their therapists definitely will color their judgments. For example, a couple's positive feelings about their therapist may cause them to rate their therapeutic experience as having been highly successful, even though a case manager or review specialist may see no observable behavior change in the identified patient's presenting problem (the husband is still depressed, has little sexual desire, and takes no initiative in his relationship with his wife).

Conversely, positive therapeutic outcomes and quantifiable behavior changes sometimes occur even though one spouse or family member expresses intense dislike of the therapist and considers the therapy to have been a total failure (for example, a spouse resents a therapist for having set limits on his or her assaultive, violent, and abusive behavior, or a teenager detests the family therapist who has been successful in teaching his parents how to resolve longstanding marital difficulties so that they are finally able to function as a more efficient parental team that can no longer be manipulated by him). Such subjective evaluations can be put in their proper perspective only if they are complemented by more objective measures and behavioral reports that specifically target the problem behaviors for which collateral contacts had been approved.

Unstructured, open-ended, and subjective self reports of client satisfaction and therapeutic outcome certainly have their place in managed mental health care settings, but they should never be the sole source of accountability, especially if no distinction is made between a client's liking his or her therapist and actual behavior change, problem resolution, symptom reduction, and so on.

Unstructured and nonstandardized outsider evaluations of therapeutic progress likewise are subject to observer/evaluator bias. This is especially true if the treating therapist is considered to be an outsider. Early on in the research studies designed to evaluate psychotherapeutic outcome, researchers questioned the validity and reliability of therapists' reports of their own success, of their clients' improvements, and of actual behavior changes (e.g. Bergin & Garfield, 1971; Garfield & Bergin, 1978, 1986; Greenberg & Pinsof, 1986; Gurman & Razin, 1977).

In reality, therefore, it can be argued that the therapist is not an outsider and that therapists' appraisals of their own effectiveness actually should be treated as subjective insiders' evaluations. Like the subjective reports of clients, therapists' reports of psychotherapeutic outcome must be balanced by more objective outcome measures. Training in the use of behavioral rating scales will be helpful for clinicians who work in managed care settings, because such training will enable them to provide case managers and review specialists with more objective evaluations of their work.

One way to improve the validity and reliability of both clients' and therapists' evaluations of clinical outcome is to teach therapists (who then can teach their clients) how to observe, record, track, monitor, and measure actual behavior changes as they occur in response to specific interventions. When behavioral reports such as these are used in conjunction with other reliable and valid measures of the clients' presenting problems (for example, depression, anxiety, stress, anger, guilt, marital satisfaction, spousal intimacy, sexual satisfaction, spousalcohesion, differentiation from family of origin, and family enmeshment) a more comprehensive and dynamic picture of change and clinical effectiveness can emerge. For example, notice the differences between the two client/therapist accounts of collateral therapy presented below:

Example I

Husband: I really liked our therapist. He was warm, caring, sensitive and sincere. He helped us learn how to communicate our feelings to each other and how to listen to each other. I feel less depressed and more hopeful about my marriage now and more satisfied with my wife.

Wife: I thought the counseling went very well. I liked my therapist. He seemed to understand our problems very well. My husband and I get along better now, and we don't fight as much as we did before we went into counseling. My husband seems happier and I feel less nervous.

Therapist: Mr. Jones appears less depressed than he was when I first saw him one year ago. Marital therapy seems to have helped considerably. He and Mrs. Jones appear to be happier and report fewer conflicts in their marriage now.

Example II

Husband: During the first week of baseline data collection, I recorded an average of 35 irrational beliefs per day. These irrational beliefs usually served as triggers for my depression. Now, after ten weeks of cognitive behavioral therapy and assertiveness training, the number of irrational beliefs averages only 2 or 3 per day.

In conjunction with individual therapy, my wife and I began marital therapy. After 8 weeks of marital therapy, which consisted of training in communication, conflict negotiation, and problem solving, serious arguments between me and my wife decreased from an average of 5 or 6 per week to about one a week. In the last two weeks, we have had only one minor disagreement.

Our sexual relationship has also improved as a result of marital/sex therapy. The frequency of our lovemaking has increased from an average of twice a month, during the baseline period, to an average of 2 or 3 times a week.

Wife: After my husband had about 4 weeks of individual therapy, I noticed that he seemed less depressed, and I began to feel less anxious about him and his emotional condition. The first week we began marital therapy, the average number of anxiety producing irrational beliefs I recorded was 9 per day. As of last week, this daily average dropped to 2 or 3 per day.

The frequency of our lovemaking has also gone up since we began sex therapy training. During the baseline period, we had sex only twice a month. Now we have sex an average of 2 or 3 times a week. My husband is much more sexually assertive now than he was when we began sex therapy. Before therapy, he rarely initiated sexual relations. Now he takes the initiative at least once a week.

Therapist: This client was initially seen on 10/1/95 for a diagnostic evaluation. He was diagnosed as suffering from a dysthymic disorder—DSM-IV 300.4. A program of cognitive behavior therapy was begun. This program consisted of a combination of individual and marital treatment. During the initial interview, the client received a score of 50 on the Beck Depression Inventory (Beck, 1978). During the first week of baseline data collection, the client reported an average of 35 irrational beliefs per day using the Irrational Beliefs Test (Jones, 1968). These irrational beliefs were said to serve as triggers for the client's depression.

During the second week of treatment, a cognitive behavior therapy program was begun. The treatments included a combination of intervention—relaxation, "stop think" procedures, cognitive restructuring, and assertiveness training.

A number of the client's irrational beliefs had to do with the client's relationship with his wife and their marriage. Therefore, during the third week of treatment marital/sex therapy was introduced as an adjunct to individual work.

After 9 weeks of combined treatment, the client reported the number of irrational beliefs that typically sparked depression to have dropped to an average of 2 or 3 per day. The client's score on the Beck Depression Inventory at this time was 17.

Cognitive behavioral marital therapy as outlined by Bagarozzi and Anderson (1989) was instituted during the fourth week of treatment. The following instruments were used to assess pretreatment–posttreatment levels of marital distress and dysfunction: Locke–Wallace Marital Adjustment Test (Locke & Wallace, 1959), Spousal Inventory of Desired Changes and Relationship Barriers: SIDCARB (Bagarozzi, 1983), and the Family Adaptability and Cohesion Scales: FACES III (Olson, Portner, & Lavee, 1985).

The couple was taught functional communication skills, conflict negotiation, problem solving, and goal setting. Pretreatment–posttreatment comparison scores are shown below.

PRETREAMENT–POSTTREATMENT COMPARISON SCORES

I. Locke–Wallace Marital Adjustment Test

	Pre	Post
Husband	79	123
Wife	87	132

II. Spousal Inventory of Desired Changes and Relationship Barriers (SIDCARB)

	Pre		Post	
	Husband	Wife	Husband	Wife
Factor I: Dissatisfaction/ Desired Changes	75	70	62	55
Factor II: Internal Barriers to Divorce	65	60	57	55

Factor III: External Barriers
           to Divorce   67   53   60   50

III. Family Adaptability and Cohesion Scales: FACES III

Husband	*Pretreatment*	*Posttreatment*
	Perceived/Ideal	*Perceived/Ideal*
	Chaotically Separated/	Flexibly Connected/
	Flexibly Connected	Flexibly Connected
Wife	*Perceived/Ideal*	*Perceived/Ideal*
	Rigidly Separated/	Flexibly Separated/
	Flexibly Connected	Flexibly Connected

The behavioral reports made by the therapist are very similar to the behavioral self reports and observations made by the client and his spouse. These self reports, coupled with the pretreatment–posttreatment scores obtained on individual measures and marital assessment instruments, provide a much more objective picture of therapeutic changes in the identified patient. The wife's behavioral report of her husband's depression also serves as an outsider's assessment of the identified patient's progress for individual therapy.

Follow-Up Evaluations: Basic Considerations

Follow-up evaluations are essential for determining the degree to which cognitive, affective, and behavioral changes made in therapy are maintained once formal treatment has been discontinued. Administration of the same instruments used in pretreatment assessment and posttreatment outcome evaluation at three-month intervals for a period of one year will provide the therapist and managed mental health care personnel with objective data concerning the long-term effects of treatment. In addition to these standardized instruments, I have developed a brief follow-up questionnaire. This questionnaire is treatment-method specific. Each client is asked to rate core aspects of treatment such as resolution of the presenting problem, symptom modification, and specific behavioral changes. In addition, clients are asked to assess the level of improvement and the maintenance of specific behavioral gains. In treatments where specific skills are taught, clients are asked to rate the degree to which these skills were learned and whether they still use these skills in their everyday lives. The questionnaires for individuals, couples, and families follow.

FOLLOW-UP QUESTIONNAIRE

Individual Treatment

1. If you sought individual psychotherapy for the relief of a specific symptom (e.g., anxiety, depression, guilt feelings, unresolved grief reaction, anger control, low self-esteem, underassertiveness, sexual desire problems, obsessive thoughts, compulsive behaviors, or another specific symptom), please specify the symptom _____ . What degree of improvement did you experience by the end of treatment? Please circle one response:

Slight Improvement				Moderate Improvement			A Great Deal of Improvement		
1	2	3	4	5	6	7	8	9	10

2. How do you rate the level of improvement for this same symptom or behavior *today?* Please circle one response:
   (a) The level of improvement has remained essentially the same.
   (b) The level of improvement has increased.
   (c) The level of improvement has decreased.
   (d) The symptom or behavior has returned.

3. If you did not seek help for a specific symptom or problem behavior, but sought help with interpersonal relationships with friends, relatives, business associates, etc., to what degree had these relationships improved by the end of our work in therapy? Please circle one response:

Slight Improvement				Moderate Improvement			A Great Deal of Improvement		
1	2	3	4	5	6	7	8	9	10

4. As a result of our work in therapy, by the end of therapy how much understanding and insight did you develop into the nature of these problems? Please circle one response:

Little Understanding				Moderate Understanding			A Great Deal of Understanding		
1	2	3	4	5	6	7	8	9	10

5. To what degree have you been able to use this understanding, knowledge, and insight to improve your current interpersonal relationships? Please circle one response:

	A Moderate Amount		A Great Deal
Very Little			
1 2 3	4 5 6 7	8 9	10

Marital/Couple Therapy

6. If you sought help *with a partner* for a marital or relationship problem, to what degree do you think you learned to use the following skills by the end of treatment? Please circle one response for each skill:

	Very Little	A Moderate Amount	A Great Deal
(a) Functional communication	1 2 3	4 5 6 7	8 9 10
(b) Problem solving	1 2 3	4 5 6 7	8 9 10
(c) Conflict negotiation	1 2 3	4 5 6 7	8 9 10
(d) Compromise	1 2 3	4 5 6 7	8 9 10
(e) Empathy (understanding your partner's feelings)	1 2 3	4 5 6 7	8 9 10
(f) Role taking (understanding how your partner perceives and experiences you)	1 2 3	4 5 6 7	8 9 10

7. To what extent do you and your partner use these same skills *today?* Please circle one response for each skill:

	Very Little	A Moderate Amount	A Great Deal
(a) Functional communication	1 2 3	4 5 6 7	8 9 10
(b) Problem solving	1 2 3	4 5 6 7	8 9 10
(c) Conflict negotiation	1 2 3	4 5 6 7	8 9 10
(d) Compromise	1 2 3	4 5 6 7	8 9 10
(e) Empathy (understanding your partner's feelings)	1 2 3	4 5 6 7	8 9 10

(f) Role taking   1   2   3   4   5   6   7   8   9   10
   (understanding
   how your partner
   perceives and
   experiences you)

8. By the end of treatment, how satisfied were you with your partner? Circle one response:

Not at All   Moderately
  Satisfied   Satisfied   Very Satisfied
  1   2   3   4   5   6   7   8   9   10

9. How satisfied are you *today* with your partner? Please circle one response:

Not at All   Moderately
  Satisfied   Satisfied   Very Satisfied
  1   2   3   4   5   6   7   8   9   10

10. By the end of treatment, how satisfied were you with your marriage? Please circle one response:

Not at All   Moderately
  Satisfied   Satisfied   Very Satisfied
  1   2   3   4   5   6   7   8   9   10

11. How satisfied are you *today* with your marriage? Please circle one response:

Not at All   Moderately
  Satisfied   Satisfied   Very Satisfied
  1   2   3   4   5   6   7   8   9   10

Family Therapy

12. If you sought help for a family problem and were seen in conjunction with other family members, to what extent was the problem that brought you into therapy resolved by the end of treatment? Please circle one response:

Slightly   Moderately   Completely
  Resolved   Resolved   Resolved
  1   2   3   4   5   6   7   8   9   10

13. How do you rate the level of improvement for this same problem
    today? Please circle one response:
(a) The level of improvement has remained essentially the same.
(b) The level of improvement has increased.
(c) The level of improvement has decreased.
(d) The problem has returned.

14. To what degree do you think you learned to use the following
    skills by the end of our family work? Please circle one response
    for each skill:

	Very Little			A Moderate Amount				A Great Deal		
(a) Functional communication	1	2	3	4	5	6	7	8	9	10
(b) Problem solving	1	2	3	4	5	6	7	8	9	10
(c) Conflict negotiation	1	2	3	4	5	6	7	8	9	10
(d) Compromise	1	2	3	4	5	6	7	8	9	10
(e) Empathy (understanding the feelings of other family members)	1	2	3	4	5	6	7	8	9	10
(f) Role taking (understanding how other family members perceive and experience you)	1	2	3	4	5	6	7	8	9	10

15. To what extent do you use these same skills *today* in your relation-
    ships with other family members? Please circle one response for
    each skill:

	Very Little			A Moderate Amount				A Great Deal		
(a) Functional communication	1	2	3	4	5	6	7	8	9	10
(b) Problem solving	1	2	3	4	5	6	7	8	9	10
(c) Conflict negotiation	1	2	3	4	5	6	7	8	9	10
(d) Compromise	1	2	3	4	5	6	7	8	9	10
(e) Empathy (understanding the feelings of other family members)	1	2	3	4	5	6	7	8	9	10

(f) Role taking   1   2   3   4   5   6   7   8   9   10
    (understanding
    how other family
    members perceive
    and experience you)

16. By the end of treatment, how satisfied were you with how your family solved problems and functioned as a unit? Please circle one response:

Not at All Satisfied				Moderately Satisfied				Very Satisfied	
1	2	3	4	5	6	7	8	9	10

17. How satisfied are you *today* with how your family solves problems and functions as a unit? Please circle one response:

Not at All Satisfied				Moderately Satisfied				Very Satisfied	
1	2	3	4	5	6	7	8	9	10

Finally, in order to avoid both positive and negative halo effects when evaluating a therapist's clinical skills and the quality of the client–therapist relationship, there are two instruments of proven reliability and validity that can be used, the Relationship Inventory (Barrett-Lennard, 1972) and the Interview Rating Scale (Anderson & Anderson, 1962).

CONCLUSIONS

In this chapter, some ways are outlined that therapists who are members of managed mental health care provider networks can work with case managers and review specialists to provide marital and family therapies to clients where relationship therapies are the treatments of record. When a therapist contracts with a managed mental health care organization, he or she must keep in mind that the focus of intervention is the individual and the goal of treatment is resolution of the presenting problem through brief, short-term therapy. Spouses and other family members are brought into the treatment process to facilitate the identified patient's progress toward his or her treatment goals and to reinforce those treatment gains that have already been accomplished. When assessment of the presenting problem clearly demonstrates that significant others are intimately involved in the identified patient's difficulties, marital and/or family intervention is used to bring about those changes in the system's structures and functioning that the therapist believes will help the identified patient achieve his or her behaviorally defined goal.

The assessment instruments and procedures discussed in this chapter are only a few of the tools that can be used to conduct brief, behavioral, problem-focused marital and family therapies. In an age of increasing medical costs and rising insurance premiums, managed mental health care organizations have stepped in and are attempting to arrest this upward spiral, but cost is not the only factor to be considered when dealing with human pain and suffering. The efficacy of any treatment and the quality of care—that is, professional accountability—must be the primary concern. Only these managed mental health care organizations that can empirically demonstrate their ability to alleviate the emotional pain and suffering of these beneficiaries through the use of short-term therapies that are economically conservative yet clinically sound and effective will survive. Those that cannot will fall by the wayside. Clinicians who are able to conduct effective short-term therapies and who are willing to participate in objective evaluations of their clinical effectiveness should have little difficulty in securing positions on provider panels. I hope that this chapter can serve as a brief orientation for how marriage and family therapists can begin to conceptualize their working relationships with managed mental health care organizations.

REFERENCES

Anderson, R. P., & Anderson, G. V. (1962). Development of an instrument for measuring rapport. In L. Litwack, R. Getson, & G. Saltzman (Eds.), *Research in counseling* (pp. 4–8). Itasco, IL: Peacock.

Bagarozzi, D. A. (1983). Methodological developments in measuring social exchange perceptions in marital dyads (SIDCARB): A new tool for clinical intervention. In D. A. Bagarozzi, A. P. Jurich, & R. W. Jackson (Eds.), *New perspectives in marital and family therapy: Issues in theory, research and practice* (pp. 79–104). New York: Human Sciences Press.

Bagarozzi, D. A. (1985). Dimensions of family evaluation. In L. L'Abate (Ed.), *Handbook of family psychology* (pp. 989–1005). Homewood, IL: Dorsey Press.

Bagarozzi, D. A. (1989). Family diagnostic testing: A neglected area of expertise for the family psychologist. *American Journal of Family Therapy, 17,* 261–274.

Bagarozzi, D. A. (1990). *Intimacy needs survey.* Unpublished instrument. Atlanta: Human Resources Consultants.

Bagarozzi, D. A. (1992). *Pragmatic marital assessment questionnaire.* Unpublished instrument. Atlanta: Human Resources Consultants.

Bateson, G. (1935). Culture, contact and schismogenesis. *Man, 35,* 178–183.

Bateson, G. (1936). *Naven.* Cambridge, England: Cambridge University Press.

Bateson, G. (1972). *Steps to an ecology of the mind.* New York: Ballantine Books.

Beck, A. T. (1979). *Beck depression inventory.* Philadelphia: Center for Cognitive Therapy.

Bergin, A. E., & Garfield, S. L. (Eds.). (1971). Handbook of psychotherapy and behavior change (1st ed.) New York: John Wiley.

Garfield, S. L., & Bergin, A. E. (Eds.). (1978). *Handbook of psychotherapy and behavior change: An empirical analysis* (2nd ed.). New York: Wiley.

Garfield, S. L., & Bergin, A. E. (Eds.). (1986). *Handbook of psychotherapy and behavior change: An empirical analysis* (3rd ed.). New York: Wiley.

Greenberg, L. S., & Pinsof, W. M. (Eds.). (1986). *The psychotherapeutic process: A research handbook.* New York: Guilford.

Gurman, A. S., & Kniskern, D. P. (1981). *Handbook of family therapy.* New York: Brunner/Mazel.

Gurman, A. S., & Razin, A. M. (Eds.). (1977). *Effective psychotherapy: A Handbook of research.* New York: Pergamon.

Haley, J. (1963). Marriage therapy. *Archives of General Psychiatry, 8,* 213–224.

Hovestadt, A. J., Anderson, W. T., Piercy, F. P., Cochran, S. W., & Fine, M. (1985). A family-of-origin scale. *Journal of Marriage and Family Therapy, 15,* 19–27.

Jackson, D. D. (1959). Family interaction, family homeostasis and some implications for conjoint family psychotherapy. In J. Masserman (Ed.), *Individual and family dynamics.* New York: Grune & Stratton.

L'Abate, L., & Bagarozzi, D. A. (1993). *Sourcebook of marriage and family evaluation.* New York: Brunner/Mazel.

Locke, H. J., & Wallace, K. M. (1959). Short marital adjustment and prediction test: Their reliability and validity. *Marriage and Family Living,* 251–255.

Moos, R. H., & Moos, B. S. (1981). *Family environment scale manual.* Palo Alto, CA: Consulting Psychologist Press.

Olson, D. H., Portner, J., & Lavee, Y. (1985). *FACES III.* St. Paul, MN: University of Minnesota.

Sauber, S. R., L'Abate, L., Weeks, G., & Buchanan, W. (1993). *Dictionary of family psychology and family therapy.* CA: Sage.

Stuart, R. B., & Jacobson, N. (1991). *Couples precounseling inventory: Psychometric properties and norms.* Seattle, WA: University of Washington, Center for the Study of Relationships.

Stuart, R. B., & Stuart, F. (1980). *Premarital counseling inventory, family precounseling inventory program and marital precounseling inventory.* Champaign, IL: Research Press.

Watzlawick, P., Beavin, J. H., & Jackson, D. D. (1967). *Pragmatics of human communication.* New York: Norton.

Weiss, R. L., & Birchler, G. R. (1983). *Areas of change questionnaire.* Eugene, OR: University of Oregon.

8

Children's Mental Health Services and Managed Care

WILLIAM L. BUCHANAN, Ph.D.

CHILDHOOD MENTAL DISORDERS AND MANAGED CARE

With the emergence of managed care for mental health services, there is an emphasis to provide services at less cost (Gray, 1991). As such, this usually means providing less service. Most mental health professionals desire to provide high quality service and there lies the dilemma; that is, how to provide high quality service that meets the needs of the patient while at the same time reducing the length of treatment and it's overall cost. Fortunately, many practitioners who work with children, adolescents, and families have been doing this type of therapy long before the advent of managed care (Haley, 1976; Watzlawick, Weakland, & Fisch, 1974).

In general, if all factors were equal, the younger the child, the easier it is to make effective interventions for the child's mental health. As a group, younger children in therapy seem to make quicker changes than adolescents. Of course all factors are not equal, and thus services must be tailor-made to meet the needs of the particular child and family. A truism most practitioners have always known is that the earlier the intervention, the better the outcome. Thus many children who don't receive early mental health services often become adolescents and adults with chronic mental illnesses or addictions. Others find themselves in the criminal justice system. Either way, billions of dollars are drained from the economy annually, not to mention lost productivity, and the unhappiness and grief that is caused. If the managed care industry truly wants to save money, then investing in children's mental health is the place to start. Of course, the practitioner is left in the position of demonstrating, on a case-by-case basis, that the mental health services provided to children are cost effective in resolving the presenting problems.

CHILDHOOD DISORDERS IN NEED OF MENTAL HEALTH SERVICES

Years ago, comprehensive reviews of the literature found support to classify childhood pathology along two dimensions, externalizing disorders and internalizing disorders (Achenbach & Edelbrock, 1978; Quay, 1979). However, since that time, there have been three new versions of the *Diagnostic and Statistical Manual of Mental Disorders* (DSM-III, DSM-III-R, and DSM-IV) by the American Psychiatric Association (APA) (1980, 1987, 1994), all of which used a multiaxial system of diagnosis instead of the externalizing–internalizing dimension. The externalizing–internalizing dimension is still very useful, although it is not comprehensive. For the purposes of providing mental health services in a managed care environment, childhood mental health problems and diagnoses can be classified as fitting into one of four broad categories. Of course these categories are not always discrete and separate. Often, an individual child will have symptoms that overlap these categories. Nevertheless, these four categories seem to be clinically useful. These include externalizing disorders, internalizing disorders, developmental disorders, and physical disorders amenable to psychological inter-ventions.

As mentioned above, childhood psychopathology has previously been classified into one of two categories, externalizing disorders and internalizing disorders (Achenbach & Edelbrock, 1978; Quay, 1979). Clearly, these two dimensions comprise most childhood mental disorders. The externalizing disorders are characterized as behaviors that are under-controlled, impulsive, noncompliant, defiant, socially disruptive, and aggressive. The externalizing disorders are classified in the DSM-IV (APA, 1994) as the attention-deficit and disruptive behavior disorders. These include attention-deficit/hyperactivity disorders, conduct disorders, and oppositional defiant disorder. Other externalizing disorders in the DSM-IV include the substance-related disorders and certain adjustment disorders. Typically, it is not the child who is suffering from his or her externalizing disorder; rather, it is others who suffer such as parents, teachers, peers, and siblings. Externalizing disorders account for the vast majority of child referrals for mental health services (Barkley, 1990).

Internalizing disorders are characterized as behaviors that are over-controlled, inhibited, anxious, withdrawn, avoidant, and depressed. The internalizing disorders are classified in the DSM-IV (APA, 1994) as a variety of disorders, most of which are not unique to childhood, and can be experienced by both children and adults. In DSM-IV, internalizing childhood disorders include the mood disorders, anxiety disorders, somatoform disorders, schizophrenia and other psychotic disorders, and some adjustment disorders. Typically, the child with an internalizing disorder is suffering more from the disorder than other people around him or her.

Developmental disorders are typically disorders with which children are born with and must cope with all of their lives. The developmental disorders are classified in the DSM-IV (APA, 1994) as mental retardation, learning disorders, motor skill disorder, communication disorders, and pervasive developmental disorders. Most developmental disorders are lifelong, although there are some exceptions; for example, new treatments have helped some patients effectively overcome stuttering, a communication disorder (DiLorenzo & Matson, 1987). However, most all other developmental disorders are typically lifelong, but with effective treatment it is possible to increase the quality of life, improve family functioning, and enhance the individual's ability to become an adult who will contribute to society. It should also be noted that an individual with a developmental disorder may simultaneously have an externalizing or internalizing disorder. Perhaps the most common examples include the child with a learning disability and an attention deficit disorder, a mentally retarded individual with an oppositional defiant disorder, and a child with a communication disorder who also has either an anxiety or a depressive disorder.

Using psychological interventions to help children with physical disorders is not new, but often it is not thought of by managed care companies as a type of mental health service. However, there is an abundance of research that clearly indicates that psychological interventions are effective for improving the quality of life, speed of recovery, and prevention of relapse for a variety of physical problems (Routh, 1988). Effective psychological interventions reduce the cost of health care; indeed, the more integrated behavioral care is to the entire health delivery system, the greater the cost offset (Cummings, 1994). Physical disorders that are amenable to psychological interventions include elimination disorders (Walker, Kenning, & Faust-Campanile, 1989), eating disorders (Buchanan & Buchanan, 1992; Foreyt & McGavin, 1989), obesity (Buchanan, 1992; Foreyt & Cousins, 1989), cancer (Stehbens, 1988), asthma (Creer, Harm, & Marion, 1988), diabetes mellitus (Johnson, 1988), failure to thrive (Drotar, 1988), brain injury (Fletcher & Levin, 1988), pain management (Dolgin & Jay, 1989), psychological sequelae of infectious diseases (Peloquin & Davidson, 1988), and chronic disabilities such as spina bifida and hemophilia (Varni & Wallander, 1988), among other physical disorders.

ASSESSMENT OF CHILDHOOD DISORDERS

Effective treatment must be based on an accurate diagnosis and an assessment that evaluates the factors that can be used to clearly identify target symptoms for therapeutic change. No single assessment technique is comprehensive, and comprehensive assessment batteries are not always needed. Therefore, the assessment must be individualized based on the presenting problem, and the circumstances in which the symptoms are produced. Because managed care companies are often reluctant to pay for psychological assessments, the practitioner may have to include an informal assessment as part of the therapy. Described below are various methods of assessment.

Typically, the first contact a practitioner has with a patient is through a telephone conversation. In the case of children and adolescents, the first contact is usually with an adult who is involved with the child or adolescent, most typically the mother. The practitioner is informally assessing the presenting problem and the context in which the problem occurs. After the initial phone contact, the practitioner should have a working definition of the problem, but it would be premature to have a diagnosis at this point. However, a working definition will allow the practitioner to decide who should be at the first interview (mother only, father only, parents only, parents and child, and so on). In general, the more people present during the first interview, the more rapid and more effective the therapy will be (Haley, 1987). However, there are times when it is useful to get background information without the child present. Additionally, parent and teacher checklists should be sent to the parents, and completed and returned by the first session.

During the first interview, the practitioner needs to assess the various contexts that affect the child and look for the contextual factors in which the problem is produced. This will include the family composition, school performance, medical condition, socioeconomic status, race, gender, and social functioning with peers. There is considerable cross-situational variation in children's behavior (Barkley, 1990). Factors that affect a child's behavior include the degree of structure, novelty, or unfamiliarity with the environment; contingencies within the environment; and the nature of what is required of the child in a given environment. Children behave differently in different environments, such as the home, the classroom, and the clinic setting. Consequently, it is important to evaluate the child's behavior in a variety of settings and to find out what behaviors are consistent in each setting and in what settings behavior is different. It is also very important to see first hand the interactions between the child and his or her parents and not to over-rely on the parents' or the child's report alone. During the interview the practitioner will want to get an understanding of the composition of the family, and who is involved in childcare. For example, if a grandparent takes care of the child after school, it will be very useful to have that grandparent routinely involved in the family therapy.

There are a variety of behavioral checklists, filled out by parents and teachers, which are useful in evaluating childhood disorders. Perhaps the most common is the Conners' Parent Rating Scale (Conners, 1973, 1989). Conners' original rating scale contained 91 items. The 48 item revision was published by Goyette, Conners, and Ulrich (1978, 1989). The Conners' Parent Rating Scale-Revised typically takes five to ten minutes to complete. Several problem areas are identified including conduct problems, learning problems, psychosomatic problems, impulsivity-hyperactivity, and anxiety. Each of these problem areas was derived through a factor analysis. Not factorially derived was a separate hyperactivity index, which is one of the more common measures for assessing Attention Deficit Hyperactivity Disorders. Normative data is available for children age three to 17.

Another very commonly used parent completed questionnaire is the Child Behavior Checklist by Achenbach and Edelbrock (1983). The Child Behavior Checklist was designed to assess both problem behaviors and adaptive competencies. Problem behaviors include social withdrawal, depression, immaturity, somatic complaints, sexual problems, hostile withdrawal, and obesity, as well as behavior that is schizoid, aggressive, delinquent, uncommunicative, obsessive-compulsive, hyperactive, and cruel. Adaptive competencies include such things as sports, friendships, clubs, and school. The Child Behavior Checklist consists of 138 items and usually requires 20 to 25 minutes for a parent to complete. Norms are available from four to 16 years of age. The checklist yields two second-order factors labeled externalizing and internalizing. The externalizing factors include undercontrol, socially disruptive conduct, and behavioral problems. The internalizing factors include over-control and inhibited, or anxious and withdrawn behaviors.

Quay developed the original Behavior Problem Checklist (1975). The checklist was later amended and entitled the Revised Behavior Problem Checklist (Quay & Peterson, 1983, 1984, 1987). The Revised Behavior Problem Checklist consists of 89 problem behaviors. Typically, it takes 15 to 20 minutes to complete. The Revised Behavior Problem Checklist derives six factors based on factor analysis. The various factors include conduct disorder, socialized aggression, attention problems (immaturity, anxiety), withdrawal, psychotic behavior, and motor excess. The first three factors tap externalizing behavior problems, the fourth factor taps internalizing problems, and the last two factors assess specific problems. Norms are available between the ages of five and 17.

The above three checklists designed for parents also have versions to be completed by teachers. Behavioral checklists are a quick and useful way to gather samples of the child's behavior in a variety of situations, specifically the home and the school. Because these are the two most important environments for children, these are the contexts in which the child's behavior must be assessed.

Most mental health treatment of children will involve the use of parent and teacher checklists and clinical interviews with the child, the family, and other important people in the child's life. Exactly who fills out the questionnaires and who attends the first session will depend on the nature of the family composition. However, there are times when a more extensive evaluation needs to be made. This is especially true when there is a developmental disorder. When there is a suspicion of a developmental disorder, certainly intellectual, academic, and neuro-psychological measures should be used in a battery of tests tailored to assess the question posed regarding the child. If the disorder is clearly an internalizing disorder, then more personality measures may also be useful. For example, if there is a question that a thought disorder may be present, then use of the Rorschach technique, using Exner's Comprehensive System (Exner, 1993), could save a great deal of valuable time in correctly diagnosing the thought disorder and prescribing the appropriate treatment for it. However, there are other times, particularly when there is an externalizing disorder, when behavioral checklists and clinical interviews will be sufficient to assess the child adequately. No single battery of tests is likely to be effective in assessing every child or adolescent, but clearly an adequate assessment is required to successfully treat children. The main point, particularly in a managed care environ-ment, is that the assessment must be very specific in order to evaluate the particular problem of a particular child at a particular time in a particular family situation.

Continuous Performance Tests (CPTs) have been around for many years, but have been used primarily by researchers and not by clinicians.

With the advent of the microcomputer, Continuous Performance Tests have become affordable and thus more common in clinical practice. The three most popular CPTs are the Gordon Diagnostic System (GDS) (Gordon, 1983), the Test of Variables of Attention (TOVA) (Dupuy & Greenberg, 1993), and the Conners' Continuous Performance Test (Conners, 1992). All three are excellent measures of attention, concentration, and impulsivity. Specifically, CPTs are of long enough duration to assess sustained attention (for example, the TOVA is 22 minutes long and the Conners' CPT is 14 minutes long). As such, these tests are extremely useful in diagnosing Attention Deficit Hyperactivity Disorder (ADHD).

Continuous Performance Tests are very useful in measuring improved performance secondary to medicine. The author uses a CPT to help titrate medication for physicians. Because the task is very simple, children's performance on CPTs tend to not improve due to practice. Thus, CPTs can be repeated before and after the administration of medication, even on the same day. In this way, a comparison can be made of the child's attention and concentration off medication versus on medication. Different dosages can be tried on different days, and the effects can be assessed with a CPT. In this way, the optimum dosage can be determined by objective data, instead of general impressions, which is usually the case with stimulants.

To standardize the testing procedure, testing using a CPT occurs 90 minutes after the medication was taken. This is typically enough time for stimulant medications such as Ritalin to begin to work. For example, it would not be a fair comparison to administer a CPT four hours after a child was given 10 mgs. of Ritalin, and then, at a later date, administer a CPT one hour after a child was given 15 mgs. of Ritalin. However, it is useful to compare the child's performance on 10 mgs. versus 15 mgs. of Ritalin when both administrations of the CPT were given 90 minutes after medication was taken.

Psychological assessment should not be a one time occurrence in treating a patient. Depending on the test, the test may be repeated several times over the course of treatment to measure progress in psychotherapy. For example, the Beck Depression Inventory and the Beck Anxiety Inventory can be given to adolescents at the beginning of each and every psychotherapy session. The Continuous Performance Tests mentioned above (the GDS, the TOVA, and the Conners' CPT) may be given each time a stimulant medication is altered or if there is some other reason to suspect that the child's dosage of medication is inadequate. Similarly, any of the behavior checklists can be given at random intervals to evaluate the progress of treatment. Thus psychological assessment is not only useful in correctly diagnosing the problem and tailoring the particular intervention for the particular person and situation, but it can also be used to assess outcome and progress over the course of treatment.

TARGETING SYMPTOMS FOR CHANGE

The goal of treatment must be specifically determined based on the specific disorder the child has and the circumstances of the child's life. For example, for most externalizing and internalizing disorders, the goal is to eliminate the presenting symptom. However, with developmental disorders, this is not the goal. Developmental disorders are generally lifelong, and thus their elimination is not possible. What is possible is to improve the quality of life for both the patient and his or her family. This also may be true for many of the physical disorders for which psychological treatment is helpful, for example, diabetes, high blood pressure, head injury, and so on. Thus, the goal is not the elimination of the disorder, but rather to help the patient and his or her family learn to cope with the disorder, improve their quality of life, and prevent relapse in the future.

In general, target behaviors selected for intervention are typically associated with one of three contexts: the family, the school, and social interactions with peers. This is typically the order in which interventions are made because there is greater control of contingencies when working with the parents, less control of contingencies in the school setting, and little or no control of contingencies in peer interactions. When a therapist is working in a managed care environment, getting results quickly is desirable, and working with the family first will help facilitate this goal.

In general, behaviors need to be conceptualized along one of three dimensions in order to bring about clear treatment goals and measured outcome. The three dimensions are frequency, duration, and intensity. When behavior is conceptualized as being discrete and measurable, a measurement can be made of how often it occurs (frequency), how long it lasts (duration), and how bothersome the behavior is to the child or others (intensity). In general, the goal of the treatment of externalizing disorders will be to decrease frequency, decrease duration, and/or decrease intensity. However, with internalizing disorders the goal might be to increase positive interactions with others (i.e., decrease withdrawal), and to increase the length of time the child interacts positively. Thus, for the three dimensions of frequency, duration, or intensity, the goal will be to either increase or decrease the behavior along one or more of these dimensions.

SERVICE DELIVERY MODELS AND MANAGED CARE

In a managed care environment, the delivery of services to children must be multilevel to produce change in multiple contexts and systems (Imber-Black, 1988). These multiple systems include the individual child, the family, peers, the school, the community, the courts, and the medical systems.

In addition to taking a multisystemic approach and working with all systems that might have some control of the contingencies in a variety of settings, child practitioners must tailor individual treatments to meet the specific target symptoms of a particular patient at a particular time in a particular context. Several excellent texts have been written in the last few years that give state-of-the-art assessment and treatment strategies for particular childhood problems. Walker and Roberts (1992) edited the second edition of the *Handbook of Clinical Child Psychology*. This handbook is very extensive and provides chapters on a variety of specific disorders including fear and anxiety, sleep disorders, tics, psychosomatic problems, depression, delinquent behavior, neurotic disorders, autism, toileting problems, attention deficit hyperactivity disorder, sexual problems, eating problems, mental retardation, school problems, learning disabilities, and language problems. Kratochwill and Morris (1991) have edited a similar text with ten chapters on specific intervention strategies for specific behavior disorders. Ammerman, Last, and Hersen (1993) edited the *Handbook of Prescriptive Treatments for Children and Adolescents*. Their book provides a summary of effective treatments derived from empirical outcome research. There are chapters for the treatment of 18 specific disorders and each chapter describes the disorder, it's diagnosis and assessment, and offers an overview of treatment options tailored for the particular problem. The practitioner has many resources available for keeping up-to-date on the most effective and efficient methods of treatments for childhood problems. In a managed care environment, documentation of providing effective treatment that meets current standards of care is mandatory.

All effective mental health treatment of children must include the family. Family therapy is a particularly effective approach, especially in a managed care environment. Historically, family therapy using strategic (Haley, 1976; Madanes, 1981; Watzlawick, Weakland, & Fisch, 1974) and structural (Minuchin, 1974; Minuchin & Fishman, 1981) approaches are very symptom focused, have clear goals for treatment, and are designed to produce specific changes in a brief period of time. Many skilled practitioners who do not consider themselves family therapists nevertheless work with families for specific problems and are able to document positive treatment outcomes through empirical research (Barkley, 1987;

Forehand & McMahon, 1981; Patterson, 1968, 1971). Regardless of a practitioner's orientation to psychotherapy, specific behavioral interventions that are effective for a variety of childhood problems should be taught to the family and the primary caretakers. These include the use of time out, contingency management, and the use of social reinforcers.

THE PRACTITIONER AS TREATMENT TEAM COORDINATOR

Not withstanding the discipline in which a practitioner was trained, the practitioner who works effectively with children must understand how to work with various systems. Taking a multisystems perspective (Imber-Black, 1988), practitioners can help produce therapeutic change by coordinating efforts between various systems, including the family, school, court, and medical system. Thus, much of the treatment for a child with a particular mental health problem will likely be focused on working with people other than the patient him- or herself; that is, much of the practitioner's time will be focused on coordinating efforts to produce multisystemic change. The advantages to this approach are not only much faster results (at a reduced cost), but also longer lasting results because the contingencies that maintain a given behavior will be altered in many contexts. Thus the effective child mental health practitioner must work as the treatment team coordinator, making sure that the various systems are working in concert with each other to resolve the presenting problems in a variety of contexts.

For example, when working with a child who has ADHD, the child practitioner will work with the family and teach parenting skills, work with the teachers to implement a behavioral or academic program in the school, and make sure the parents and the school personnel communicate clearly with one another. Additionally, the child practitioner will communicate with the pediatrician to evaluate the effectiveness of stimulant medication. In this example, the family, school, and medical systems were coordinated by the child practitioner. By having all the systems work together in a coordinated fashion, the presenting problem will likely be resolved and maintenance will be increased. It should also be noted that coordinating these various systems to produce effective therapeutic change in the child often occurs without the child actually being present in the practitioners' office.

INDIVIDUAL CHILD PSYCHOTHERAPY

Historically, most individual child psychotherapy has been psychodynamic and has had little involvement with the parents (for example,

Gardner, 1986). Furthermore, a great deal of individual child psychotherapy has been play therapy (Schaefer, 1979). However, more recently individual child therapy has become more cognitive-behavioral in nature (Kendall, 1991). Kendall provides chapters about using cognitive-behavioral therapy for children with internalizing disorders, externalizing disorders, developmental disorders, and chronic illnesses. Cognitive behavioral interventions for children have been explicitly guided by theory. For example, Meichenbaum and Goodman (1971) cited the work of several Russian psychologists, such as Vygotsky and Luria, proposing that in normal development children acquire self-regulated behavior through the internalization of guided speech. Specifically, adult verbal demands initially direct the young child's behavior. Over time, such directions eventually become internalized and covert, which facilitates self-control.

Many inattentive and impulsive children fail to follow the normal progression through which self-guiding private speech regulates their cognition and behavior. Meichenbaum and Goodman's (1971) intervention strategy is to explicitly instruct children to "talk to themselves" in order to slow down, approach a task logically, analyze its components, mediate careful performance, and self-reward. Kendall and Braswell (1985) wrote a book based on this approach entitled *Cognitive-Behavioral Therapy for Impulsive Children*. In the back of the book is a treatment manual for developing self-control in children. Individual psychotherapy with children has become much more cognitive-behavioral than psychodynamic, focused more on self-control and other behavioral skills, than on gaining insight or resolving intrapsychic conflicts.

FAMILY GROUP THERAPY

Conducting group therapies with families is a very efficient method of therapy. This is especially helpful in teaching parenting skills. There are several structured parenting programs on the market that can be used effectively to improve parenting skills. These programs include *STEP—Systematic Training for Effective Parenting* (Dinkmeyer & McKay, 1976) and *Active Parenting* (Popkin, 1983, 1990, 1993). Other family group therapies focus on a variety of different problems; there are family group therapies for dealing with divorce, remarriage, death of a parent, death of a child, drug addiction in a parent, and drug addiction in child, just to name a few. Whenever there are a few families suffering from the same type of issue, combining them in group therapy may be an efficient and effective intervention.

A word of caution is needed here. There is a huge difference between an educational class and group therapy. For example, in a parenting class, the leader is typically a parent or teacher who organizes the class, plays an audio or videotape, and then leads a structured discussion with exercises based on a course outline. Group therapy is led by a licensed mental health professional who may or may not play an audio or video-tape, and also leads a discussion. The difference is that the discussion would be more focused on directly applying the principles learned for the particular family, so that the principles are tailored to meet the specific needs of each family. Additionally, in group therapy for families, there is professional help present to deal with the painful experiences the families were having that led them to the group in the first place. Typically, participants in parenting classes are more superficial with each other than in group therapy, and the information learned is more likely to be intellectual rather than a behavioral skill that is readily applied at home. A skilled group therapist will facilitate more personal interactions and provide role playing opportunities with extensive feed-back, from both the therapist and other participants. Thus, group ther-apy participants are much more likely to learn behavioral skills that then can be applied at home to produce changes in family functioning. Parenting classes are helpful for well-functioning families who want to learn more about parenting; however, families who have a child with a mental disorder typically require therapy in order to effectively apply the principles learned.

CHILD GROUP THERAPY

Group therapy has shown some promise in working with children. Typically, group therapies with children are structured such that chil-dren are grouped with peers of approximately the same age. Typically the children are grouped within one or two academic grades of each other. Thus the successful group therapy may have second and third graders together, but is unlikely to be successful if it includes children from first grade through fourth grade. Although this is not always the case, the practitioner needs to be sensitive to developmental issues, particularly with younger children. Five simple divisions, which need to be evaluated depending on the particular individuals involved in the group, include younger elementary school students, older elementary school students, middle school students, younger high school students, and older high school students. Of course, some children will be placed in a group not because of their age or grade placement but because of their maturity level. Group therapies with children also need to be problem specific so that children are dealing with the same types of issues. Different topics for group therapy include divorce adjustment, death of a parent, social skills training, having a parent with alcohol or drug dependence, anxiety disorders, groups for children with self-control problems, and anger control.

Perhaps the most helpful group therapy for the largest number of children is group therapy that teaches social skills. Children who do not develop adequate social skills are at much higher risk for developing mental disorders later in life. Thus having a deficit in social skills does not in and of itself constitute a DSM-IV diagnosis, but it appears to be the foundation for many mental disorders. Social skills training has a wide applicability to a variety of disorders. Depressed children, children with anxiety, children with Attention Deficit Disorder, and children with development disabilities can show considerable improvement in their behavior as they develop competency in social skills.

Most often, effective group therapies with children will be specific and time limited. A specific theme will be developed (for example, adjusting to parental divorce) and, as already mentioned, a specific age group will be established. Children typically need to be interviewed individually prior to starting the group to make sure that they are appropriate for the group therapy and that the group therapy is appropriate for the child. The goals of the group therapy must match the child's individual treatment goals.

PSYCHOPHARMACOLOGY AND CHILDHOOD DISORDERS

Clearly, most parents view psychopharmacology as an undesirable treatment for their child. Furthermore, most psychologists, social workers, marriage and family practitioners, and professional counselors also view medication for the treatment of a mental disorder in children as undesirable, but, at times, necessary. Most practitioners prefer to intervene through the use of psychotherapy and family therapy prior to initiating medical intervention. However, some disorders clearly need medication as an integral part of treatment.

It should be clearly stated, however, that medication should never be the primary intervention for a child's mental disorder and that other types of psychological treatment should always be the primary focus of therapy. It is the author's belief that treating a child's mental disorder through medication alone is unethical. Many parents, for example, hope that Ritalin alone will be enough to treat their child who has Attention Deficit Hyperactivity Disorder. Nothing could be further from the truth. The family who has a child with Attention Deficit Hyperactivity

Disorder needs increased structure, routine, and consistency in both the school and the home environments. This is not accomplished by medication alone. Thus family therapy, which focuses on structuring the home environment to bring healing to the child and his or her family, needs to be the primary focus of treatment. At best, medication should be considered an adjunct to treatment and should not be considered the primary treatment for a child with a mental disorder. However, medication clearly is needed for many children with mental disorders. For example, children with a psychotic disorder definitely need an antipsychotic, children with an Attention Deficit Hyperactive Disorder usually need a stimulant medication, and children with an accurately diagnosed bipolar disorder will need Lithium or an alternative to Lithium. To deprive such a child of medication is tantamount to depriving a diabetic child of insulin. For these children medication is a necessity, and to withhold medication from a child who truly needs it is unethical. Parents and practitioners need not get trapped into the either/or argument, but rather should see the issue of treating children with mental disorders as a both/and proposition. For the above-named disorders (psychosis, bipolar disorder, ADHD), to ask if one should treat children with these disorders by *either* psychotherapy *or* medication is tantamount to asking if maintaining an automobile requires the owner *either* to make sure the car has gas *or* to make sure the oil is changed regularly. Clearly, what is needed is to do *both*.

A potential conflict exists between the desires of the parents and the managed care company. Typically, parents do not want their children to be medicated, whereas most managed care companies want the quickest results, and medication may help. Psychologists are often caught in the middle between wanting to have enough time to adequately process this issue with the parents and knowing that the managed care company does not want to pay for any more treatments until the child is on medication. Clearly, prescribing the medication is inadequate if the parents refuse to give it to their children. Managed care companies need to allow adequate time for the practitioner to process with the parents the child's need to take medication. Unless this happens, there will be noncompliance, which will delay adequate treatment and thus increase the cost of treatment to the managed care company.

For other disorders, particularly anxiety disorders and to a lesser extent depressive disorders, the practitioner should be very careful before referring the child for medical intervention. Phenothiazines such as Xanax can become very addictive and it is not advised to have a child on Xanax or any of the Phenothiazines except under extreme circumstances. Anxiety disorders in particular can be handled much better through psychotherapy than through medication. Likewise, children with depressive disorders will very seldom need medication. Psychotherapy and family therapy, by and large, will adequately treat depression in children. The exception to this is the child with a bipolar disorder, a form of depression, who will very likely need Lithium or some other antidepressant.

The childhood disorders that will require medication in most cases are Attention Deficit Hyperactivity Disorder, Tourette's disorder, childhood psychosis, and bipolar disorder. There are occasions where increased structure, routine, and consistency, improved parenting skills, and psychotherapy are effective in treating these disorders, but in most cases medication will be a very useful adjunct to treatment. Depression is a childhood disorder that most typically will *not* require medication, although in a some cases, medication also may be a useful adjunct to therapy. In other cases, it is ill advised to use medication. This would be true for anxiety disorders with children, mental retardation, learning disabilities, and general family problems. This is not to say that the person who has mental retardation should not be on medication, but it is to say that no medication should be prescribed merely because a person is mentally retarded. Rather, if any medication is prescribed at all, it should be for some other problem, not for the mental retardation in and of itself.

HOSPITALIZATION

Hospitalizing adolescents for mental disorders, along with alcohol and drug abuse treatment, has become one of the most expensive problems in mental health treatment. Clearly the system has been abused in the past, when hospitals would admit a patient because he or she had good insurance coverage, not because he or she truly needed inpatient treatment. This problem became so rampant in Texas that a statewide investigation took place in all Texas psychiatric hospitals. Additionally, in the 1980s hospitals discovered that psychiatric hospitals were exempted from dealing with DRGs (Diagnostically Related Groups). As a result, between 1986 and 1990 the number of psychiatric hospitals in the United States doubled. Clearly a profit bonanza occurred for hospital corporations at the expense of the insurance companies and more importantly, at the expense of the consumer (Cummings, 1995).

As a result of the abuses of the late 1980s and early 1990s, managed care companies have been especially diligent in trying to decrease the utilization of hospitals, not only for the treatment of adolescents but for all people receiving mental health treatment. Clearly there was much fraud and abuse in the hospitalization arena, which unfortunately is making practitioners in the outpatient arena suffer. Nevertheless, it is a reality that must be dealt with.

Despite the fraud and abuse of the 1980s in regard to adolescent hospitalization, there still is a need for hospitalization for some children and some adolescents. The need for hospitalization typically occurs for two reasons, crisis intervention and the treatment of severe mental disorders.

In regard to crisis intervention, hospitals may play a very useful part in treating a child or an adolescent with a mental disorder because it has the resources to provide the logical and natural consequences of the child's behavior, but without involving the legal system. Crisis intervention hospitalization should be short term, typically less than 10 days. At the end of the hospitalization, the child should return to the family, or to a relative in the extended family, a residential school, or another treatment (nonhospital) setting. There are also a certain percentage of children who will need intensive or recurrent hospitalization over the course of childhood and adolescence because he or she suffers from a severe mental disorder.

The percentage of children seen in the outpatient treatment who will need hospitalization is probably less than two percent, and thus will be the distinct minority of cases in the practitioner's office. However, hospitalization needs to remain a viable option for families when the child is: a) psychotic, b) suicidal, c) homicidal, d) abusing alcohol or drugs, or e) behaviorally out of control, or when f) other treatment programs have not been successful in altering the presenting symptoms. Although adolescent inpatient hospitalization has been abused, one should not "throw the baby out with the bath water" and deny all hospitalization. It is true that the vast majority of adolescents and children can be treated on an outpatient basis without hospitalization; however, those children who truly need it should be able to get inpatient treatment services.

ALTERNATIVES TO HOSPITALIZATION

When the child needs to live outside the home for a period of time, alternatives to hospitalization ought to be considered. Reasons for a child needing to live outside the home include alcohol and drug addiction, a single parent who has no control over an acting-out adolescent, behavior problems secondary to mental retardation, an attachment disorder, or some other difficulty in the child developing adequate self-control. Alternatives to hospitalization include intensive outpatient treatment programs, partial hospitalization programs, residential treatment facilities, and therapeutic foster homes.

Historically, insurance companies have paid for either weekly outpatient psychotherapy or inpatient hospitalization. Over the last 20 years, insurance companies typically have paid for inpatient hospitalization at a higher rate than outpatient services. For years, because of these two policies, parents were faced with trying to get treatment for their children on an outpatient basis with only 50% of the fees covered by insurance or having the patient in the hospital with virtually 100% of the fees paid by insurance. Many parents, faced with these alternatives, chose hospitalization, not because it was the best treatment but because it was the only treatment they could afford. Although this has changed to some degree, managed care companies have been slow to pay for alternative treatment programs. If the goal is to provide mental health services at the lowest possible cost, then managed care companies will need to consider paying for other alternative treatment programs, something in between traditional outpatient and traditional inpatient treatment. A great deal of money could be saved by paying for intensive outpatient treatment programs (2 to 20 hours of treatment a week), or partial hospitalization programs (20 to 40 hours of treatment a week) instead of hospitalization (24 hours a day). Because insurance companies historically have paid for either one hour of therapy a week or inpatient hospitalization, they have refused to pay for any treatment that was in between. Clearly this is penny wise but pound foolish. Not only have the insurance companies' own policies driven up the cost of health care, but also people have been denied less disruptive and intrusive treatments because of these policies.

A variety of alternatives to hospitalization can be found throughout the country. Such programs include therapeutic outdoor wilderness programs, therapeutic foster homes, and intensive outpatient programs. The advantage of having intensive outpatient programs is that the program can be designed specifically for each child's particular problem. Most hospitalization programs are general psychiatric programs divided along three lines: inpatient adult programs, inpatient adolescent programs, and inpatient adult alcohol and drug abuse psychiatric programs. The advantage of intensive outpatient and partial hospitalization programs is that the program can be designed specifically for the individual. For example, intensive outpatient programs and partial hospitalization programs have been designed for the following: eating disorders for adults, eating disorders for adolescents, adults with depression, adults with anxiety, children with Attention Deficit Hyperactivity Disorder, children with reactive attachment disorders, adults with bipolar disorder, adults with schizophrenia, adults with mental retardation, children with mental retardation, adolescents with substance abuse problems, and so on. Thus the advantages of intensive outpatient and partial hospitalization programs are that the patient's treatment can be tailored made, providing better treatment, and it is less expensive than hospitalization.

A variety of residential treatment programs exists but historically have been denied reimbursement by insurance companies. Accreditation by the Joint Commission of Accreditation of Health Care Organizations (JCAHO) has been used by some insurance companies to determine the program's eligibility for reimbursement. However, many such programs not accredited by JCAHO provide quality services through these alternative programs. Such programs include independent partial hospitalization programs not associated with an inpatient hospital, intensive outpatient programs, therapeutic foster homes, outdoor therapeutic programs, and other forms of residential treatment. Therapeutic outdoor programs have been shown over the years to be extremely effective, although the average length of stay is between one and three years. Such alternatives need to be available to families and to children because it is clear that treating children at a younger age will save a great deal of money over the course of lifetime. The advantage to a managed care company is that some of these programs cost as little as $100 to $300 a day, which is much less than $800 to $1500 a day most adolescent hospitals were charging a few years ago.

PARENT AND TEACHER CONSULTATION

Sometimes the most effective therapy is not with the child but is to consult with the parents or teacher without the child being present. Some insurance companies have refused to pay a practitioner unless the child was present in session. It is true that in physical medicine the patient must be present to receive the treatment. What seems logical to a business person ("How can people receive treatment if they are not present?") is not necessarily true in mental health treatment, especially with children. Often, the most effective, quickest, and least expensive treatment is *not* to have the child present, but to meet with the parents or teachers instead. The goal is to teach the parents or teachers therapeutic interventions to apply in the home or school. Such interventions may include the dry bed procedure (Azrin, Sneed, & Foxx, 1974), a time-out procedure (Green, Budd, Johnson, Larg, Pinkston, & Rudd, 1976), designing a token economy to use in the home or school (Ayllon & Azrin, 1968), or creating a list of chores and responsibilities that the child or adolescent needs to take care of both daily and weekly.

For example, the author takes three weeks (three one-hour sessions) to teach parents a very specific form of time out (see Figure 8-1). Although time out can be discussed in a few minutes, the author has the parents memorize the procedure to the point where they can recite it flawlessly, and then practice the procedure to the point of mastery (the practitioner plays the part of the child, and the parents must effectively send the practitioner to time out). The parents also learn

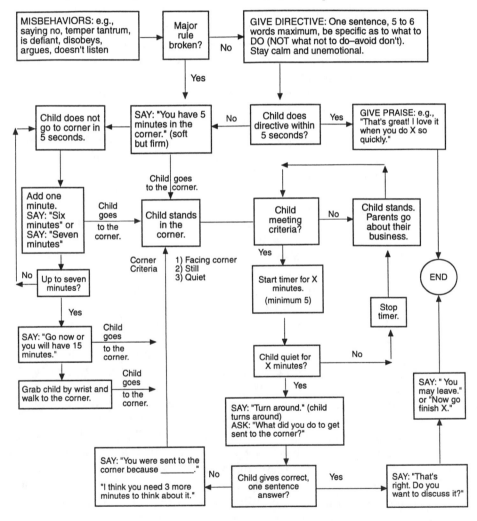

FIGURE 8-1

Time-Out Flowchart for the School-Age Child.

and practice the nonverbal aspects of effectively implementing the intervention, such as body language, tone of voice, timing, rhythm, and so on. This is rehearsed over and over again until the parents are adept at implementing the intervention. At this point, the practitioner has the parents practice handling the child being oppositional at every step in the procedure, thereby teaching them how to handle a variety of unexpected twists and turns. To develop mastery of the intervention, it is quicker and more efficient if the children are *not* present while the parents learn and practice the intervention. Of course, once the parent has mastered the intervention the practitioner uses the next session to teach time out to the child, and for the parents and child to practice it in session.

Other times, parent consultation is very helpful in providing information to them about their child. Telling parents that their child has mental retardation, a severe learning disability, or a developmental disorder is best done with the parents and the doctor alone, without the child present, and without other parents (as in a group therapy). The practitioner needs to be able to answer all of the parents' questions, and to deal with their emotional reactions. In such situations, it is inappropriate to have the child present.

Systems-oriented practitioners also understand how conflict in a marriage can at times create behavioral problems in children. The opposite is also true, behavioral problems in a child can create a great deal of marital disagreement and strife. Either way, the child's behavioral and emotional problems will likely continue until the parents can agree upon a way to deal with the child. The best behavioral intervention is likely to fail miserably if the parents are divided. For example, many families show a very divisive difference in what they think the child needs: one parent insists that the child needs more love, understanding and compassion; the other parent insists the child needs more firmness, discipline, and control. Any intervention will fail if the parents are divided in this manner. Therefore before an intervention is implemented, the practitioner must get the parents more united. Often an intervention needs to be somewhere in the middle so that both parents are right, the child needs *both* more love and understanding *and* the child needs more firmness, discipline, and control. The task of the practitioner is to persuade the parents that the intervention will allow both things to happen. Needless to say, the practitioner will be most effective in this effort by talking to the parents without the children present. This approach also teaches proper boundaries in the family; that there are times when the parents need to talk and make decisions without the children present.

FAMILY EDUCATION AND SUPPORT GROUPS

Several interventions that have not been traditionally considered psycho-therapy are nevertheless very useful in the treatment of mental disorders in children. Such is the case of family education and enrichment, which will include parent education programs. Parenting and family enrich-ment can be facilitated through providing parents with education regard-ing parenting and family and marital dynamics. Additionally, parent support groups that deal with specific mental disorders (for example, Attention Deficit Hyperactivity Disorder, attachment disorders, drug abuse, alcohol abuse, mental retardation, divorce adjustment, coping with sexual abuse, coping with physical abuse, and so on) are extremely helpful in reducing stress in a family, improving family functioning, and diminishing the mental disorder within the child. Thus, these alternatives need to be available to parents and are very efficient in treating the child's disorder and decreasing long-term difficulties, thus reducing mental health costs over the course of several years.

There are several national support groups that have local chapters throughout the country. Perhaps two of the oldest are Alanon and Ala-teen, two support groups for spouses and children of alcoholics. A newer, but rapidly growing support group is CHADD, the association for Chil-dren and Adults with Attention Deficit Disorder. Other support groups include helping patients and their families who suffer from Tourette's syndrome, mental retardation, severe mental illness such as bipolar disor-der and schizophrenia, and learning disabilities, among others.

Support groups offer information regarding the disorder, how the dis-order affects the family, what to expect throughout the life of the individ-ual, and, perhaps most importantly, they offer a forum for families to hear how other families have dealt with the problem. It is very comforting for families to know others have struggled with the same problems; it reduces their feelings of being alone and different from others.

In general, families should be informed of the existence of such groups and encouraged to attend them. Although such groups should not be considered a substitute for therapy, they are a very good adjunct to therapy and fit the managed care philosophy.

COMPREHENSIVE SERVICES IN A MANAGED CARE ENVIRONMENT: THE EXAMPLE OF THE TREATMENT OF ATTENTION DEFICIT/HYPERACTIVITY DISORDER (ADHD)

The treatment of ADHD is an excellent example of efficient, compre-hensive and cost-effective treatment of a childhood mental disorder.

The model proposed here is useful not only in treating ADHD but several other disorders as well (for example, mental retardation, drug abuse, attachment disorders, children of divorce, etc.). An approach that is very effective is the Family Psychology model (L'Abate, 1983; Sauber, L'Abate, Weeks, & Buchanan, 1993), which is similar to the family medicine model, with the idea that both family medicine and family psychology treats an individual over the life span. Thus, in family medicine a family practitioner will follow the health care of infants, children, adolescents, adults, and the elderly. The family psychology approach is very similar in that treatment does not terminate as it does in psychodynamic psychotherapy. Instead, there is an open door approach to families over the course of the family life cycle. Thus using a family psychology model, a child may be treated for a specific difficulty at one point in his or her life, and later return to the practitioner as other twists and turns occur in his or her life. Thus the patient may have brief, intermittent therapy throughout the life cycle (Cummings, 1991, Cummings & Sayama, 1995).

Applying this approach to the treatment of ADHD, the author initially treats families on a short-term basis, typically six to eight sessions. The treatment usually includes parent training, family therapy, and school consultation. In the treatment of ADHD, this is a very good start. However, since ADHD is like a developmental disorder in that symptoms are not cured but must be managed, treatment will likely need to occur over the course of a life span. This does not mean weekly psychotherapy, but it does mean that the family should have access to the practitioner over the course of the life span.

During the first six to eight sessions of therapy for a child who has ADHD, very specific interventions are instituted. The first session should be a thorough evaluation to diagnose if the child really has ADHD. Often parents, teachers, or pediatricians will make the diagnosis of Attention Deficit Hyperactivity Disorder, but this does not mean that their diagnosis is accurate. Children are often labeled ADHD inappropriately. Attention Deficit Hyperactivity Disorder is a neurological disorder that child psychologists who have training in neuropsychology are best able to evaluate; parents, teachers, and physicians can be terribly inaccurate in making this diagnosis. Indeed, it is inappropriate, and in most states illegal, for parents and teachers to diagnose a mental disorder; for parents or teachers to do so is to practice medicine and psychology without a license. However, just because someone has a license doesn't mean he or she is competent to accurately make the diagnosis. Physicians, social workers, marriage and family therapists, and counselors also are often inaccurate in making this diagnosis. This is because there can be several reasons a child is inattentive, impulsive, and/or hyperactive. For example, depressed or anxious children often display these symptoms. Making a differential diagnosis is always the place to start, and this needs to be done by a properly trained professional, preferably a clinical child psychologist.

Once the diagnosis of ADHD has been made accurately, the most efficient, helpful, and pragmatic approach is to train the parents to increase structure, routine, and consistency in the home and school environments. An important component of this is to teach the parents how to give directives so that children are most likely to comply. A handout given to parents to assist in their skill development is presented in Table 8-1.

Parents need to follow basic rules when giving directives. This includes: a) making a statement as opposed to asking a question, b) making the statement a maximum five or six words, c) telling the child what to do as opposed to what not to do, and d) staying calm and unemotional.

Children with ADHD (and all children for that matter) need to have very clear and precise instructions as to how they should behave. Therefore, parents need to give directives instead of asking questions. Often, parents in an attempt to be polite, kind, or soft hearted, will ask a question as opposed to making a direct statement. Thus, instead of a parent saying, "Go get ready for bed," he or she will ask, "Don't you think it is getting late?" This is not helpful in disciplining children. Parents need to state very clearly, without asking a question, what it is they expect the child to do. A mistake that parents often make is that instead of making a short and precise statement about what they want, they ask questions, make roundabout statements of what they want, or give a lot of detail by explaining why a behavior is not good for the child. Such a tactic is a mistake with children who have ADHD, or for that matter any child.

The practitioner spends three sessions teaching the parents how to give directives correctly and how to implement time out. This will include behavioral rehearsal (role play) in which the parents practice giving directives and sending the child to the corner in session, with the practitioner playing the role of the child. Once the parents have mastered the technique in session, the practitioner then teaches the intervention to all the children in the family during the next session. By the end of the session, the children have practiced going to time out many times, not only with the therapist but with all the parents as well. The family is then sent home, and the time out procedure is instituted.

It is often very useful to teach how to give directives and how to use time out to more than just the parents. For example, if grandparents

TABLE 8-1

Giving Directives so That Children Will Comply

Often, parents complain that their children just won't do what they tell them to do. Before we assume that the problem is with the child, parents are advised to make sure that they are giving directives in a way that will increase the likelihood that the child will comply. Four basic principles are important when giving directives to children:

1. **Make your directive a statement instead of a question.** Often, parents will ask a question instead of clearly stating what it is they want the child to do. For example, instead of saying, "Go take your bath," a parent will say, "Don't you think it is time to take your bath now?" The difficulty with this is that the child might genuinely believe that the answer is "No." Parents should not ask a question if they are not prepared to accept the answer. Parents should also learn to feel more comfortable in making clear statements.

2. **Make the directive no more than five or six words.** Often parents get into too much explaining. Children's attention spans usually are limited, and thus the longer a parent spends time giving explanations and details, the more lost the child gets and the more the child tunes the parents out. Thus, directives need to be short and simple; for example, "Go take your bath," "Come to the table," "Turn off the TV," and so on.

3. **Tell a child what to *do* instead of what *not* to do.** Parents frequently get into the habit of saying "Don't, don't, don't." The trouble with this is that kids get sick of hearing the word "don't" and parents get sick of saying the word "don't." "Don't" is negative. It is much better to be positive by telling children what you want them to do *instead of* what not to do. For example, if a child is running through the house, instead of saying, "Don't run in the house," say "Slow down, walk."

4. **When giving directives stay calm and unemotional.** Parents often mistakenly believe that if they become emotional, it will provide the necessary emphasis for children to know that the parents really mean business. Instead, what it does most often is escalate hostility and negativity. Parents must model for children what it is they want their children to do. Upset parents will not be effective when telling their children to calm down. Becoming emotional when dealing with a child's misbehavior is like trying to put out a fire by pouring gasoline on top of it. The best way to discipline and to give directives is for the parent to do so in a businesslike manner, one that is respectful, calm, and in control.

are involved in child care, they will also need these interventions. The more consistent all the adults are with each other in implementing the intervention, the more effective the intervention. The multisystems therapist will use the three sessions to teach all parent figures the interventions. The author has taught the above interventions to as many as 12 people at one time, all of whom were present to intervene in the behavior of one severe ADHD child. Thus for this child, not only did his mother and father learn how to give directives correctly and how to properly implement time out, so did his step-mother, step-father, parental grandparents, three aunts, an adult cousin, a teacher, and their minister. From a systems perspective, having all the parental figures in the family together and learning one intervention is a structural-strategic intervention. However, to effectively use this type of intervention, the practitioner needs to have skill in managing many family members with various agendas so they stay on task and learn to implement the intervention. Needless to say, having all these people use the same intervention consistently with each other was an extremely powerful and effective intervention.

Often, the procedure, taught and practiced in the manner described above, will produce significant changes in the child's behavior and in family interactions. Once this procedure is in place, future sessions will evaluate the effectiveness of the intervention, and make adjustments in the protocol as necessary. The next intervention is likely to be to increase structure, routine, and consistency in the home. This will include establishing or improving the family's routine throughout the day: mornings, after school, study hall, meals, after dinner, bath, and bedtime. Chores need to be addressed, and children need to have age-appropriate responsibilities. Helping the parents establish routine and consistency in family life is one of the most important things a practitioner can do to help the family of an ADHD child.

Next is to improve school functioning in both academics and behavior. Part of this is to establish a routine homework hour in which the child does something academic for a set amount of time, regardless of whether or not he or she has homework assigned that night. Sending home a daily assignment sheet, signed by all teachers, is often very helpful in improving the child's academic functioning. Additionally, the child's behavior can be rated by each teacher, and contingencies established at home for appropriate behaviors. Often these interventions can be implemented by working with the parents and child in session and talking to the teachers and principle over the telephone. However, there are times when the best intervention is for the practitioner to go to the school in person, and meet with the parents and teachers together. This is an example of a multisystems intervention.

Having everyone involved with an intervention in the same room at the same time often is necessary to implement the intervention effectively. When the author has explained this intervention to various managed care companies, usually it has approved two to three hours of reimbursement for the intervention.

An adjunctive procedure that will help the ADHD child, particularly with school, is medication. Medication does not have to be prescribed by a psychiatrist and often is prescribed by pediatricians and family practitioners. Typically, the medication is prescribed initially based on the child's weight (0.5 mg/kilograms/dose). Behavioral checklists filled out by the parents and teachers and a Continuous Performance Test such as the TOVA are very helpful in titrating medication so that children are given the appropriate dosage to maximally improve their attention, concentration, and behavior.

The practitioner using the family psychology model will then follow the child over time, but decrease the frequency of the sessions. The author has followed several ADHD children for up to nine years (the length of time he has practiced in his present location), but may only see a child and his or her family for a total of 10 to 15 sessions during that time. Children with ADHD often have difficulty adjusting to change, and thus there are predictable times when the ADHD child will have problems (e.g., beginning of the school year, winter holidays, end of the school year, starting middle school, etc.). At these times, the family may return for one or two sessions. Because the practitioner knows the child and the family, and a variety of interventions are already in place, one or two sessions may be all that is needed to help the child and family adjust to these transitions. Providing brief, intermittent therapy over the life span in this manner is not only conducive to working in a managed care environment, it also provides the type of service that best meets the needs of the ADHD child and his or her family.

REFERENCES

Achenbach, T. M., & Edelbrock, C. S. (1978). The classification of child psychopathology: A review and analysis of empirical efforts. *Psychological Bulletin, 55,* 1275–1301.

Achenbach, T. M., & Edelbrock, C. S. (1983). *Manual for the Child Behavior Checklist and the Revised Child Behavior Profile.* Burlington, VT: University of Vermont, Department of Psychiatry.

Achenbach, T. M., & Edelbrock, C. S. (1986). *Manual for the Teacher's Report Form and Teacher Version of the Child Behavior Profile.* Burlington, VT: University of Vermont, Department of Psychiatry.

American Psychiatric Association. (1980). *Diagnostic and statistical manual of mental disorders* (3rd. ed.). Washington, DC: Author.

American Psychiatric Association. (1987). *Diagnostic and statistical manual of mental disorders* (3rd. ed., Rev.). Washington, DC: Author.

American Psychiatric Association. (1994). *Diagnostic and statistical manual of mental disorders* (4th. ed.). Washington, DC: Author.

Ammerman, R. T., Last, C. G., & Hersen, M. (Eds.). (1993). *Handbook of prescriptive treatments for children and adolescents.* Boston: Allyn & Bacon.

Ayllon, T., & Azrin, M. H. (1968). *The token economy: A motivation system for therapy and rehabilitation.* New York: Appleton.

Azrin, M. H., Sneed, T. J., & Foxx, R. M. (1974). Dry-bed training: Rapid elimination of childhood enuresis. *Behavior Research and Therapy, 12,* 147–156.

Barkley, R. A. (1987). *Defiant children: A clinician's manual for parent training.* New York: Guilford.

Barkley, R. A. (1990). Foreword. In M. J. Breen & T. S. Altepeter, *Disruptive behavior disorders in children* (pp. vii–ix). New York: Guilford.

Breen, M. J., & Altepeter, T.S. (1990). *Disruptive behavior disorders in children.* New York: Guilford.

Puchanan, L. P., & Buchanan, W. L. (1992). Eating disorders: Bulimia and anorexia. In L. L'Abate, J. E. Farrar, & D. A. Serritella (Eds.), *Handbook of differential treatments for addictions* (pp. 165–188). Boston: Allyn & Bacon.

Buchanan, W. L. (1992). Eating disorders: Obesity. In L. L'Abate, J. E. Farrar, & D. A. Serritella (Eds.), *Handbook of differential treatments for addictions* (pp. 189–210). Boston: Allyn & Bacon.

Conners, K. C. (1973). Rating scales for use in drug studies with children. *Psychopharmcotherapy Bulletin, Special Issue: Pharmacotherapy with children, 9,* 24–84.

Conners, K. C. (1989). *Conners' Rating Scales.* North Tonawanda, NY: Multi-Health Systems, Inc.

Conners, K. C. (1992). *Conners' Continuous Performance Test.* North Tonawanda, NY: Multi-Health Systems, Inc.

Creer, T. L., Harm, D. L., & Marion, R. J. (1988). Childhood asthma. In D. K. Routh (Ed.), *Handbook of pediatric psychology* (pp. 162–189). New York: Guilford.

Cummings, N. A. (1991). Brief intermittent therapy throughout the life cycle. In C. S. Austad, & W.H. Berman (Eds.), *Psychotherapy in managed care: The optimal use of time and resources.* Washington, DC: American Psychological Association.

Cummings, N. A. (1994). The successful application of medical offset in program planning and delivery. *Managed Care Quarterly, 2* (2), 1–6.

Cummings, N. A. (1995). Behavioral healthcare after managed care: The next golden opportunity for professional psychology. *Register Report, 20* (3), 1, 30–33.

Cummings, N. A., & Sayama, M. (1995). *Focused psychotherapy: A casebook of brief, intermittent psychotherapy throughout the life cycle.* New York: Brunner/Mazel.

DiLorenzo, T. M., & Matson, J. L. (1987). Stuttering. In M. Hersen & V. B. Van Hasselt (Eds.), *Behavior therapy with children and adolescents* (pp. 263–278). New York: John Wiley and Sons.

Dinkmeyer, D., & McKay, G. D. (1976). *Systematic training for effective parenting.* Circle Pines, MN: American Guidance Service.

Dolgin, M. J., & Jay, S. M. (1989). Pain management in children. In E. J. Mash and R. A. Barkley (Eds.), *Treatment of childhood disorders* (pp. 383–404). New York: Guilford.

Drotar, D. (1988). Failure to thrive. In D. K. Routh (Ed.), *Handbook of pediatric psychology* (pp. 71–107). New York: Guilford.

Dupuy, T. R., & Greenberg, L. M. (1993). *Test of Variables of Attention computer program.* Los Alamitos, CA: Universal Attention Disorders.

Exner, J. E. (1993). *The Rorschach: A comprehensive system. Volume 1: Basic Foundations* (3rd ed.). New York: John Wiley.

Fletcher, J. M., & Levin, H. S. (1988). Neurobehavioral effects of brain injury in children. In D. K. Routh, (Ed.), *Handbook of pediatric psychology* (pp. 258–295). New York: Guilford.

Forehand, R. L., & McMahon, R. J., (1981). *Helping the noncompliant child.* New York: Guilford.

Foreyt, J. P., & Cousins, J. H. (1989). Obesity. In E. J. Mash and R. A. Barkley (Eds.), *Treatment of childhood disorders* (pp. 405–422). New York: Guilford.

Foreyt, J. P., & McGavin, J. K. (1989). Anorexia nervosa and bulimia nervosa. In E. J. Mash and R. A. Barkley (Eds.), *Treatment of childhood disorders* (pp. 529–558). New York: Guilford.

Gardner, R. A. (1986). *The psychotherapeutic techniques of Richard A. Gardner.* Cresskill, NJ: Creative Therapeutics.

Gordon, M. (1983). *The Gordon Diagnostic System.* Dewitt, NY: Gordon Systems.

Goyette, C. H., Conners, C. K., & Ulrich, R. F. (1978). Normative data for Revised Conners Parent and Teacher Rating Scales. *Journal of Abnormal Child Psychology, 6,* 221–236.

Gray, B. (1991). *The profit motive and patient care.* Cambridge, MA: Harvard University Press.

Green, D. R., Budd, K., Johnson, M., Larg, S., Pinkston, E., & Rudd, S. (1976). Training parents to modify problem child behaviors. In E.J. Mash, L.C. Handy, & L. A. Hamerlynck (Eds.), *Behavior modification approach to parenting* (pp. 3–18). New York: Brunner/Mazel.

Haley, J. (1976). *Problem solving therapy.* San Francisco: Jossey-Bass.

Haley, J. (1987). *Problem solving therapy.* (2nd. ed.). San Francisco: Jossey-Bass.

Imber-Black, E. (1988). *Families and larger systems.* New York: Guilford.

Johnson, S. B. (1988). Diabetes mellitus in childhood. In D. K. Routh (Ed.), *Handbook of pediatric psychology* (pp. 9–31). New York: Guilford.

Kendall, P. C. (Ed.). (1991). *Child and adolescent therapy: Cognitive-behavioral procedures.* New York: Guilford.

Kendall, P. C., & Braswell, L. (1985). *Cognitive-behavioral therapy for impulsive children.* New York: Guilford.

Kratochwill, T. R., & Morris, R. J. (Eds.). (1991). *The practice of child therapy* (2nd ed.). New York: Pergamon Press.

L'Abate, L. (1983). *Family psychology: Theory, therapy, and training.* Washington, DC: University Press of America.

Madanes, C. (1981). *Strategic family therapy.* San Francisco: Jossey-Bass, Inc.

Meichenbaum, D. H. & Goodman, J. (1971). Training impulsive children to talk to themselves: A means of developing self-control. *Journal of Abnormal Psychology,* 77, 115–126.

Minuchin, S. (1974). *Families and family therapy.* Cambridge, MA: Harvard University Press.

Minuchin, S., & Fishman, H. (1981). *Family therapy techniques.* Cambridge, MA: Harvard University Press.

Patterson, G. R. (1968). *Living with children: New methods for parents and teachers.* Champaign, IL: Research Press.

Patterson, G. R. (1971). *Families: Applications of social learning to family life.* Champaign, IL: Research Press.

Peloquin, L. J., & Davidson, P. W. (1988). Psychological sequelae of pediatric infectious diseases. In D. K. Routh (Ed.), *Handbook of pediatric psychology* (pp. 222–257). New York: Guilford.

Popkin, M. H. (1983). *The Active Parenting video-based discussion program.* Atlanta, GA: Active Parenting Press.

Popkin, M. H. (1990). *The Active Parenting for teens.* Atlanta, GA: Active Parenting Press.

Popkin, M. H. (1993). *Active Parenting today: For parents of two to twelve year olds.* Atlanta, GA: Active Parenting Press.

Quay, H. C. (1975). *Manual for the Behavior Problem Checklist.* Coral Gables, FL: Author (University of Miami).

Quay, H. C. (1977). Measuring dimensions of deviant behavior: The Behavior Problem Checklist. *Journal of Abnormal Child Psychology,* 5, 277–287.

Quay, H. C. (1979). Classification. In H. C. Quay & J.S. Werry (Eds.), *Psychopathological disorders in childhood* (2nd ed., pp. 1–42). New York: John Wiley.

Quay, H. C., & Peterson, D. R. (1983). *Revised Behavior Problem Checklist.* Coral Gables, FL: Author (University of Miami).

Quay, H. C., & Peterson, D. R. (1984). *Appendix I for the Revised Behavior Problem Checklist.* Coral Gables, FL: Author (University of Miami).

Quay, H. C., & Peterson, D. R. (1987). *Manual for the Revised Behavior Problem Checklist.* Coral Gables, FL: Author (University of Miami).

Routh, D. K. (1988). (Ed.) *Handbook of pediatric psychology.* New York: Guilford.

Sauber, S. R., L'Abate, L., Weeks, G. R., & Buchanan, W. L. (1993). *The dictionary of family psychology and family therapy.* Newbury Park, CA: Sage Publications.

Schaefer, C. (Ed.). (1979). *The therapeutic use of child's play.* Northvale, NJ: Jason Aronson.

Stehbens, J. A. (1988). Childhood cancer. In D. K. Routh (Ed.), *Handbook of pediatric psychology* (pp. 135–161). New York: Guilford.

Varni, J. W., & Wallander, J. L. (1988). Pediatric chronic disabilities: Hemophilia and spina bifida as examples. In D. K. Routh (Ed.), *Handbook of pediatric psychology* (pp. 222–257). New York: Guilford.

Walker, C. E., Kenning, M., & Faust-Campanile, J. (1989). Enuresis and encopresis. In E. J. Mash and R. A. Barkley (Eds.), *Treatment of childhood disorders* (pp. 423–448). New York: Guilford.

Walker, C. E., & Roberts, M. (1992). *Handbook of clinical child psychology* (2nd ed). New York: John Wiley and Sons.

Watzlawick, P., Weakland, J., & Fisch, R. (1974). *Change: Principles of problem formation and problem resolution.* New York: W.W. Norton.

9

Adjustment Disorders and Brief Treatment

DANIEL L. ARAOZ, Ph.D.
MARIE A. CARRESE, Ph.D.

INTRODUCTION

A brief review of the DSM-IV explanation of the mental condition labeled Adjustment Disorder (AD) will make what follows easier to understand.

For the diagnosis of AD, the following conditions are required:

1. an identifiable psychosocial stressor
2. a maladaptive reaction to (1)
3. reaction that starts within three months after the onset of (1) and
4. (2) lasts no longer than six months.

If these four conditions are met, we have a patient with AD.

The maladaptive reaction manifests itself in many forms, although it is always a culturally perceived overreaction to the stressful event with impairment in social or occupational functions and in interpersonal relations in general.

A culturally perceived overreaction is one that is considered exaggerated in the patient's culture. For instance, in some cultures a normal

216

expression of grief includes loud crying and sobbing, tearing the clothes, and pounding the head and chest with the fists. All these behaviors are considered strange and abnormal in our society.

Stressful psychosocial events are classified as single (divorce), multiple (financial problems), recurrent (yearly holidays), or continuous (chronic illness of self or family member); affecting the individual (inability to drive due to poor eyesight or age), the family (dysfunctional behavior), or the community (floods, earthquakes, fires, or hurricanes), or merely developmental (leaving home for college, retirement, and so on).

We emphasize that the nature of the stressor—for example, the death of a pet—does not determine a person's reaction to it—one person might react with prolonged depression, another with the determination to get another pet.

One main set of conditions, following the above four, is used regardless of the classification of the stressor according to the six types or categories of AD listed in the DSM-IV. These conditions are:

1. A defined, identifiable psychosocial stressor,
2. that took place within three months of when the symptoms started.
3. Overreaction to (1) measured by cultural norms and
4. affecting normal social and/or occupational functioning.
5. The disturbance has manifested itself in more than one instance
6. but it has lasted less than six months.
7. and will probably cease when stressor is no longer present.

All six categories of AD are *passing disturbances* by definition, and managed care companies recognize this. Brief therapy is most effective with AD and there is no indication whatsoever for using medication with people suffering from AD. As a matter of fact, sometimes medication is contraindicated because it may make the patient less motivated to assume responsibility for the AD and to do something constructive about it in order to produce change. It is particularly important for nonmedical providers to keep this in mind, because these patients need the therapist's direct guidance. Adjustment disorders are among the few DSM-IV categories that need psychological counseling rather than medication, and the referral of AD patients to *medical* health service providers is questionable. (Other DSM-IV categories seldom requiring medical intervention are *Relational Problems* (V61.9, etc.), some of the *Problems Related to Abuse or Neglect* (V61.21, etc.) and many of the *Additional Conditions That May Be a Focus of Clinical Attention* (V15.81, etc.).)

In three to eight sessions, patients should experience marked improvement of their disturbance. In recalcitrant cases, a maximum of 12 sessions will be necessary to alleviate the condition and give the patient effective means of coping with it in the future. However, care should be taken to recognize personality disturbance or psychotic symptoms that might be triggered by the stressor in the life of the patient.

DIAGNOSIS

Practical points to keep in mind:

1. *Define:* What has changed in the patient's behavior and become burdensome since the stressful event was experienced?
2. *Affirm and connect:* In what way is her or his life less productive, enjoyable, or effective than it had been before?
3. *Tracking behavior:* How has the person handled his or her symptoms since they started and before seeking treatment?
4. *Goal:* What does the person expect to get from treatment?
5. *Obstacles to overcome:* Are the symptoms exaggerations of normal reactions within her or his culture or are they out of touch with reality (hearing messages from aliens)?

The clinician must be sure that the patient is not suffering from a Personality Disorder, especially of Cluster C in the DSM-IV, or from a schizophrenic or paranoid condition.

Clinicians should note that patients with the following conditions may not benefit from the brief, solution-oriented approach proposed:

1. Personality Disorders (Axis 2)
2. Mental retardation
3. Cognition impairment, including memory dysfunction
4. Inability to focus on concrete and specific goals
5. Psychotic symptoms (no reality testing).

In all these cases the AD diagnosis must be reviewed. In (4) and (5), referral to a psychiatrist for possible medication should be made immediately.

Once these conditions are excluded, the AD diagnosis is safe. The general checklist shown in Exhibit 9-1 is useful for an accurate diagnosis of AD.

EXHIBIT 9.1

General Checklist for Adjustment Disorders

Directions: Check as many as apply. The more checks on the two right columns ("Often," "Much") the more accurate is the AD diagnosis.

KEY

N = Never
S = Somewhat
O = Often
M = Much

	N	S	O	M
1. Thinks of stressor				
2. Wastes time with the thought				
3. Depressed				
4. Tearful				
5. Hopeless				
6. Nervous				
7. Worrying				
8. Jittery or other physical symptom (specify)				
9. Angry				
10. More dependent TBS (Than Before Stressor)				
11. Ambivalent				
12. Truancy				
13. Vandalism				
14. Reckless driving				
15. Fighting				
16. Defaulting in legal responsibilities				
17. Poorer work performance TBS				
18. Poorer academic performance TBS				
19. Less concentration TBS				
20. Withdraws from social activities				
21. Avoids people				
22. Avoids fun activities				

NOTES FOR GENERAL CHECKLIST

The patient's responses lead to one of the nine specific categories listed in the DSM-IV under AD. Remember that there is no AD diagnosis without a specific category or type, except 309.90, the catch-all "Unspecified," which should be used only when the predominant symptoms following the stressor cannot be coded in any of the eight specific categories

The responses of the General Checklist must be elucidated when they fall under "Often" and "Much."

309.24 Adjustment Disorder with Anxiety

"Often" and "Much" responses to # 1, 5, 6, 7, 8, 17, or 18 and 19 on the General Checklist elicit the these *or similar* follow-up questions:

1. When is your hopelessness worse?
2. How do you cope with it?
3. How do you experience your nervousness?
4. What do you worry about?
5. How do you cope with your physical symptoms?
6. How has what you do in order to cope helped you?
7. Give details of your poorer work or academic performance.
8. How are you not able to concentrate as you did before?
9. When do you specifically think more of the stressor?
10. What happens then? (e.g. "I become anxious")
11. What do you do then? (coping strategies)

309.0 Adjustment Disorder with Depressed Mood

"Often" and "Much" responses to #1, 3, 4, 5, 9, 11, 20, and 22 elicit these *or similar* follow-up questions.

1. What happens to you physically when you feel depressed?
2. What events, thoughts, or people make you tearful?
3. How do you describe your feelings of hopelessness?
4. When do you feel especially angry?
5. How do you describe your ambivalence?
6. What social activities have you withdrawn from?

7. What fun activities have you avoided?
8. When do you think of (stressor) more, or more intensely?

309.3 Adjustment Disorder with Disturbance of Conduct

"Often" and "Much" responses to 12, 13, 14, 15, and 16 elicit these *or
similar* follow-up questions.

1. What circumstances trigger your (specific) conduct?
2. What goes through your mind before you decide to do or engage
   in _____ ?
3. Do you think that you could stop yourself from doing _____ ?
4. What reasons do you use in your thinking *not* to stop yourself?
5. Why do you think you want to change this conduct now, by coming
   to therapy?

309.4 Adjustment Disorder with Mixed Disturbance of Emotions and Conduct

"Often" and "Much" responses for #2, 9, 10, and 19 elicit these *or similar*
follow-up questions as for the last three categories, because the diagnosis
of 309.4 is based on a combination of the three previous diagnoses.

309.9 Adjustment Disorder Unspecified

This is a maladaptive reaction to psychosocial stress triggering symptoms
not listed in the five previous subtypes. Thus, the old categories from
DSM-III-R that the new edition does not list any longer—AD with emotional features, AD with physical complaints, AD with withdrawal and
AD with work (or academic) inhibition—will now be subsumed by this
all-embracing category.

An example of AD unspecific is a 29-year-old man who a month ago
broke up with his girlfriend of three years and says that he does not
care; that he never really cared about her. However, his mood is less
cheerful in general and he frequently refers to women in anger and
with negative and sarcastic talk. His boss recommended that he enter
therapy "to get back into shape."

Another example is a 61-year-old widow who was fired from the
secretarial job she had done well for the last 18 years. Always with a

pleasant smile, she tells her friends and family that she does not care about the lost job. Nevertheless, she now spends much time window shopping in the mall and going to the movies. She also calls her children daily, talking incessantly over the phone. She came to therapy at the request of her children.

A third example is a 12-year-old child who shows marked changes for the worse in her schoolwork since the family moved to a new town. She, too, now needs to be listed under this general category.

Finally, a 39-year-old, overweight, college-educated diabetic woman, who refuses to change her diet and lifestyle, saying that she feels great and that doctors exaggerate, was referred by her physician who was concerned about her lack of compliance with his prescriptions and treatment.

Responses of "Somewhat" or "Often" to twelve or more of the General Checklist items may be indicative of a 309.9 diagnosis. The main task of the therapist is to find the origin of the denial and the thoughts regarding the stressor that occupy the patient's mind.

DIAGNOSTIC VIGNETTES

Before proceeding with the actual treatment of AD, we believe that the following three diagnostic vignettes will help you in its differential diagnosis. Therefore, test your skill by establishing a specific AD diagnosis in each of these clinical cases. The answers appear at the end of the chapter.

Case # 1: Elizabeth

Elizabeth is a 40-year-old married woman who is enrolled in a doctoral program in psychology. Throughout her life she has experienced periods of low self-esteem, followed by general lethargy. Five months ago, she took a leave of absence from her job to complete her clinical internship. She recently learned that her job may not be available to her, as was previously agreed upon before she took her leave of absence. Although she has had a positive experience with her internship, she still is two years away from completing her degree. The change in her financial situation, due to her separation from a good paying job combined with the pressure resulting from the nature of her internship in a psychiatric hospital, has created exceptional stress in her daily life. She has frequent headaches and severe stomach cramps, which her physician has been unable to diagnose medically. She has little energy left at night when she returns from her internship and often falls asleep after dinner. Her husband, although supportive of her educational pursuits, is beginning to resent their inability to spend time together. She tells her friends that she feels sick to her stomach and emotionally empty.

Her clinical supervisor complained to her that her work is not as satisfactory as it was in the beginning of her internship and advised her to go into therapy in order to "get herself together."

Case # 2: Lucy

Lucy, 26 years old, moved from Milwaukee to New York City with her husband four months ago. Both she and her husband wanted to experience life in the big city. Neither had jobs before leaving their home town, but both managed to find work with a temp agency. After two months in New York, Lucy's husband met another woman and began seeing her, using the excuse that he had to work overtime. Lucy subsequently became aware of his relationship with the other woman and moved out. She is now living alone, as she feels she needs time to sort things out. Her husband tells her that he loves her and promises to stop the relationship with the other woman. Recently Lucy began experiencing difficulties falling asleep, and she has been tense and nervous. She is afraid of staying in the apartment alone and is frightened of noises she hears at night. She finds herself biting her fingernails and constantly talking to coworkers about her situation. She tells herself that she needs to get this off her chest, and because she has no real friends in New York City, she feels that her coworkers are the only people she can talk to about her problems. One of her coworkers related to her that she, too, had a similar problem with her boyfriend and is now going to therapy to make changes in her life. She told Lucy how therapy has helped her to focus on the positive aspects of her life and recommended that Lucy make an appointment to see a therapist.

Case # 3: Ed

Ed is an office manager who has been involved in a homosexual relationship for the past four years. However, in the last two months this relationship has become strained due to his lover's desire to date other men without leaving Ed. Prior to this relationship Ed was married for two years, but because his ex-wife wanted to return to her country of origin they decided to divorce—he had no intention of living in a foreign country. Although he was not unhappy in his marriage; he stated that he felt more comfortable in the present relationship, which has lasted longer than his marriage. When asked about his lifestyle, he stated that he was relatively happy but in the last two months he often felt anxious and depressed about his homosexuality, the choice he has made, and how it will affect his future. He feels that there are some issues he still needs to resolve, like getting married and having children. Therefore, he is not sure if he should continue in this relationship and lead an alternate lifestyle. He feels anxious about turning 40 and wakes up in the middle of the night thinking about his life. Because Ed has been to therapy before to resolve issues related to his family background—both of his parents were alcoholics—he has decided to return to therapy to discuss his present dilemma.

TREATMENT PLAN

An overall view of managed care treatment for AD includes:

1. Diagnosis
2. Immediate intervention
3. Homework assignments
4. Environmental changes
5. Building support network
6. Overcoming obstacles and resistance
7. Therapist availability

The *immediate goal* is to start experiencing relief right away, immediately after the first session with the therapist.

The *intermediate goal* is to teach the patient effective ways, both mental and behavioral, of reacting to the stressful event, as opposed to the ineffective manner in which he or she has handled the identifiable psychosocial stressor to date.

The *ultimate goal* is to provide new ways of reacting to stressful situations and events in the future.

Treatment

The steps involved in the therapy for AD are basically the following:

1. Define the problem; affirm its existence; and connect the symptoms to the stressor.

2. Set tentative goal for improvement with patient, using resources (personality, mental and social) to overcome effects of stressor.
3. Identify strengths and personal resources.
4. Form a plan of action.
5. Overcome obstacles, including patient's resistance
6. Practice plan and foresee possible difficulties.
7. Evaluate plan and elicit commitment from patient.

Out of these steps emerges the *general outline* of treatment, presented here before the *detailed session-by-session* explanation of psychotherapeutic strategies for AD. This general outline of treatment may be used as a quick point of reference by the busy clinician, who might ask him- or herself where the patient is in treatment and what comes next.

GENERAL OUTLINE OF TREATMENT

First Session

Objectives:

- Define problem.
- Formulate (or confirm) diagnosis.
- Develop therapeutic relationship.
- Establish goals (solutions).
- Teach and practice cognitive restructuring.
- Assign specific practice as home task.

Strategies:

- Help patient define clearly the presenting problem.
- Establish accurate diagnosis (see previous section).
- Question strategically to elicit essence of problem.
- Assign therapeutic practice to reinforce positive feelings and avoid problem-related ones.

Prescription:

- Perform daily repetition of practice learned and done in office.
- Keep written record of practice.
- Make appointment for following week.

Second Session

Objectives:

- Confirm diagnosis.
- Review compliance with prescription.
- Encourage constructive behaviors moving toward solution.

Strategies:

- Check patient's reactions to practice.
- Track behavior toward solution.
- Review prescription, goals, and plans.

Prescription:

- Continue home practices, including written record.

Third Session

Objectives:

- Evaluate progress to date.
- Reinforce positive effort to improve.
- Reframe therapy as learning and growth experience.
- Encourage more solution-oriented behaviors.

Strategies:

- Discuss last prescription.
- Review progress toward goals.
- Review negative situations to avoid.

Prescription:

- Prepare written statement on learning and growth experience.
- If progress is good, make appointment for two weeks later.

Fourth Session

Objectives:

- Solidify gains.
- Prepare patient for possible setbacks.
- Prepare patient for continuing own work without therapy.

Strategies:

- Review compliance with prescriptions.
- Address possible setbacks.

Prescription:

- Contact positive people in patient's life.
- Make next appointment for at least two weeks.

Fifth Session

Objectives:

- Reinforce gains from previous sessions.
- Practice active mental rehearsal of fulfilled life without therapy.
- Evaluate and commit to continue practices without therapist.

Strategies:

- Review prescriptions from previous sessions.
- Review setbacks, if any, and repeat practices learned so far.
- Practice visualization projecting "new" life—with family, at work, with friends, others.

Prescription:

- Practice visualization exercise everyday.
- Schedule next appointment for two or three weeks later.

Sixth Session

Objectives:

- Reinforce patient's ability to be own "therapist" in overcoming AD.
- Review gains made since previous session.
- Apply learning experiences from therapy to other areas of patient's life.

Strategies:

- Encourage practice of do-it-yourself therapy.
- Focus on positive gains.
- Discuss mechanisms of adjustment learned so far in order to generalize gains made to date.

Prescription:

- Practice mind and behavioral exercises to rehearse new attitudes and beliefs in different areas of life.
- Make new appointment for, at least, three weeks later.

Seventh Session

Objectives:

- Follow up on previous session.
- Provide new mental technique to facilitate adjustment to similar new situations.

Strategies:

- Discuss setbacks; analyze patient's ways of handling them with new strategies learned in therapy.
- Teach BRIMS as new mental technique to abort psychological problems due to adjustment situations in the future.
- Give patient audiotape of BRIMS

Prescription:

- Practice BRIMS at least every other day.
- Give new appointment for, at least, three weeks later.

Eighth Session

Objectives:

- Solidify gains.
- Terminate therapy.

Strategies:

- Review adjustment to original stressor and other aspects of patient's life.
- Review practice of BRIMS. (Repeat practice of technique if needed.)
- Arrange for possible future telephone contact; discuss fees for this service.
- Refer to support group if warranted.
- Confirm termination within framework of gains made to date.

DETAILED SESSION-BY-SESSION OUTLINE

First Session

Objectives:

1. Formulate diagnosis, at least tentatively.
2. Begin the building of trust and rapport: "Your problem is not unique. There is an effective cure. Treatment involves your cooperation. I'm here to help you to resolve your problem and go back to living your life fully."
3. Address the AD problem giving patient valid sense of moving toward a solution: thoughts to foster; actions to take and avoid.

Strategies:

1. Help patient clarify and define problem of AD.
2. Establish diagnosis.
3. Ask, "What comes to mind when you think of a stressful event?" In patient's answer, remark on the negative, self-defeating statements. Then ask, "What mental images come to mind when you say to

yourself (such and such)"? In patient's reply, identify negative elements.

4. Then ask, "How can you change what you say to yourself and the images that you allow in your mind to make them more positive?" If patient does *not* come up with any positive elements, you suggest a statement and an image (both related to the original, negative ones he or she gave you earlier) that are positive, constructive and, of course, in agreement with the patient's values, beliefs and lifestyle. For instance, if patient said in step 2, "I can't take this any longer" and visualized in step 3 becoming sleepless and sick to his or her stomach, the therapist may suggest this alternative statement: "I have gone through many difficult things in the past and survived!" Then, the therapist suggests a peaceful image— mountains, seashore, a quiet room in a museum, etc.—where patient keeps saying to self, "I have survived! I can survive this too!"

5. Then, guide him or her to practice in the office, under your direction, until he or she does it smoothly.

Prescription:

1. To practice this mind exercise once a day until the next session.
2. To keep a daily record of practice and of his or her reactions to it. (If you prefer, make an audiotape of the practice and prescribe its daily use).

NOTE: Because the first therapy session is crucial in establishing rapport, make sure that you are able to give patient your full attention, without any other worries in your mind. Objective 2, the building of trust, depends greatly on your positive firmness, your professionally friendly attitude, and your assurance that AD is not an indication of mental illness or craziness but a frequent reaction, painful and disturbing to be sure, of the human organism (body, mind, and spirit) in an effort to adapt to a new situation.

In many cases, it is useful to explain AD in Rational Emotive Therapy (RET) terms: It's not what happens to us, but the way we react to the difficult situation, that produces the problem. The solution lies in changing our reaction. Therapy teaches us to use new reactions to the same situation.

Second Session

Objectives:

1. Confirm diagnosis.
2. Help patient realize importance of own thinking in the way he or she feels based on last session's home assignment.
3. Encourage patient to increase the activities that diminish symptoms of presenting problem by effecting necessary environmental changes.

Strategies:

1. Check on the patient's compliance with the prescription given during the first session.
   (a) If the patient has complied, at least every other day, proceed to step b.
   (b) If the patient did not comply, say something like this: "You practiced the mind exercise with me the last time you were here and I understood that you felt it could help you to learn to do it on your own. What stopped you from doing it?"
   • If the patient has a good reason, renew your previous prescription, guide him or her through the practice again, and proceed to the next step.
   • If patient does not have a good reason, review the diagnosis, or
2. Didactically explain that AD is a function of a person's inner reaction to a stressor.
   (a) Reaction can be changed if the person chooses effective thoughts.
   (b) There is no pill or magic to do this: everyone has to do it him- or herself.
   (c) Obtain commitment to practice previous prescription until next week.
   (d) Guide patient through same practice in the office as in the first session and proceed to step 3.
3. Ask the patient if he or she has any change in symptoms.
   (a) If things are better, proceed to step 4.
   (b) If symptoms are the same or worse, find out how patient practiced the prescribed mind exercise.
   • If practice was adequate (frequent enough, without distractions, following the method taught last session) encourage continued practice and proceed to step 4.

- If practice was *not* adequate, explain again how to do it and lead patient through the same mind exercise again, as in the first session.
4. Review patient's environment
   (a) Ask about
      - Daily schedule: workdays, weekends, last vacation.
      - Interpersonal relations: at work, at home, friends.
      - Interests and hobbies.
      - General dietary habits.
      - Physical activities.
      - Any other aspect of patient's world/environment.
   (b) Rate the above in terms of situations, activities or people that are pleasant, enjoyable, and positive as well as those that are stressful, unpleasant, and difficult. Ask, "Which of these make your symptoms worse? Which make them better?"
   (c) Discuss *practical* means to engage the patient in more nurturing behaviors and interactions and in less toxic ones until the next therapy session.

Prescription:

1. Obtain patient's commitment to do (c) above and to keep a written record of the performance. Explain to patient how to do it.

Third Session

Objectives:

1. Evaluate progress made so far.
2. Reinforce patient's efforts to improve.
3. Reframe the whole therapy experience as a learning and growth opportunity.
4. Encourage continued work on the part of the patient.

Strategies:

1. Check the written record kept by the patient since last visit.
   (a) If the patient kept adequate records, proceed to step 2.

(b) If patient did *not* keep adequate records, do the same as in Second Session, under Strategies, 1 (b).
2. Ask the patient about progress made. Praise any little progress and encourage continuation of the patient's efforts.
3. Ask the patient what lessons about self he or she is learning from this whole AD experience: the event that triggered the adjustment disorder, the initial reactions to it, the beginning of therapy, the progress made, the current feelings about the entire experience. Pay special attention to the patient's associations of the identifiable stressful event with other aspects of his or her life. Always take a positive attitude toward whatever progress has been made so far. This attitude conveys the message that in spite of other difficult situations in the past, the patient is moving forward and not using them as excuses in the current case.

NOTE: The third session is important because by now the patient must be thoroughly committed to therapy. At this point, the prognosis can be determined. If the prognosis is negative, this is the time to discontinue treatment. This may be done by informing the patient that treatment cannot be continued without his or her serious and active cooperation. If the patient insists on continuing, the therapist must firmly assert that the following week will be a test: if he or she does not fulfill his or her part, therapy cannot go on. Continue as follows.

4. Ask the patient again to review people, activities, and places (as in Second Session, step 3) so that the patient can continue to avoid negative situations.

Prescription: For next time

1. Patient writes an introspective statement about strategy 3.
2. Continues the daily practice of the mind exercise and keeps a written record of it, as before.
3. If progress is good, make next appointment for two weeks later. If progress is not satisfactory, make an appointment for the following week.

Fourth Session

Objectives:

1. Solidify the gains made.
2. Prepare the patient for possible setbacks.

3. Prepare the patient for continuing own therapy, without therapy by a provider.

Strategies:

1. Review compliance with prescriptions 1 and 2 from last session.
   (a) If patient wrote statement about what this experience taught her or him and how it has been indeed a growth experience, go to 3, below.
   (b) If patient did not write statement, inquire about reasons.
      • If reasons are acceptable, request that the statement be mailed to you before the next session so you have it when you see her or him again.
      • If reasons are not acceptable, go to 1(d).
   (c) Ask about patient's keeping written record.
      • If patient kept record, go to 2.
      • If patient did not keep it, go to (e).
   (d) Assuming a secondary gain for patient's lack of compliance, explain that therapy will be discontinued at the next session if patient does not cooperate; that therapy necessitates the patient's taking responsibility for progress.
   (e) Ask if the patient wants to work now in the rest of this session.
      • If "Yes," repeat what was done in Third Session.
      • If patient says "No," dismiss until next session, repeating prescriptions of last session.
2. Address yourself to the issue of possible setbacks. Expect them; consider them as detours or parentheses, so that patient can get back on the right track as soon as possible.
   (a) Rehearse with patient: "Assume that you go back to the previous symptoms." What would patient think and say to self; do and not do, and so on. His or her need to go back to practices learned so far in therapy.
3. Establish network of nurturing/positive people that the patient can contact without difficulty. Encourage patient to come up with a list of positive people (*at least* three).

Prescription:

1. Continue previous prescriptions as a preventive measure for possible setbacks.
2. Compose a list of positive people.

3. Give new prescription: "Contact your positive people and let them know that you would like to keep in touch, especially when you need encouragement in order to continue your personal growth." Obtain promise from patient that new prescription will be honored.
4. Make next appointment for double the interval that existed between sessions so far; if you saw patient once a week, make it for two weeks, and so on.

Fifth Session

Objectives:

1. Reinforcement of the previous session's gains
2. Active mental rehearsal of a fulfilled life without the help of a therapist.
3. Commitment to be his or her own therapist by taking full responsibility for self-recovery from AD by practicing all prescriptions between sessions.

Strategies:

1. Get patient's report on practice of prescriptions given last time (visualizing, with written record; listing positive people; getting in touch with those positive people).
   (a) If done, go on to strategy 2.
   (b) If not done, find out why.
   • If reasons are acceptable, go to strategy 2.
   • If reasons are not acceptable, ask patient to reverse roles with you: What would he or she think, say, or do, if the patient were the therapist? Discuss patient's response and obtain commitment to continue therapy. If not, dismiss. If Yes, go to strategy 2.
2. Review issue of setbacks from last session. Repeat practice of Fourth Session, 2(a).
3. Review patient's network of positive people. Has he or she new people to add to the list?
4. Ask patient to visualize a fulfilled life. Go slowly over different areas: family, work, friends, when being alone, on special occasions, and so on.

Pay attention to any constructive, positive elements in what the patient says and encourage the patient to linger on the daydream of those situations that the patient envisions as being fulfilling, enjoyable, and rewarding. Reframe this practice as "do-it-yourself-therapy."

Prescription

1. Prescribe the practice of the above mind exercise to be done once a day until the next session. Request that the patient keep a written record, scoring it with "A" for very good, "B" for good, "C" for not good and "O" for not done that day.
2. Again, make an appointment for at least two weeks from date of this session.

Sixth Session

Objectives

1. Strengthening of patient's readiness to continue without therapy from a provider.
2. Reviewing gains made in the previous sessions.
3. Applying what was learned from therapy to other areas of patient's life that may benefit from better adjustment.

Strategies

1. Inquire about the practice of "do-it-yourself-therapy." Answer questions, and go over practice once more with the patient. Encourage the patient to continue practicing on her or his own.
2. Ask the patient to tell you how things have improved in her or his life in the last eight or nine weeks. Give patient credit for what she or he has done, following the prescriptions of therapy.
3. Because the patient has found new ways of adjusting to the situation that triggered his or her symptoms, discuss the mechanisms of adjustment (thoughts, beliefs, and attitudes; behaviors; things, places or people to avoid, etc.) that have produced the current good results.

Then, suggest the possibility of using the same mechanisms in other areas of his or her life that could benefit from better adjustment.

Prescriptions:

1. Patient will have long conversation with one of his or her positive people about 3, above.
2. Patient will continue the practice of visualization and keep a written record of it.
3. Make a new appointment for at least three weeks from this session.

Seventh Session

Objectives

1. Follow up on previous session to take care of any setbacks.
2. Provide patient with new mental technique to facilitate adjustment to new situations.

Strategies

1. Discuss any setbacks experienced by the patient. Ask "Could you have done anything different? What more effective thoughts, words, or actions could you have used?"
   Mentally rehearse with the patient a situation in which he or she could have responded differently.
2. Introduce and practice BRIMS and provide audiotape published by the Long Island Institute of Ericksonian Hypnosis. (See Appendix at the end of this chapter.)

Prescription:

1. Practice BRIMS and keep written record.
2. Make last appointment for at least one month

Eight Session

Objectives

1. Solidify gains made
2. Terminate therapy

Strategies

1. General review of how patient is adjusting to the original stressor and, in general, to other life situations.
2. Review patient's practice of BRIMS and, if need be, lead patient through it once more.
3. Arrange for possible telephone contact in the future: when patient can call you; fee, if any, that you charge for phone consultation; and so on.
4. Depending on the patient and his or her situation, consider possibility of the patient joining a support group.
5. Explain why you believe therapy has been completed and say goodbye.

Prescription: Continue practice of BRIMS every day.

THE PROCESS OF THERAPY IN A CASE OF ADJUSTMENT DISORDER

Mr. D., who had run his own company for over 20 years, decided to sell it when he was about to retire at the age of 63. After a big party in his honor and a wonderful sailing vacation in the Caribbean, he returned home with grand plans for enjoying his "golden years," as he was fond of calling them. He had more than ten books that he wanted to read and was planning a three-month trip to Europe with his wife. She had retired at about the same time as Mr. D. from a long and satisfying teaching career.

However, two weeks after his return from the Caribbean trip, Mr. D. started to feel very anxious, insecure, afraid, restless, and unable to concentrate on anything. He would wake up several times each night and worry about finances, although rationally he knew that there was nothing to worry about. At night he worried about his worrying during the day.

Finally he called a physician who had been his high school friend and with whom he had been close ever since. Over the phone, he was prescribed antianxiety drugs, which did very little, if anything, for his condition. His wife, who had been in psychotherapy on and off for the previous 12 years, kept insisting that he go into therapy. Mr. D. repeated that he did not believe in "shrinks." However, two months after his Caribbean sailing vacation he was feeling so awful, and all his symptoms were becoming so much worse, that he agreed to see a therapist—but only for three sessions.

The psychotherapist, a Fellow of the Academy of Counseling Psychology who had many years of experience, also had some consulting experience with corporations. This made Mr. D. feel less of "a mental case." In spite of it, he started the first session with an air of aloofness, boasting about his wisdom and worldly knowledge and the help he had been to others, since he was about twice the age of the psychologist. But he was impressed by the fact that Dr. Y. asked what came to mind when he thought of his problem. He had never paid attention to that. He realized that his thoughts were very negative: growing old, feeling alone, bored, useless, and being afraid of his wife dying. Dr. Y. encouraged him to think differently and to focus on what he could do with the rest of his life, both to enjoy himself and to be useful to others in any possible way he could. Mr. D. talked about his dream of playing the clarinet and became enthusiastic about the idea. Dr. Y helped him make concrete plans to stop dreaming about it and start learning how to do it. Dr. Y. also encouraged Mr. D. to plan ways in which he could benefit others. Mr. D. came up with two things he could do: He could offer some form of consulting to young business people through his church, in which he was active, and he could give free sailing lessons to poor youngsters in Florida, where he lived six months of the year.

When Mr. D. asked Dr. Y. what his condition was, he was told that it was a common reaction to retirement, technically called "adjustment disorder with anxiety." In the first session, Mr. D. also learned to identify his negative thoughts, which Dr. Y. called "negative self-hypnosis," and to replace them with constructive, positive thoughts, which Dr. Y. labeled "power thoughts." Dr. Y. also suggested a book, *Reengineering Yourself,* and Mr. D. wasted no time procuring it. Dr. Y. had suggested that he start reading this book before the second visit. To his surprise, Mr. D. realized that he was looking forward to continuing his meetings with Dr. Y.

During the seven days between the first two visits, Mr. D. started reading *Reengineering Yourself* and took many notes, mostly positive, about his reaction to the book. He caught himself many times doing "the negative self-hypnosis thing" and made a special effort to change his thoughts. He also inquired about clarinet lessons and, through his church, offered to teach sailing to deprived youngsters.

In the second session he told Dr. Y. that he did not need to come back because he felt all better. Dr. Y. congratulated Mr. D. on all the positive things that he had done in only one week, but also warned him that they should watch such quick progress and recovery in order to make sure that the gains were solid and lasting. He invited Mr. D. to practice visualization, and Mr. D. did it well. In his mind, he saw himself in his boat, playing the clarinet, with his wife smiling at him. He could also visualize himself teaching sailing to the deprived youngsters.

Dr. Y. told him that he should do this mind exercise every day for the next two weeks, and he should continue reading *Reengineering Yourself.* Mr. D. was asked to call Dr. Y. in two weeks to let the doctor know how he was doing, and Dr. Y. requested that he keep a daily written record of his moods and activities.

Two weeks later, Mr. D. called Dr. Y. and said that he wanted another appointment. At the session, Mr. D. reported enthusiastically on his tremendous improvement, his continuing the positive activities he had started, and the benefits he obtained from reading the book and doing some of the practices suggested in it. Only on three occasions in the last two weeks had he started to feel a little gloomy, and, he added, he had been able to short-circuit the negative mood without too much effort. He also asked Dr. Y. if he could hire him as "my personal consultant" and call on him at least once a month. According to Mr. D. this was a recommendation he had taken from the book, and it would allow his progress to be monitored by an expert. Dr. Y. agreed to do so.

Even though this case sounds artificially simple, dramatic progress in AD cases is rather frequent when the therapeutic approach is the solution-oriented brief therapy—cognitive, behavioral and self-hypnotic—that Dr. Y. used with this patient. The main point to keep in mind is to ascertain that the patient has a healthy, functioning personality and is going through a crisis-like situation in the process of adapting to a stressful new set of circumstances.

This case also shows that a directive, strategic approach works well in cases of AD. Rather than spend the first session gathering unnecessary information or attempting to interpret the reasons for the disturbance, an immediate call to action functions both as a messenger of hope for the patient and as a diagnostic indicator for the clinician. Had Mr. D. not been able to put into action what he discussed with Dr. Y. during the first session, his diagnosis would have been changed. Probably he would have been diagnosed with either a personality disorder or a more specific anxiety or depressive disorder.

The case is presented to encourage clinicians to involve the AD patient in his or her recovery from the very first therapeutic contact. However, clinicians should also avoid the mistake of trying to shortcut the process by merely alleviating the symptoms, as Mr. D's. old physician friend tried to do.

Because AD patients find themselves in a new set of unfamiliar, stressful circumstances, they need a new structure and framework to operate in safety. This is what Dr. Y. provided. The new framework included cognitive and behavioral elements to which Mr. D. responded positively. A nonpositive response on the part of the patient is always a warning to review the diagnosis and the expectations of the patient.

The impairment severity of an AD patient may be very acute. The case should be presented to managed care companies for approval of treatment on this basis of behavioral impairment whether it is acute or mild. The truth is that, untreated, these patients are in serious danger of deteriorating and becoming permanently disabled. As a bad cold can turn into pneumonia, a person diagnosed with AD can end up with a personality disorder or one of the depressive or anxiety disorders, which are all much more serious than AD.

For the certification of treatment that managed care companies need, the wise clinician details the impairment that AD is producing in the patient's functioning, knowing quite well that the treatment, after the proper diagnosis, has a favorable prognosis.

DIAGNOSES FOR THE VIGNETTES

Case # 1: Elizabeth

Diagnosis

Adjustment Disorder Unspecified (309.9)

Rationale

The patient, Elizabeth, clearly expresses physical symptoms, such as headaches and stomach cramps. These symptoms have no medical cause. The onset of these physical manifestations was brought about after the patient realized the potential loss of her job (the identified psychosocial stressor). Prior to that event, there were no indications of unusual stressors. General lethargy and low energy are also experienced as a physical manifestation in this case.

The symptoms began within the three months time-frame required by the DSM-IV diagnostic category for AD. In view of all this, other AD categories are excluded because the physical symptoms are predominant and in the DSM-IV the new code is "unspecified."

Case # 2: Lucy

Diagnosis

Adjustment Disorder with Anxiety (309.24)

Rationale

The essential features of AD with anxious mood category are symptoms such as nervousness, worry, and trouble falling asleep. Lucy reports nail biting, which is a common physical manifestation of nervousness. She feels compelled to keep talking to her coworkers about her problem, another indication of anxiety. These symptoms appeared after the estrangement from her husband, which happened approximately two months after her arrival in New York City.

Because there is no evidence of any other mental disorders, such as compulsive personality disorder or borderline personality disorder, and because the reaction was brought about by her husband's unfaithfulness (the psychosocial stressor), this is the AD category that is appropriate to this case.

Case # 3: Ed

Diagnosis

Adjustment Disorder with Mixed Disturbance of Emotions and Conduct (309.4)

Rationale

This category combines symptoms found in both AD with anxious mood and AD with depressed mood, accompanied by feelings of decreased self-esteem and worthlessness.

The fact that Ed reports often feeling anxious and depressed, awakening in the middle of the night and thinking morosely about his life, is indicative of the predominant features associated with this category.

The "disturbance of emotions" has affected his "conduct," as the case indicates. The confusion about his homosexual lifestyle and preoccupation about his future and the choices he needs to make underlie issues of poor self-esteem. These issues have become more apparent to him as he approaches 40, a significant developmental step, coupled with the new estrangement between him and his lover. Both these events are the psychosocial stressors that have manifested themselves at this time in his life.

Because there are no indications of other mental disorders, the AD category "with mixed disturbance of emotions and conduct" is the most appropriate for this case.

APPENDIX

The BRIMS audiotape referred to in the text of the chapter was made by the senior author and can be obtained from the Long Island Institute of Ericksonian Hypnosis, 66 Gates Avenue, Malverne, NY, 11565–1912.

REFERENCES

American Psychiatric Association. (1987). *Diagnostic and statistical manual of mental disorders,* 3rd. edition, Revised (DSM-III-R). Washington, DC: American Psychiatric Association.

American Psychiatric Association. (1994). *Diagnostic and statistical manual of mental disorders,* 4th. edition. (DSM-IV). Washington, DC: American Psychiatric Association.

Araoz, D.L., & Sutton, W.S. (1994). *Reengineering yourself: A blueprint for personal success in the new corporate culture.* Boston: Bob Adams, Inc.

Brown, J. (1991) *The quality management professional's study guide.* Pasadena, CA: Managed Care Consultants.

Goodman, M., Brown, J., & Deitz, P. (1992). *Managing managed care.* Washington, DC: American Psychiatric Press, Inc.

Reid, W.H., & Wise, M.G. (1989). *DSM-III training guide.* New York: Brunner/Mazel.

10

Managed Care and Treatment
of Depression

MARK MAYS, Ph.D., J.D.
JAMES CROAKE, Ph.D.

Managed care is the new environment in which mental health care will be delivered. In biology, environments determine which species flourish and thrive, and which dwindle and decline. Harsh environmental changes may cause some species to disappear altogether, as has the dinosaur and the snail darter. Ecological environments nurture and support certain species but not others. Some species thrive on what an environment provides, and others cannot adapt to the sustenance available. Survival is a dance between the environment and the organism. Compatibility defines survival.

This applies as well to health care. Managed care becomes the environment and sets the ecology for the delivery of health care services. Some species of mental health care will flourish and others will fade. Managed care is an environment that supports those approaches that focus on change, define goals, allow flexibility of treatment approach, and achieve measurable results. Theories and therapies in mental health care that support these treatment approaches will grow. Other therapies seek less measurable results, embracing more subjective and intrapsychic changes. Such treatment may take years in some therapeutic approaches, which strive to explore character restructuring and modification of global patterns of personal organization in the context of a slowly evolving therapeutic relationship. Perhaps sadly, these theories will not be compatible with the health care milieu and will not gain the reimbursement necessary to continue. Some therapies will thrive. Some will merely survive. Others will die.

MORE THAN ABBREVIATED TREATMENT

Managed care is different. It is a mistake to view it as merely abbreviated treatment. The changes in treatment go far beyond brevity. Managed care prompts a different way of conceptualizing patients, involves different mechanisms for interventions, and defines different results. Even the office support and technology necessary to support managed mental health care is different than that of more traditional therapeutic approaches. If information is the byword, and if time is money, technology that speeds the flow of relevant information in a timely way will be necessary for the managed care provider. Handwritten notes in paper charts and cumbersome methods conveying information to others on a treatment team will be eliminated.

GOALS

Establishing treatment goals that seek to remedy all diagnostic conditions might be a major task of therapy for the traditional therapist, but some diagnoses might only provide a road map of treatment for the managed care provider. Personality disorder diagnoses may even serve primarily to encourage or discourage the practitioner from choosing certain interventions to help a patient respond to disorders of mood or problems with anxiety. Mental health professionals will be dissuaded from seeing patients primarily as individuals with intrapsychic difficulties, and encouraged to see them more as social beings who live with varying degrees of adaptiveness in a social context that influences them and is influenced by them. Insight and understanding historical antecedents of a patient's problems will more often be seen as interesting but irrelevant, potentially even a distraction from the true therapeutic goal of encouraging change and increasing the patient's level of adaptive functioning. Rule-bound procedures will be frowned upon and practical solutions will be applauded. It is going to be a new manner of treatment world.

THE "D" EMPHASIS

Managed care will demand changes that can be viewed as emphasizing "The Six Ds." There will be an emphasis on *diagnostic* skills. Treatment will be *directed*. *Didactic* and educational interventions will be increasingly employed. Treatment will be more detailed and entail greater *documentation,* and some interventions will be *delegated* to others who serve as part of a treatment team. Finally, therapy will be *delimited* in duration and goal.

Managed care demands accurate diagnoses on a variety of dimensions. On the one hand, clinical diagnoses are important in terms of both treatment and administration. Utilization review, outpatient tracking of diagnostically related groups, authorization for treatment of certain conditions and not others, and legal and regulatory demands to avoid fraud by misrepresentation all require precision in use of diagnostic nomenclature. Reimbursement often will hinge upon a patient's diagnoses. Case review and monitoring and quality assurance programs will necessitate validation for such diagnoses. Knowledge of the current diagnostic system, such as the DSM-IV, will be familiar references to practicing clinicians. Even twenty years ago the occasional mental health professional could gain reimbursement by describing a patient as "nervous." Now the therapist might need to diagnose a major depressive disorder, severe without psychoses, and differentiate it from an adjustment disorder with depression, dysthymia, simple bereavement, or mere unhappiness associated with a life circumstance problem or as a residual of a behavioral disorder best diagnosed on Axis II. Different managed care programs might reimburse differentially for different diagnoses, and some diagnoses might receive no reimbursement.

ASSESSMENT

Assessment in managed care goes beyond mere labeling and reliance upon treatment protocols. The person working in the managed care environment not only will assess an individual's psychological multiaxial diagnosis, but will need to make practical assessments, as well. A clinician will assess a patient's social support, family context, vocational adjustments, social skills, personal strengths, and other resources, so that he or she can develop a practical treatment plan tailor-made for this individual in a certain environmental social context. Various patient resources will be appraised so the clinician can draw upon them to bring about a return to equilibrium and the previous level of adaptive functioning.

The managed care mental health professional might be compared to a traveling mechanic who goes from garage to garage, repairing different cars as they arrive. There will be an assessment of the problem with the vehicle, such as the failure of the diodes in the alternator or a problem with the intake valve, and an appraisal of the tools in the local garage that are available for fixing this and other problems. If some tools are missing, other solutions will have to be found. If other tools are available, they can be called upon. Unavailability of a replacement part may require special recalibration of the engine system so the part in place continues to function within the limits of its impairments. A mechanic in such a situation, to be helpful, makes assessments that go beyond diagnosing the problem with the car. A truly helpful mechanic must also know the availability of parts and tools, consider the climatic conditions in which the auto is used, maintain an attentiveness for the driving conditions that may cause such a breakdown, and be able to give advice about altering driving habits to prevent future trouble. In like manner, assessment of psychological problems in managed care involves an expanded view of assessment.

THERAPIST RESPONSIBILITY

Psychotherapeutic approaches differ in terms of the degree of therapist responsibility and therapist activity that different approaches demand. Managed care will involve very active therapist involvement. Some therapeutic approaches seem analogous to the gardener in the greenhouse. In the greenhouse the gardener creates the right circumstances for plants and flowers to grow and thrive. The role of the gardener is creating the appropriate environment in which the plants can grow themselves. While there is some tending and removal of weeds, the blueprint for change and growth lies within the genetic structure of the plant's seed. A gardener given new seeds might plant them, nourish them, and watch with great interest as they unfold. Growth may take many seasons.

MECHANIC

Managed care on the other hand, draws much more upon the metaphor of the mechanic. Here the customer's complaint defines the scope of intervention. The customer with wheels slightly misaligned, a rear power window not operational and a noise from the alternator might come to the mechanic's shop concerned about none of these problems, but wanting the ignition fixed since the car occasionally won't start. The mechanic would be confined to the dictates of the consumer's request for involvement. The helpful mechanic might notify the owner of other problems that could use attention, including repairs the customer could do unassisted, but it would be surprising for mechanic in such a situation to intervene beyond the initial request for repairs.

Most importantly, few mechanics would claim that the repair wasn't possible because "the starter was resistant." There might be very justifiable reasons for the car not being fixed. Repairs could require a major engine overhaul that the local mechanic is not equipped to complete. It could be that the problem is not mechanical and resides somewhere else in the system—perhaps it is poor fuel—and the owner may leave with suggestions to look for other causes and remedies.

The analogy does not suggest that people are machines, but more that managed care will certainly assume special skills, knowledge, experience, and training that the professional brings to the relationship that makes the mental health consultation more than a visit with a well-meaning friend. Managed care seeks to achieve specific results. These are not merely subjectively defined but, more often than not, objectively measurable. Further, interventions are not focused on personal discovery, self-knowledge, or personal growth.

Treatment is designed to correct specific signs and symptoms that are so personally unacceptable to the patient or the social context in which the patient lives that a diagnosis of a mental and emotional condition is made. Treatment is defined as reducing the presence of symptoms and making their recurrence less likely over time. Managed care exists to manage appropriate treatment, and appropriate treatment is that which is found to be effective and potent in achieving specific results. While results are often implied in a diagnosis, the explicit concern in managed care remains on achieving articulated results. Managed care itself is actively directed towards achieving specific system results in health care, and this creates a ripple-down effect in which the therapist will be quite active in achieving dependent variables.

EXPLICIT GOALS

Though some results may be implicit in diagnoses, managed care encourages treatment goals to be explicit as well as specific. Patient reports of "I think I'm feeling better" will be replaced by specific measures of targeted signs and symptoms. As is said in the vocational counseling literature "if you don't know where you're going, you'll end up some place else." So, too, does this apply in managed care.

FLEXIBILITY

Given that there are explicit goals and the inherent demand to achieve them efficiently, the most effective therapist in this environment will use a multitude of tools and resources to move toward therapeutic goals. The therapist will be accountable for achieving results by whatever mechanisms and resources are appropriate, and he or she may be seen more as a change manager than an individual change agent. Change does not need to occur in the therapeutic session—it merely needs to occur. The therapist administers and creates plans that rely upon ancillary resources, monitors change, and coordinates further efforts towards additional changes. The therapist is the person who makes sure that change is accomplished, not necessarily the person who accomplishes the dependent variables. One gets no extra points for therapeutic progress that occurs as a result of psychotherapy in a psychotherapeutic relationship. One only gets credit if the changes occur. The most laudable of psychotherapeutic relationships, the most exquisite of insights and understandings, and a powerful patient re-experiencing of emotionally charged events can be a deepening and a rewarding experience. It will not be applauded, rewarded, or even considered relevant to the process of managed care if it does not produce measurable progress towards specifically defined treatment goals.

The managed care therapist delegates and coordinates aspects of the change process. The managed care provider is almost always a member of a team, though not necessarily in a geographically proximate group practice. There are many resources that can be seen as part of the "therapeutic alliance" or "treatment team." These may include a primary care physician, family members, resources in the community such as teachers and ministers, and specific programs with certain apparent benefits for specific situations. In no context more than the context of managed care does the therapist need to be able to develop such complex relationships and coordinate such a range of resources.

MODELS

Some of these resources are didactic and educational. Viewing treatment in a component model certainly opens the door to such educational modalities as audio and videotapes that explain signs and symptoms, demonstrate skills, and provide models for alternative responses. Explanations as to the reasons and justifications for interventions are often more explicit and conscious than experiential. Written materials can enhance understanding and thus compliance and participation, involving the patient more in the partnership of change. Workbooks, monitoring programs, and checklists are all a part of the managed care environment. Didactic resources can be very helpful, particularly to the therapist who adopts the change manager paradigm.

EXTERNAL REVIEW

Managed care is subject to external review by those who ensure quality; hence, documentation is important. Managed care is collective care. Information will be recorded so that it can be easily and quickly reviewed and communicated to the treatment team. For the effective managed care therapist, the skill will be to know which information is relevant to the treatment team. This is different from the information that might be relevant to the therapist in the therapeutic context. Extensive information documenting a diagnosis may be required for regulatory and quality assurance purposes. It could be even counterproductive to treatment. Extensive material may not be reviewed by a very busy physician, for example, who also might participate in the care.

CONFIDENTIALITY

Differing policies about confidentiality and privacy will be articulated in the managed care context. Some informal standards will evolve that will serve as the "minimal standard of care" and charted. Similarly "maximal standards" in terms of the personal information will not go beyond providing to others. It is to be remembered that patient records are always best viewed as potential public documents. Maintaining balance between privacy and appropriately informing other treatment providers is a tension between competing goals that is likely to persist.

  Fortunately, the task focus of managed care helps resolve this tension. While it is clear that communication about a patient must occur, the information that is usually most relevant to others and that is documented in durable records is more clinical than private and personal. Services, symptoms, and interventions are noted. A diagnosis and a basis for treatment will be documented. Documentation that ensures conformity to the limits and boundaries of treatment authorization will be maintained to show that the clinician is not primarily treating other problems, such as marital discord, when treatment has only been authorized for a major depressive disorder. Information about private or embarrassing past experiences may be relevant to clinical understanding, but perhaps not important for managed care records. Coordination and administration of care requires documentation in a different domain. Data included will be that which is relevant to others on the treatment team who approach the patient from very different perspectives.

Time Limits

Managed care is usually delimited in time or number of sessions. This implies that there are limits not only to the extent of treatment, but to what can be achieved in treatment as well. A patient is looking at an enhancement of his or her current capacity to function with a lessening of distress, not at character restructuring. Treatment usually focuses more on Axis I syndromes, which may wax and wane and are more remediable than Axis II conditions. A therapist does not open doors or start therapeutic tasks that will be difficult to complete within the time constraints of authorized care. Managed care insists that therapists define achievable goals that take the realities of limited resources into account from the onset.

THE SIX Ds AND THE TREATMENT OF DEPRESSION

Diagnosis

Nowhere more than in the treatment of depression under managed care does this approach to treatment apply. Diagnosis is vital with depressive disorders. Studies (Duffy, 1994; Gullick & King, 1979; Johnson, 1974; Magruder-Habib et al., 1989) show a high rate of misdiagnosis on both the primary care and the mental health level in terms of mood disorders. There is much data about the prevalence of depression in various studies (Barrett, Barrett, Oxman, & Gerber, 1988; Blacker and Clare, 1988; Coulehan, Schulberg, Block, Janosky, & Arena, 1990; Kessler, Cleary, & Burke, 1985; von Korff, Shapiro, Burke, et al. 1987). Up to one in four people may require treatment for major depressive disorder alone at some point during their lives. When this baseline expectation is contrasted to the rate of diagnoses of depressive disorder in medical charts, there is wide variance among primary care physicians. Their ability to diagnose depressive problems in their patients ranges from excellent to poor. Managed care encourages the primary care physician to be more attentive to the presence of depression in medical patients, because undiagnosed depression is often reflected in overutilization of primary medical care resources.

Estimates of the costs of major depressive disorders are startling. One study estimated costs, including costs of lost productivity, at $16 billion in 1980 dollars (Stoudemire, Frank, Hedemark, Kamlet, & Blazer, 1986). A reanalysis of this data to assess costs for treatment, morbidity, and increased mortality resulted in an estimated cost of almost $44 billion (Greenberg & Stiglin, 1993). Up to 38 percent of patients with major depressive disorder show significant restrictions in activity. Disability days for those with depression were almost five times that of the general population (Broadhead, Blazer, George, & Tse, 1990; Wells, Golding & Burnham, 1986). Health care utilization is increased in depressed populations and is significantly greater than for others in general outpatient medical settings (Regier, Hirschfeld, & Goodwin, 1988).

Accurate diagnosis of mood disorders on the primary medical care level is particularly difficult given the wide range of manifestations of depressive signs and symptoms. Pain, somatic symptoms, and complaints of fatigue and of general malaise are often indicative of depression rather than physical illness. Some studies show that a majority of patients with psychiatric syndromes, particularly depressive disorders, have physical complaints. Other studies show that a majority of depressed patients report significant pain complaints. It has even been noted that complaints of more than one pain problem correlate with between a six and an eightfold increase in the likelihood of a diagnosis of depression (Bridges & Goldberg, 1985; Dworkin, von Korff, & LeResche, 1990; Katon, 1987; Katon, Kleinman, & Rosen, 1982; Katon, Ries, & Kleinman, 1984).

Accurate diagnosis of mood disorders is also a problem on the mental health level (Abou-Saleh & Coppen, 1983; Beckham and Leber, 1985; Marseille, Hirschfeld, & Kate, 1987; Tyler & Brittlebank, 1993). Depression is a term that is casually used by many, yet the diagnostic manuals are quite clear. Through all of their revisions, the manuals show that there are qualitatively different depressive disorders, rather than merely degrees of severity of depression. Most researchers believe that a dysthymic disorder is different qualitatively as well as quantitatively from a major depressive disorder (Beckham & Leber, 1985; Depression Guideline Panel, 1994). There is also a difference between a major depressive episode and a bipolar disorder, as there is between depression secondary and an organic problem, medical illness, iatrogenic effect, or adjustment disorders with depressive features; and differences between depressive disorders in children and in adults. Each of these qualitatively different depressive entities may warrant a different therapeutic response. It should also be recalled that unhappiness is distinct from depression. Depression is a mood disorder, not merely an appropriate and limited reaction to a dissatisfying situation (Spaner, Bland, & Newman, 1994; Zisook and Shuchter, 1991). Depression indicates either a reaction that is so extreme and excessive as to impair functioning, or a reaction that is more or less independent of a patient's situation.

A clinician must be sure that he or she is treating a disorder of mood and not a disguised medical condition. Many physical conditions and the side effects of some medicines can mimic emotional symptoms of depression (Bant, 1978; Coulehan, Schulberg, Block, Janosky, & Arena, 1990; Goodwin & Bunny, 1971; Hall, Gardner, Stickney, LeCann, & Popkin, 1980; Whitley, 1991). Some cardiovascular drugs, certain hormones and steroids, psychotropics, and anticancer agents, as well as some anti-inflammatory and anti-infective medicines can lead to depression (Bant, 1978; Goodwin & Bunny, 1971; Herzberg & Coppen, 1970; Pope & Katz, 1988). Certain medical disorders, cancers, infections, and toxic environmental agents may show an overlap of symptoms with depression. These commonly include low energy, weight loss, weight gain, and decreased activity or cognitive inefficiency. The cause of signs and symptoms resulting from a medical problem could be life-threatening if a primary mood disorder is the principal diagnosis. Complicating the picture even further is the frequent comorbidity of depression with such medical conditions as early dementia, mononucleosis, Crohn's disease, thyroid disfunction, diabetes, and coronary artery disease, calling for separate diagnosis of a disorder of mood and physical illness, each receiving appropriate, yet different, treatments.

Nosology

Major depressive disorder is the most well researched depressive condition. Though some revisions are found in the new diagnostic manual, DSM-IV, it is not substantially different from the DSM-III in terms of diagnostic criteria for major depression (American Psychiatric Association, 1994). A patient must have at least five of the included symptoms during a two-week period, and the symptom presentation must be a change from a previous level of functioning. There must be either a depressed mood or the loss of interest or pleasure in his or her activities. The patient must also experience specific symptoms, such as significant weight loss or gain, sleep problems, and physical slowing or agitation. There may also be some cognitive symptoms, such as a diminished ability to think or concentrate, indecisiveness, or recurrent thoughts of death or suicide, or feelings of worthlessness or excessive guilt.

Medications

Major depressive disorders respond to antidepressant medicines in half to two-thirds of people (Cohn & Wilcox, 1985; Coppen, Mendelwicz, & Kielholz, 1986; Guze & Gitlin, 1994; Rush, 1986). A slightly lower percentage of patients has been found to benefit from psychotherapy alone (Beck, Rush, Shaw & Emery, 1979; Elkin et al., 1989; Gallagher & Thompson, 1983; Klerman & Weissman, 1987; McLean & Hakistian, 1979; Nezu, 1986; Thompson, Gallagher, & Breckenridge, 1987). Psychotherapy combined with medicines has generally been found to benefit half to 80 percent of patients diagnosed with major depressive disorder. There is some suggestion in the research that psychotherapy combined with medicine makes future depressive symptoms less likely to recur (Blackburn, Bishop, Glen, Whalley, & Christie, 1981; Blackburn, Eunson, & Bishop, 1956; Murphy, Simmons, Wetzel, & Lustman, 1984; Rush, Beck, Kovacs, & Hollon, 1977; Wessman, 1979).

Clearly, antidepressant medicines are a resource to consider in the treatment of major depressive problems; particularly newer antidepressant medicines, called selective serotonin reuptake inhibitors (SSRIs). The SSRIs can help many people with major depressive disorders gain benefit without some of the problematic and irritating side effects found in the older tricyclic antidepressants. The same is true of patients who cannot or will not follow the tyramine restrictions necessary when using monamine oxidase inhibitors (MAGIs)—it would be very risky to trust that a teenager would not eat any pizza (Guze & Gitalin, 1994). The decision about use of medicines involves an assessment of a variety of factors rather than merely a clinical diagnosis of depression. Medical status must be evaluated. Assessing alcohol use and substance abuse is important for a variety of treatment, health, and compliance issues.

An assessment of sleep disruption is important in selecting antidepressants, because the side effect profile of some antidepressants, particularly the tricyclics, may make certain medicines much more desirable than others. Sleep apnea, awakening due to physical pain, and too much sleep can be primary causes of depression. Early morning awakening may be nature's method for treating depression. This idea follows the finding that most depression improves when the patient who normally sleeps about eight hours is deprived of the last four hours of sleep.

A history of depression in a person's biological family will both help support this diagnosis and provide possible suggestions for the selection of biological interventions (medications and electric shock). Depressive disorders are increasingly thought to have a genetic component. A medication that worked well for a close relative may be the drug of choice for this patient.

Medications will work only when the patient takes them as prescribed. Quite often, when prescriptions do not relieve depression it is not due to incorrect diagnosis or choice of medication. The physician may have the correct diagnosis and drug, but give it at the lower level suggested in the PDR. A referral to a psychiatrist who then increases the amount of medication might find success. A failure at that point, the upper limits recommended by the PDR, would result in a referral to a university department of psychiatry, which would find results by increasing the drug beyond that recommended by the PDR. Compliance with prescription regimens, sometimes referred to as adherence to prescription schedules, is vital. The therapist in managed care may play a pivotal role in biological therapy by enhancing the likelihood of compliance. Research indicates that compliance with treatment using antidepressants is quite poor, even less than patients report to their prescribing health care provider. One study showed that only 40 percent of general medical patients took more than 75 percent of prescribed medications, and almost 25 percent did not even get their prescriptions filled (Zoega, Barr, & Barsky, 1991). A study using patients prescribed antidepressants, and using measures of blood serum antidepressant levels rather than the patient's reports, found that 45 percent of those prescribed certain medicines (amitriptyline and imipramine) were noncompliant, but only one in twelve of those prescribed a medicine with a more benign side effect profile (desipramine) were noncompliant (Boza et al., 1989). Another study found that more than half of a group of Southeast Asian patients had no detectable antidepressant blood levels despite their reports of compliance (Kroll et al., 1990).

Although the rate of compliance with medicines is possibly quite low, it can be improved by effective and directed therapeutic efforts that acknowledge and attempt to resolve adherence difficulties. Verbal and written commitments by the patient to adhere to prescription regimens improve the likelihood that this will occur (Putnam, Finney, Barkley, & Bonner, 1994). Reducing the complexity of prescription schedules, for example, from three times a day to nightly, might increase compliance (Conn, Taylor, & Kelly, 1991). Providing simpler instructions, adopting communication styles that are sensitive to patient attitudes, rewarding patients' compliance, and providing them with reminders to take medicines increase compliance (Holloway, Rogers, & Gershenhorn, 1992; Spilker, 1992; Woody, 1990). Education regarding medicines is highly effective in enhancing compliance (Peet and Harvey, 1991; Youssel, 1983). Use of compliance- and adherence-enhancing strategies are effective. They reduce noncompliance more than 50 percent even in long-term patient populations (Lee, 1993). A continuing relationship with someone who monitors the medicine, explains the monitoring, reinforces, supports, inquires, and encourages is key to studied adherence enhancement strategies. The managed care therapist can certainly fill this role.

Suicide Risk

An assessment of suicide risk is important in depression, particularly in major depression. Depressed patients are clearly more likely than nondepressed patients to attempt suicide and to complete it (Hirschfeld & Davidson, 1988). Factors such as hopelessness, male gender, Caucasian race, advanced age, and social isolation are statistical predictors of suicidal risk (Bent et al., 1988; Beck et al., 1985). Prior suicide attempts, a family history of suicide, and a family history of substance abuse also increase the risk of suicide attempts and completions. Psychosis, involvement with substances, and severe medical illnesses and chronic pain are other risk-enhancing factors. The presence of future plans, a patient's commitment and promise not to commit suicide, and a sense of meaning in a patient's life, as well as emotional attachments to other people or causes, tend to reduce the risk of suicide (Quinette, 1992).

Consistency of inquiry is helpful in assessing suicidal risk. Standardized procedures, such as structured interviews and computer-based questionnaires, are better at predicting suicidal risk than even trained and experienced clinicians because the structured procedures inquire about suicide with each and every patient (Beckham & Leber, 1985). Clinicians usually inquire only if depression seems severe or if the patient appears to be at some risk due to hints of suicide or indications of poor levels of functioning.

An additional variable may well be the fact that patients answer drug and alcohol questions, for example, more honestly on a computerized form than in a face-to-face interview with a clinician (Butcher, 1987). Consistency of inquiry with all who have major depressive illness will improve accuracy in predicting suicidal behavior.

Bipolar

Major depressive symptoms are to be assessed further. The distinction between a bipolar disorder and a major depressive disorder is the next step. A bipolar disorder refers to mood cycles with psychotic features or extremely retarded movement, and excessive highs that can last from several days to months. These highs are psychotic because they grossly violate social norms or because the behavior is no longer in concert with common sense to the point where it has disabled the patient. This disorder is less common than major depression, affecting perhaps one in a hundred people (APA, 1994). Some studies suggest that more than 20 percent of us experience a major depression at any one time (Kessler, 1994). The likelihood is that a patient will have a major depression and not a bipolar disorder. The implications for treatment are quite important. Different medicines and different strategies are appropriate in treating these different conditions.

Mania

With a bipolar disorder the feelings of elation and euphoria are quite intense. There is a diminished need for sleep, increased creativity and incisive thinking, and a great increase in activity. The patient's thoughts are more distractible and there is a flight of ideas. People report a pressure to keep talking, and they become overly talkative, typically exhibiting excessive and grandiose views of themselves and their present and future plans. They may be excessively involved in activities that give them pleasure but may have long-term painful consequences, such as sexual indiscretions, impulsive decisions regarding spending, socially unacceptable behavior, and excessive drug use. A clinician should look specifically for these symptoms, and not be satisfied with a patient's report of "mood cycles."

Unipolar

People with unipolar depression have mood cycles vary from depressed to normal. They may report that at times they feel elevated and expansive, when they are merely referring to feeling appropriately happy during those periods when they are not experiencing a recurrent depressive problem.

Bipolar Medications

If a bipolar disorder is present, differing medicine considerations come into play. Lithium carbonate is certainly one consideration, though not the panacea or cure for a bipolar disorder that some believe it to be. Studies have shown Lithium to be useful in 60 to 80 percent of cases. Carbamazepine, valproic acid, Resperidone, and Clozapine are useful mood stabilizers. Carbamazepine and valproic acid are both anticonvulsants; Resperidone and Clozapine are both antipsychotic medications. Carbamazepine or valproic acid are usually the first-line drugs for bipolar disease in adolescents (Winstead, 1994). Some with an accurately diagnosed bipolar disorder do not respond to mood-stabilizing medications (Nelsen & Dunner, 1993).

Although the research is a bit confusing given the variable reliability of clinical diagnoses and various ways of measuring depression, the difference between acute versus chronic problems, studies combining patients who have single episodes with those who have recurrent depression, and conditions that vary on the basis of severity, the research generally does show that there are different entities that should be treated differently. The major depressive disorders and the bipolar disorders demand consideration of medicines. To have some knowledge of resource and medicines is incumbent upon even the nonmedical psychotherapist.

Dysthymia

Some people are diagnosed as depressed when they have a more chronic and enduring depression called dysthymia, perhaps more often viewed as milder in degree as well as qualitatively distinct from major depression. To receive this diagnosis a patient must be in a depressed mood most of the time, more days than not, either by their reports or by other people's observations, for at least two years. When they are depressed, patients have some of the symptoms found in a major depression, such as poor appetite or overeating, sleep problems, diminished energy, poor concentration, and low self-esteem. There can be, however, no evidence of an unequivocal major depressive episode during the first two years of the disturbance.

The use of antidepressant medicines have a smaller role in treatment of dysthymic problems. Talking therapy is more effective. There is also a more minor variant of a bipolar disorder called a cyclothymic disorder. This, too, is best treated with talking therapy. For these conditions, talking therapy, behavioral or life changes, and other interventions are indicated.

The recurrence of depressions, whether they are unipolar or bipolar, is more common than not. Recurrent disorders of mood are best responded to differently than single-episode conditions. Recurrent major depressions indicate the need for continuing maintenance on antidepressants. The most recent study suggests that if a patient has a second occurrence of major depression, or is over fifty years old, he or she would do better if left on an antidepressant drug.

The possibility of a seasonal mood disorder is part of any history. Certain specialized light therapy treatments may be helpful with these conditions.

ECOLOGY OF THE PATIENT

The managed care therapist also assesses absence or presence of a patient's social supports. Involving family members and significant others certainly reinforces positive change. Recommendations for changes that are ecologically incompatible with the patient's current situation will be unlikely to occur. Involving a patient's spouse in treatment is usually quite worthwhile. Diagnosing a patient's skill repertoire is particularly helpful. Articulate and verbal patients make better use of certain cognitive forms of psychotherapy. Less intellectually skilled or schooled patients may require more directive treatment. The patient's strengths are assessed and used as building blocks in therapy: How has the patient maintained functioning heretofore? What has he or she done well? How can the current strengths, either still present or easily resurrected, serve as a fulcrum to add leverage to other life changes? What are the patient's enjoyable activities and social involvements? What is the patient's spiritual or religious focus? What is the patient's cultural background? Knowing the condition of the patient and the patient's context and situation is a prerequisite to further treatment.

Assessing the role of alcohol and substance abuse is important in treating any psychiatric condition, particularly disorders of mood. The Ecological Catchment Area studies (Helzer and Pryzbeck, et al, 1988) have found approximately a 5 percent rate of alcoholism. Most studies have found that alcoholism is an unlikely outcome of depression (Deykin, Levy, & Wells, 1987; Hasin, Read, et al, 1987). However, alcoholics do tend to become depressed over time, with studies finding between 10 and 30 percent of them also having some form of diagnosable mood disorder (Petty, 1992; Depression Guideline Panel, 1994). This suggests that the primary intervention for a substance-involved depressed patient might likely be behavioral efforts to effect abstinence. Once that is achieved the depression can be better evaluated.

FAMILY INVOLVEMENT

Even if a clinician is treating a depression as a biochemical condition, that condition exists in an individual who has specific skills and resources and lives within a certain social context. Mobilizing family resources to encourage treatment compliance in a way that does not embarrass or cause resistance makes it more likely that a patient will take medicines as prescribed. It is well to remember that the prescription of medicine does nothing. The patient must actually take the medicines for them to have a positive biochemical effect.

Monitoring suicidal risk, educating the patient about depressive symptoms to allow early detection of a recurrence, and monitoring major life decisions so that future choices are not minimized during a current depressive problem are important ingredients to the short-term treatment of any depression.

Family members brought into treatment as allies of the treatment team can help with these matters. The managed care therapist assesses many factors to manage improvement in the patient's depressive disorder, and family responses are one avenue for such data. Depression is significantly related to family distress. Relapse of depression is often preceded by marital discord (Bothwell & Weissman, 1977; Brown & Harris, 1978).

DIRECTIVE THERAPY

Treatment of depression in managed care is quite directive. The therapist is active in the treatment of depression, as much or more than with other clinical syndromes. Goals are cooperatively targeted by both the patient and the therapist after assessment of the condition, patient, and context. For example, the patient may be somewhat socially isolated with few social supports following a move to a new community. There may be a depressive condition that exceeds a mere adjustment reaction with depression following the move. There may even be a history of recurrent major depressive episodes.

Medicines might help with some depressive problems, although social withdrawal, often a component of depression, indicates increasing the patient's level of social interaction. Social support is important in reducing the risk and magnitude of depression. Deficits in social skills are frequently encountered in depressed patients. Attending to interpersonal skills is an important treatment consideration (Beach, Arias & O'Leary, 1983; Bellack, Hersen, & Himmelhoch, 1983; Lewisohn et al., 1984). Both social skills training and direct intervention programs for shyness are available as adjuncts to the treatment of depression (Zimbardo, 1982; Becker, Heimberg & Bellack, 1987).

GOAL ALIGNMENT

The patient and therapist target a goal, such as increasing social interaction, they create by cooperative game plan and strategy to help the patient to become more socially involved. Assessing a patient's social skill level might help decide which social opportunities are most likely to lead to reinforcement and continuation of social activity. For example, a patient who is not socially skilled might benefit from gradual involvement with other people through sharing a task such as a volunteer activity. A patient with a high level of social skills who has become depressed might do better in a more socially focused context, as with a church dinner.

The therapist directs treatment by guiding changes that might be ameliorative. However, patient cooperation is essential to achieving those changes. A well-formed intervention will likely lead to behavioral change. The patient's failure to make progress towards mutually chosen goals indicates that the strategy can be altered rather than seen as a failure on the patient's part. Recalling that therapy is always done *with* a patient, not *to* a patient, helps the therapist adopt a cooperative and mutual approach to treatment. The patient's perception of control over health-related matters is important in compliance, patient satisfaction, and therapeutic success (Barlow, Macy, & Struthers, 1993; Obrien, Petrie & Raeburn, 1992).

PHYSICAL ACTIVITY

An increase in physical activity is another goal to be mutually targeted. The therapist's skill will make consistent increases in physical activity more likely to occur and persist. Exercise often significantly reduces depression and anxiety (Byrne & Byrne, 1993; Gleser & Mendelberg, 1990; Rosscher, 1993). Exercise even enhances the effect and metabolism of antidepressant medicines (de Zwann, 1992).

The managed care therapist will realize the need for out of session therapy efforts and will be familiar with strategies for increasing patient adherence to behavior change strategies such as exercise programs. Some studies suggest that people are far more likely to start and maintain an exercise program if they participate with at least one other person known to them (Dishman, 1992; Martin & Dubbert, 1982; Spevak, 1982).

SOCIAL CONTRACT

The social contract encourages behavioral change (Obrien, Petrie, & Raeburn, 1992). This is particularly true with depressed patients. Involving family members in such things as an evening walk, with such commitment cooperatively made, will be far more potent as a directive strategy than merely advising a patient to "exercise for a half hour a day three times a week." The patient's selected goals will be effective to the extent that the therapist knows most likely and effective ways to achieve them (Bandura, 1977).

HOLISM

It is the therapist who will know the research that indicates that decreased assertiveness, limited risk-taking ability, social avoidance and loneliness, decreased physical activity, and behavioral habits that complicate sleep are all potential access points in a directive treatment of depression. Additional interventions abound in the research literature on depression. The managed care therapist considers various therapeutic interventions for the specific patient, choosing those most likely to succeed in a specific situation.

By considering various mechanisms to achieve targeted component goals that can help bring about a reduction in patient symptomatology, a therapist can delegate aspects of the therapy process. Many programs and life efforts effect therapeutic change. With accurate diagnoses and relevant information clearly and yet briefly communicated to primary medical care providers by nonmedical therapists, a quick assessment can be made and medicines appropriate for a patient's care can be provided. Medicines play a role in treatment provided by nonphysicians.

REFERRALS

The same is true with other resources, as well. A therapist may refer the patient for other interventions. As medicines supplement the ongoing therapy process, patients with mild or chronic depression profit from an assessment of their skills and deficits in assertiveness. Developing assertive skills through formal training may be a treatment emphasis (Coyne, 1976).

Assertiveness can be discussed in the therapy session. The patient also can be referred to assertiveness classes offered through community colleges, women's centers, churches and synagogues, or a variety of other social service agencies. These classes might be quite inexpensive, and perhaps more effective than individual instruction. Opportunity to practice assertiveness in a group situation furthers patient socialization and cooperation. Those who specialize in teaching such classes may be more effective than the individual practitioner.

Other programs can be seen as bringing about therapeutic benefit outside of the therapy context. Outward Bound programs show very positive results for a variety of people, including mildly depressed adolescents. Situations that offer physical exertion, team-based efforts, and the development of a sense of competency are beneficial with depression and are integral to wilderness survival classes. These programs promote a shift in the patient's perception of control from external to internal. The same is true with physical education and skill classes.

A situation in which a discouraged child is somewhat distant from his father might be improved by a car-repair class that father and adolescent son can take together. Parenting classes or support groups for parents of children with specific problems, such as attention deficit disorders, will provide skills to aid in the challenges with which they are confronted daily.

SELF-HELP PROGRAMS

Self-help programs such as Alcoholics Anonymous certainly have a role in treatment of dual disorders, as do specific programs for eating disorders and other behavioral and limited problems that may be combined with depression. (See Gould & Clum, 1993, and Powell & Cameron, 1991 for reviews of self-help programs in mental health treatment.) Marital enrichment classes reduce social isolation and strengthen attachment and ties between well-functioning adults who find some distance in their marriages. Self-help programs that follow the outline of Recovery Incorporated can be very beneficial even for those with chronic and severe disorders. Respite care programs for the aged provide help to family and others who are responsible for the care of the aging. Counseling that directly addresses the client's financial situation serves as a metaphor for dealing directly with other problems. This reduces the sense of helplessness that accompanies a patient whose financial fortunes are problematic. Massage helps those who have muscular tension and provides socially appropriate human contact. Self-defense classes enhance the feeling of power and protection for people who see themselves as vulnerable in a world full of danger.

SELF-DIRECTION

Considering a host of corrective alternatives, regardless of what they are, helps define a problem as solvable. They change the perception of a patient's problems to those that they can potentially control (Kanfer, 1977; Rehm, 1979). Many patients see their depression like the weather, something that they must merely suffer through but cannot affect or control. It is encouraging to explore with them various ways to build skills, solve problems, and generate new experiences that challenge their past ways of viewing themselves, their relationships, and their prospects. It is a statement that things can be different.

Viewing depression as having a behavioral component and indicating that a person can develop skills to change behavior changes the social role of the patient from medically ill to untrained. The implications for family relationships shift a patient's view of him- or herself and redefines how others in the family view him or her. Reduction in the subtle, inadvertent social reinforcement of depression by overly caretaking families may be altered by defining a patient's problems as a skill deficit rather than an illness. Behavioral and adjunctive programs may be more appropriate for milder than more chronic depressive problems, but they serve as a reminder that there are many paths up the mountain to patient change.

DIDACTIC SOURCES

Patient change also occurs through didactic information. Depression is a syndrome that can be explained to people. Such books as the U.S. Department of Health and Human Services' *Depression Is a Treatable Illness: A Patient's Guide* provide an inexpensive, understandable, and almost indisputable explanation of depression. Information of this type enhances compliance with medications, evokes cooperation with patients, and allows alternatives in explorations for further change. Self-help books and bibliotherapy are helpful in a variety of conditions with very little risk to a patient. Advice in books may be quite irrelevant to a patient's current circumstances, but the involvement in reading furthers hope in the patient. Bibliotherapy may be a powerful component to treatment (Quackenbush, 1991; Scogin, Jamison, & Davis, 1990; Wollersheim & Wilson, 1991). Recent research has indicated the importance of homework and bibliotherapy—there are over 300 references in the professional literature, almost all added within the last few years (PsychoInfo, APA, 1994).

Informing a patient about a clinical syndrome that can be explained and treated enhances the patient's sense of control over the disorder. Educational and didactic resources also reduce the sense of power-lessness and encourage a patient's perception of having control over life's satisfactions. Objective information explains his or her problems. This changes self-image from the passive patient to an active problem solver. Increasing the patient's participation and responsibility for thera-peutic gain enhances the success of any treatment process.

Didactic information on medicines is particularly helpful. Patients are alerted to the symptoms of depression and can recognize problems that recur after treatment. Compliance occurs with informed patients who actively participate in the decision to pursue medicines. Risk of side effects, drug misuse, and drug and alcohol interactions are mini-mized when patients understand risks and benefits. Understanding med-icines helps the patient develop realistic expectations that are more likely to be met, and discourages unrealistic expectations that may result in discontinuing the medicine.

MONITORING MEDICATION

Documentation requirements for quality assurance are combined with monitoring the effects of medicine. Rating scales that can be adminis-tered quickly and inexpensively provide better and more specific infor-mation on the effects of medicine than does a patient's more global and casual self-report (Faravelli, Albanesi, & Poli, 1986; Margo, Dewan, Fisher, & Greenberg, 1992). Such measures as the Symptom Checklist 90-Revised, by Dergotis (1975), provide a standardized measure to medi-cines used over time.

The Beck Depression Rating Scale (Beck et al, 1961) is another quick and consistent measure of change in depressive symptoms. Administer-ing questionnaires every other week for the first two months of treat-ment will provide trends in sign and symptom change. They help alert the clinician to possible suicidal risk that may have rekindled since intake. Specificity of response reduces halo affects. Questionnaires are a constant reminder that the treatment context is one that seeks improvement rather than merely discussion.

POSTTREATMENT

Subsequent letters and after-treatment responses from patients are very useful in time-limited care, and particularly when seeing patients for problems that may recur after posttreatment consultation (Beach, Arias, & O'Leary, 1983; Last, Thase, Hersen, Bellack, & Himmelhoch, 1985). Letters sent two and four months after treatment can be seen as something of a safety net for those who have improved to the point of discontinuing treatment, but who have had problems recur or found improvement to be brittle. Communicating with patients following treatment defines a continuance of the therapeutic relationship and reminds patients that a resource is available to help should the need arise. Information from former patients helps the clinician know what worked and what hindered, so that treatment might improve with others in the future.

BRIEF REPORTS

Documentation includes initial diagnosis, comments on useful and less effective interventions, problems encountered, and specific signs and symptoms. Limited and briefer reports sent to those who are cotreating a patient assists physicians with medication effectiveness and assures the appropriateness of a referral to specialized treatment programs. Records are historical documents. Patients with a depressive problem might be likened to those having a sprained ankle—the ankle, once injured, is more easily sprained again in the future. Knowledge of appropriate treatment and problems with treatment can help others who might later provide more treatment. To be effective, the report should be very brief and to the point. Longer reports are rarely read.

DELIMITING

Managed care is delimited. These limits are acknowledged from the outset. Some issues are best only diagnosed and not addressed given time limits. Discussion of emotionally charged historical issues is best deferred to another treatment context. Clinicians are well advised to maintain referral resources that provide treatment for more enduring problems for conditions not covered by this brief therapy.

TIME LIMITS

Time limits to treatment are integrated into initial treatment planning and are understood by both therapist and patient. If there is some thought that problems will persist over time and only a certain number of visits are authorized, it is often useful to save a few visits after the initial treatment. Titrating the contact over time, after a series of initial diagnostic and treatment planning sessions, will facilitate work with persistent problems. There is an increasing body of knowledge that even one visit can be of benefit even for major problems (Talmon, 1993). A series of individual and fairly autonomous consultations about an ongoing problem can be a viable model in a time-limited treatment context.

CONCLUSIONS

Managed care is here and it is different. It means alternative approaches to the treatment of depression. It does not necessarily mean that the therapeutic results will be different. Creativity and flexibility will allow for adaptation in this new environment. Patients can still get help and therapists can still help them, but the manner in which this is accomplished will be quite different. Different problems require different responses. Available contexts determine what approaches are possible. There is hope and there is possibility in managed care; the managed care system is designed to bring about change in patients. It will also promote behavioral change in those treating the patients.

REFERENCES

Abou-Saleh, M., & Coppen, A. (1983). Classification of depression and response to antidepressant therapies. *Br J Psychiatry, 143*, 601–603.

Adler, G., & Gattaz, W. (1993). Pain perception threshold in major depression. *Biological Psychiatry, 34*(10), 687–689.

Akiskal, H. (1985). A proposed clinical approach to chronic and "resistant" depressions: Evaluation and treatment. *J Clin Psychiatry, 46*, 32–36.

Allen, A., & Skinner, H. (1987). Lifestyle assessments using microcomputers. In J. Butcher (Ed.), *Computerized psychological assessment*. New York: Basic Books.

Altamura, A., & Mauri, M. (1985). Plasma concentrations, information and therapy adherence during long-term treatment with antidepressants. *Br J Clin Pharmacol, 20*(6), 714–716.

American Psychiatric Association (1987). *Diagnostic and statistical manual of mental disorders* (3rd ed., rev.). Washington, DC: American Psychiatric Association.

American Psychiatric Association (1994). *Diagnostic and statistical manual of mental disorders* (4th ed.). Washington, DC; American Psychiatric Association.

Amsterdam, J., Brunswick, D., & Mendels, J. (1980). The clinical application of tricyclic antidepressant pharmacokinetics and plasma levels. *Am J Psychiatry, 137*, 653–662.

Anthony, D. (1992). A retrospective evaluation of factors influencing successful outcomes on an inpatient psychiatric crisis unit. *Research on Social Work Practice,* 2(1), 56–64.

Bandura A. (1977). *Social learning theory.* Englewood Cliffs, NJ: Prentice-Hall.

Bant, W. (1978). Antihypertensive drugs and depression: A reappraisal. *Psychol Med, 8,* 275–283.

Barlow, J., Macy, S., & Struthers, G. (1993). Health locus of control, self-help and treatment adherence in relation to ankylosing spondylitis patients. Special issue: psychosocial aspects of rheumatic diseases. *Patient Education & Counseling, 20*(2–3), 153–166.

Barrett, J. E., Barrett, J. A., Oxman, T., & Gerber, P. (1988). The prevalence of psychiatric disorders in a primary care practice. *Arch Gen Psychiatry, 45,* 1100–1106.

Beach, S., Arias, I., & O'Leary, K. (1983). Risk for depression as a factor of social support. Paper presented at the Eastern Psychological Association, Philadelphia.

Beasley, C., Sayler, M., Cunningham, G., Weiss, A., & Masica, D. (1990). Fluoxetine in tricyclic refractory major depressive disorder. *J Affect Disord, 20,* 193–200.

Beck, A., Rush, A., Shaw, B., & Emery, G. (1979). *Cognitive therapy of depression.* New York: Guilford Press.

Beckham, E., & Leber, W. (1985). *Handbook of depression: Treatment, assessment, and research.* Homewood, IL: Dorsey Press.

Bellack, A., Hersen, M., & Himmelhoch, J. (1983). A comparison of social-skills training, pharmacotherapy and psychotherapy for depression. *Behav Res Ther, 21*(2), 101–107.

Berg-Cross, L., Jennings, P., & Baruch, R. (1990). Cinematherapy: Theory and application. 96th Annual Meeting of the American Psychological Association, Psychotherapy supervisions: professional and ethical issues (1988, Atlanta, GA). *Psychotherapy in Private Practice, 8*(1), 135–156.

Berndt, S., Maier, C., & Schutz, H. (1993). Polymedication and medication compliance in patients with chronic non-malignant pain. *Pain, 52*(3), 311–339.

Bielski, R., Major, J., & Rice, J. (1992). Phototherapy with broad spectrum white florescent light: A comparative study. *Psychiatry Research, 43*(2), 167–175.

Black, D., Bell, S., Hulbert, J., & Nasrallah, A. (1988). The importance of axis II in patients with major depression: a controlled study. *J Affect Disord, 14*(2), 115–122.

Blackburn, I., Bishop, S., Glen, A., Whalley, L., & Christie, J. (1981). The efficacy of cognitive therapy in depression: A treatment trial using cognitive therapy and pharmacotherapy, each alone and in combination. *Br J Psychiatry, 139,* 181–189.

Blackburn, I., Eunson, K., & Bishop, S. (1986). A two-year naturalistic follow-up of depressed patients treated with cognitive therapy, pharmacotherapy and a combination of both. *J Affect Disord, 10,* 67–75.

Blacker, C., & Clare, A. (1988). The prevalence and treatment of depression in general practice. *Psychopharmacology, 95,* 514–517.

Blazer, D. (1993). *Depression in later life.* St. Louis, MO: Mosby-YearBook.

Blumenthal, J., Williams, R., Wallace, A., Williams R. Jr., & Needles, T. (1982). Physiological and psychological variables predict compliance to prescribed exercise therapy in patients recovering from myocardial infarction. *Psychosom Med, 44*(6), 519–527.

Bosscher, R. (1993). Running and mixed physical exercises with depressed psychiatric patients. Special issue: Exercise and psychological well-being. *International Journal of Sport Psychology, 24*(2), 170–184.

Bothwell, S., & Weissman, M. (1977). Social impairments four years after an acute depressive episode. *Am J Orthopsychiatry, 47,* 231–237.

Bourin M., Kergueris, M., & Lapierre, Y. (1989). Therapeutic monitoring of treatment with antidepressants. *Psychiat J Univ Ottawa, 14,* 460–462.

Boza, R., Milanes, F., Hanna, S., Kaye, J., et al. (1989). Noncompliance in chronic depression: Assessment of serum antidepressant determination with the enzyme-innunoassay method. American Academy of Clinical Psychiatrists Meeting (1988, Seattle, WA). *Annals of Clinical Psychiatry, 1*(1), 43–49.

Bridges, K., & Goldberg, D. (1985). Somatic presentation of DSM-III psychiatric disorders in primary care. *J Psychosom Res, 29*(6), 563–569.

Broadhead, W., Blazer, D., George, L., & Tse, C. (1990). Depression, disability days, and days lost from work in a prospective epidemiologic survey. *JAMA, 246*(19), 2524–2528.

Buchanan, A. (1992). A two-year prospective study of treatment compliance in patients with schizophrenia. *Psychological Medicine, 22*(3), 787–797.

Burns, D., & Auerbach, A. (1992). Does homework compliance enhance recovery from depression? *Psychiatric Annals, 22*(9), 464–469.

Byrne, A., & Byrne, D. (1993). The effect of exercise on depression, anxiety and other mood states: A review. *Journal of Psychosomatic Research, 37*(6), 565–574.

Caillard, V. (1990). Syndromes depressifs et antidepresseurs [Depressive syndromes and antidepressants] *European Psychiatry, 5*(6), 355–362.

Cantwell, D. (1994). Depression in adolescents/comorbidity in mania. *Audio Digest, 23,*(9).

Cohn, J., & Wilcox, C. (1985). A comparison of fluoxetine, imipramine, and placebo in patients with major depressive disorder. *J Clin Psychiatry, 46*(3, Part 2), 26–31.

Conn, V., Taylor, S., & Kelley, S. (1991). Medication regimen complexity and adherence among older adults. *IMAGE: Journal of Nursing Scholarship, 23*(4), 231–235.

Coppen, A., Mendelwicz, J., & Kielholz, P. (1986). *Pharmacotherapy of depressive disorders: a concensus statement.* Geneva: World Health Organization.

Coulehan, J., Schulberg, H., Block, M., Janosky, J., & Arena, V. (1990). Medical comorbidity of major depressive disorder in a primary medical practice. *Arch Intern Med, 150,* 2363–2367.

Covi, L., & Lipman, R. (1987). Cognitive behavioral group psychotherapy combined with imipramine in major depression. *Psychopharmacol Bull, 23*(1), 173–176.

Dean, C., & Kendell, R. (1981). The symptomatology of postpartum illness. *Br J Psychiatry, 139,* 128–133.

Depression Guideline Panel (1994). *Depression in primary care: Detection, diagnosis, and treatment. Technical report Number 5.* Rockville, MD: U.S. Department of Health and Human Services, Public Health Services.

Deykin, E., Levy, J., & Wells, V. (1987). Adolescent depression, alcohol and drug abuse. *Am J Public Health, 77*(2), 178–182.

de Zwann, M. (1992). Exercise and antidepressant serum levels. *Biological Psychiatry, 32*(2), 210–211.

DiGiacomo, S. (1992). Metaphor as illness: Postmodern dilemmas in the representation of body, mind and disorder. Special issue: the application of theory in medical anthropology. *Medical Anthropology, 14*(1), 109–137.

Dishman, R. (1982). Compliance/adherence in health-related exercise. *Health Psychology, 1*(3), 237–267.

Dobgson, K. (1985). An analysis of anxiety and depression scales. *J Pers Assess, 49*(5), 522–527.

Dornseif, B., Dunlop, S., Potvin, J., & Wernicke, J. (1989). Effect of dose escalation after low-dose fluoxetine therapy. *Psychopharmacol Bull, 25*(1), 71–79.

Dorus, W., Kennedy, J., Gibbons, R., & Ravi, S. (1987). Symptoms and diagnosis of depression in alcoholics. *Alcoholism: Clin Exp Res, 11*(2), 150–154.

Draine, J., & Solomon, P. (1994). Explaining attitudes toward medication compliance among a seriously mentally ill population. *Journal of Nervous & Mental Disease, 182*(1), 50–54.

Duffy, J. F. (1994). Psychologist defends dispensing of prozac. *Psychiatric Times*. April, p. 50.

Dworkin, S., von Korff, M., & LeResche, L. (1990). Multiple pains and psychiatric disturbance. *Arch Gen Psychiatry, 47*, 239–244.

Eaton, W., Holzer, C. III, von Korff, M., Anthony, J., Helzer, J., George, L., Burnam, M., Boyd, J., Kessler, L., & Locke, B. (1984). The design of the Epidemiologic Catchment Area surveys. *Arch Gen Psychiatry, 41*, 942–948.

Eaton, W., Regier, D., Locke, B., & Taube, C. (1981). The Epidemiological Catchment Area Program of the National Institute of Mental Health. *Public Health Rep, 96*, 319–325.

Elixhauser, A., Eisen, S., & Romeis, J. (1990). The effects of monitoring and feedback on compliance. American Public Health Association Conference (1988, Boston, MA). *Medical Care, 28*(10, 882–893.

Elkin, I., Shea, T., Watkins, J., Imber, S., Sotsky, S., Collins, J., Glass, D., Pikonis, P., Leber W., Docherty, J., Fiester, S., & Parloff, M. (1989). National Institute of Mental Health Treatment of Depression Collaborative Research Program: General effectiveness of treatments. *Arch Gen Psychiatry, 46*, 971–982.

Endicott, J., & Spitzer, R. (1978). A diagnostic interview: The schedule for affective disorders and schizophrenia. *Arch Gen Psychiatry, 35*, 837–844.

Faravelli, C., Albanesi, G., & Poli, E. (1986). Assessment of depression: A comparison of rating scales. *Journal of Affective Disorders, 11*(3), 245–253.

Fawcett, J., Scheftner, W., Clark, D., Hedeker, D., Gibbons, R., & Coryell, W. (1987). Clinical prospective study. *Am J Psychiatry, 144*, 35–40.

Feldman, E., Mayou, R., Hawton, K., Ardern, M., & Smith, E. (1987). Psychiatric disorder in medical inpatients. *O J MED, 63*, 405–412.

Fingeret, M., & Schuettenberg, S. (1991). Patient drug schedules and compliance. *Journal of the American Optometric Association, 62*(6), 478–480.

Finnegan, D., & Suler, J. (1985). Psychological factors associated with maintenance of improved health behaviors in postcoronary patients. *Journal of Psychology*, *119*(1), 87–94.

Finney, J., Hook, R., Friman, P., Rapoff, M., et al. (1993). The overestimation of adherence to pediatric medical regimens. *Children's Health Care, 22*(4), 297–304.

Fishbain, D., Goldberg, M., Meagher, B., Steele, R., & Rosomoff, H. (1986). Male and female chronic pain patients categorized by DSM-III psychiatric diagnostic criteria. *Pain, 26* 181–197.

Frank, E., & Kepfer, D. (1987). Efficacy of combined imipramine and interpersonal psychotherapy. *Psychopharmacol Bull, 23*(1), 4–7.

Frank, E., Kupfer, D., Perel, J., Cornes, C., Jarrett, D., Mallinger, A., Thase, M., & Grochocinski, V. (1990). Three-year outcomes for maintenance therapies in recurrent depression. *Arch Gen Psychiatry, 47,* 1093–1099.

Frank, E., Perel, J., Mallinger, A., Thase, M., et al. (1992). Relationship of pharmacologic compliance to long-term prophylaxis in recurrent depression. 30th Annual Meeting of the American College of Neuropsychopharmacology (1991, San Juan, PR). *Psychopharmacol Bull, 28*(3), 231–235.

Gallagher, D., & Thompson, L. (1982). Treatment of major depressive disorder in older adult outpatients with brief psychotherapies. *Psychotherapy: theory, research, and practice, 19*(4), 482–490.

Gallagher, D., & Thompson, L. (1983). Effectiveness of psychotherapy for both endogenous and nonendogenous depression in older adult outpatients. *J Gerontol, 38*(6), 702–712.

Gallagher-Thompson, D., Hanley-Peterson, P., & Thompson, L. (1990). Maintenance of gains versus relapse following brief psychotherapy for depression. *J Consult Clin Psychol, 58*(3), 371–374.

Geiselmann, B., & Linden, M. (1991). Prescription and intake patterns in long-term and ultra-long-term benzodiazepine treatment in primary care practice. *Pharmacopsychiatry, 24*(2), 55–61.

Giblin, P. (1989). Use of reading assignments in clinical practice. *American Journal of Family Therapy, 17*(3), 219–228.

Giles, D., Jarrett, R., Biggs, M., Guzick, D., & Rush, A. (1989). Clinical predictors of recurrence in depression. *Am J Psychiatry, 146*(6), 764–767.

Gleser, J., & Mendelberg, H. (1990). Exercise and sport in mental health: a review of the literature. *Israel Journal of Psychiatry & Related Sciences, 27*(2), 99–112.

Goodwin, F., & Bunney, W., Jr. (1971). Depressions following reserpine: A re-evaluation. *Sem Psychiatry, 3*(4), 435–448.

Gould, R., & Clum, G. (1993). A meta-analysis of self-help treatment approaches. *Clinical Psychology Review, 13*(2), 169–186.

Green, P., Stiglin., Finkelstein, S., & Berndt, E. (1993). Depression: A neglected major illness. *Journal of Clinical Psychiatry, 54*(11), 419–424.

Greenberg, P., Stiglin, L., Finkelstein, S., & Berndt, E. (1993). The economic burden of depression in 1990. *Journal of Clinical Psychiatry, 54*(11), 405–418.

Gullick E., & King, L. (1979). Appropriateness of drugs prescribed by primary care physicians for depressed outpatients. *J Affect Disord, 1*(1), 55–58.

Guze, G., & Gitlin, M. (1994). New antidepressants and the treatment of depression. *Journal of Family Practice, 38*(1), 49–57.

Haley, W., Turner, J., & Romano, J. (1985). Depression in chronic pain patients: Relation to pain, activity, and sex differences. *Pain, 23,* 337–343.

Hall, R., Gardner, E., Stickney, S., LeCann, A., & Popkin, M. (1980). Physical illness manifesting as psychiatric disease: II. Analysis of a state hospital inpatient population. *Arch Gen Psychiatry, 37,* 989–995.

Hamilton, M. (1960). A rating scale for depression. *J Neurol Neurosurg Psychiatry, 23,* 56–62.

Hamilton, M. (1968). Development of a rating scale for primary depressive illness. *Br J Soc Clin Psychol, 6,* 278–296.

Hecht, H., von Zerssen, D., & Wittchen, H. (1990). Anxiety and depression in a community sample: The influence of comorbidity on social functioning. *J Affect Disord, 18,* 137–144.

Hill, M. (1992). Light, circadian rhythms, and mood disorder: A review. *Annals of Clinical Psychiatry, 4*(2), 131–146.

Hinkle, J. (1992). Aerobic running behavior and psychotherapeutics: Implications for sports counseling and psychology. *Journal of Sport Behavior, 15*(4), 263–277.

Holloway, R., Rogers, J., & Gershenhorn, S. (1992). Differences between patient and physician perceptions of predicted compliance. *Family Practice, 9*(3), 318–322.

Joffe, R., & Regan, J. (1988). Personality and depression. *J Psychiatr Res, 22,* 279–286.

Johnson, D. (1974). Study of the use of antidepressant medication in general practice. *Br J Psychiatry, 125,* 186–212.

Katon, W. (1987). The epidemiology of depression in medical care. *Int J Psychiatry Med, 17*(1), 93–112.

Katon, W. (1988). Depression: Somatization and social factors. *J Fam Pract, 27*(6), 579–580.

Katon, W., Kleinman, A., & Rosen, G. (1982). Depression and somatization: A review. Part I. *Am J Med, 72*(1), 127–135.

Katon, W., Ries, R., & Kleinman, A. (1984). Part III: a prospective DSM-III study of 100 consecutive somatization patients. *Compr Psychiatry, 25,* 305–314.

Katz, G., & Watt, J. (1992). Bibliotherapy: the use of books in psychiatric treatment. *Canadian Journal of Psychiatry, 37*(3), 173–178.

Kaufmann, C. (1993). Roles for mental health consumers in self-help group research. Special issue: Advances in understanding with self-help groups. *Journal of Applied Behavioral Science, 29*(2), 257–271.

Kearns, N., et al. (1982). A comparison of depression rating scales. *Br J Psychiatry, 141,* 45–49.

Kessler, L., Cleary, P., & Burke, J. (1985). Psychiatric disorders in primary care. *Arch Gen Psychiatry, 42,* 583–587.

Kessler, R., (1994). *Prevalence and comorbidity of major psychiatric disorders.* Ann Arbor: University of Michigan Survey Research Center.

Klerman, G., DiMascio, A., Weissman, M., Prusoff, B., & Paykel, E. (1974). Treatment of depression by drugs and psychotherapy. *Am J Psychiatry, 131*(2), 186–192.

Klerman, G., & Weissman, M. (1987). Interpersonal psychotherapy (IPT) and drugs in the treatment of depression. *Pharmacopsychiatry, 20,* 3–7.

Klerman, G., Weissman, M., Rounsaville, B., & Chevron, R. (1984). *Interpersonal psychotherapy of depression.* New York: Basic books.

Klingle, R. (1993). Bringing time into physician compliance-gaining research: Toward a reinforcement expectancy theory of strategy effectiveness. *Health Communication, 5*(4), 283–308.

Kornblith, S., Rehm, L., O'Hara, M., & Lamparski, D. (1983). The contribution of self-reinforcement training and behavioral assignments to the efficacy of self-control therapy for depression. *Cognitive Ther Res, 7*(6), 499–528.

Kovacs, M. (1981). Rating scales to assess depression in school-aged children. *Acta Paidopsychiatrica, 46*(5–6), 305–315.

Kovacs, M., Rush, A., Beck, A., & Hollon, S. (1981). Depressed outpatients treated with cognitive therapy or pharmacotherapy: A one-year follow-up. *Arch Gen Psychiatry, 38,* 33–41.

Kramlinger, K., Swanson, D., & Maruta, T. (1983). Are patients with chronic pain depressed? *Am J Psychiatry, 140*(6), 747–749.

Kroll, J., Linde, P., Habenicht, M., Chan, S., et al. (1990). Medication compliance, antidepressant blood levels, and side effects in Southeast Asian patients. *Journal of Clinical Psychopharmacology, 10*(4), 279–283.

Kupfer, D., Frank, E., & Perel, J. (1989). The advantage of early treatment intervention in recurrent depression. *Arch Gen Psychiatry, 46,* 771–775.

Kupfer, D., Frank, E., Perel, J., Cornes, C., Mallinger, A., Thase, M., McEachran, A., & Grochocinski, V. (1992). Five-year outcome for maintenance therapies in recurrent depression. *Arch Gen Psychiatry, 49* 769–773.

Large, R. (1986). DSM-III diagnoses in chronic pain. *J Nerv Ment Dis, 174*(5), 295–303.

Last, C., Thase, M., Hersen, M., Bellack, A., & Himmelhoch, J. (1985). Patterns of attrition for psychosocial and pharmacologic treatments of depression. *J Clin Psychiatry, 46*(9), 361–366.

Lee, C. (1992). Getting fit: A minimal intervention for aerobic exercise. *Behavior Change, 9*(4), 223–228.

Lee, S. (1993). The prevalence and nature of lithium noncompliance among Chinese psychiatric patients in Hong Kong. *Journal of Nervous & Mental Disease, 181*(10), 618–625.

Lehofer, M., Klebel, H., Gersdorf, C., & Zapotoczky, H. (1992). Running and motion therapy for depression. 7th Psychiatric Forum: Actual aspect of depression (1991, Salzburg, Austria). *Psychiatria Danubina, 4*(1–2), 149–152.

Lenkowsky, R. (1987). Bibliotherapy: A review and analysis of the literature. *Journal of Special Education, 21*(2), 123–132.

Lewisohn, P., Antonuccio, D., Steinmetz, J., & Teri, L. (1984). *The coping with depression course: A psychoeducational intervention for unipolar depression.* Eugene, OR: Castalia Press.

Lindsay, P., & Wyckoff, M. (1981). The depression-pain syndrome and its response to antidepressants. *Psychosomatics, 22*(7), 571–577.

Luke, D., Roberts, L., & Rappaport, J. (1993). Individual-group context, and individual-group fit predictors of self-help group attendance. Special issue: Advances in understanding with self-help groups. *Journal of Applied Behavioral Science,* 29(2), 216–238.

Lynch, D., Birk, T., Weaver, M., Gohara, A., et al. (1992). Adherence to exercise interventions in the treatment of hypercholesterolemia. *Journal of Behavioral Medicine, 15*(40), 365–377.

Magni, G., Schifano, F., & de Leo, D. (1985). Pain as a symptom in elderly depressed patients: Relationship to diagnostic subgroups. *Arch Psychiatr Neurol Sci, 235*(3), 143–145.

Magruder-Habib, K., Zung, W., Feussner, J., Alling, W., Saunders, W., & Stevens, H. (1989). Management of general medical patients with symptoms of depression. *Gen Hosp Psychiatry, 11* 201–206.

Mahalik, J., & Kivlighan, D. (1988). Self-help treatment for depression: Who succeeds? *Journal of Counseling Psychology, 35*(3), 237–242.

Malan, D. (1976). *The frontier of brief psychotherapy.* New York: Plenum Press.

Mann, J. (1973). *Time-limited psychotherapy.* Cambridge, MA: Harvard University Press.

Margo, G., Dewan, M., Fisher, S., & Greenberg, R. (1992). Comparison of three depression rating scales. *Perceptual & Motor Skills, 75*(1), 144–146.

Marsella, J., Hirschfeld, R., & Katz, M. (1987). *The measurement of depression.* New York: Guilford Press.

Martin, J., & Dubbert, P. (1982). Exercise and health: The adherence problem. *Behavioral Medicine Update, 4*(1), 16–24.

Maruta, T., Vatterott, M., & McHardy, M. (1989). Pain management as an antidepressant: Long-term resolution of pain-associated depression. *Pain, 36,* 335–337.

Marx, J., Gyorky, Z., Royalty, G., & Stern, T. (1992). Use of self-help books in psychotherapy. *Professional Psychology: Research and Practice, 23*(4), 300–305.

Matinsen, E., & Medhus, A. (1989). Adherence to exercise and patients' evaluation of physical exercise in a comprehensive treatment programme for depression. *Nordisk Psykiatrisk Tidsskrift, 43*(5), 411–415.

McLean, P., & Hakistian, A. (1979). Clinical depression: Comparative efficacy of outpatient treatments. *J Consult Clin Psychol, 47*(5), 818–836.

McLean, P., Ogston, K., & Grauer, L. (1973). A behavioral approach to the treatment of depression. *J Behav Ther Exper Psychiatry, 4,* 323–330.

Miklowitz, D. (1992). Longitudinal outcome and medication noncompliance among manic patients with and without mood-incongruent psychotic features. *Journal of Nervous & Mental Disease, 180*(11), 703–711.

Mintz, J., Mintz, L., Arruda, M., & Hwant, S. (1992). Treatments of depression and the functional capacity to work. *Arch Gen Psychiatry, 49*(10), 761–768.

Murphy, G., Simmons, A., Wetzel, R., & Lustman, P. (1984). Cognitive therapy and notriptyline, singly and together, in the treatment of depression. *Arch Gen Psychiatry, 41,* 33–41.

Myers, E., & Calvert, E. (1984). Information, compliance and side-effects: A study of patients on antidepressant medication. *Br J Clin Pharmacol, 17,* 21–25.

Myers, E., & Branthwaite, A. (1992). Out-patient compliance with antidepressant medication. *Br J Psychiatry, 160,* 83–86.

Neimeyer, R. & Feixas, G. (1990). The role of homework and skill acquisition in the outcome of group cognitive therapy for depression. *Behav Ther, 21,* 281–292.

Nezu, A. (1986). Efficacy of a social problem-solving therapy for unipolar depression. *J Consult Clin Psychol, 54,* 196–202.

Nezu, A., & Perri, M. (1989). Social problem-solving therapy for unipolar depression: an initial dismantling investigation. *J Consult Clin Psychol, 57*(3), 408–413.

NIMH Consensus Development Conference Statement. (1985). Mood disorders: Pharmacologic prevention of recurrences. *Am J Psychiatry, 142,* 469–476.

Norcross, J., Alford, B., & DeMichele, J. (1992). The future of psychotherapy: Delphi data and concluding observations. Special Issue: The future of psychotherapy. *Psychotherapy, 29*(1), 150–158.

Obrien, M., Petrie, K., & Raeburn, J. (1992). Adherence to medication regimens: updating a complex medical issue. *Medical Care Review, 49*(4), 435–454.

Oren, D., & Rosenthal, N. (1992). Seasonal affective disorders. In E. Paykel (Ed.), *Handbook of affective disorders (2nd ed, pp. 551–567).* London: Churchill Livingstone.

Pardeck, J. (1991). Using books in clinical practice. *Psychotherapy in Private Practice, 9*(3), 105–119.

Partonen, T., & Lonnqvist, J. (1993). Effects of light on mood. *Annals of Medicine, 25*(4), 301–302.

Partonen, T., Partonen, M., & Lonnqvist, J. (1993). Frequencies of seasonal major depressive symptoms at high latitudes. Special issue: Genetic epidemiology of psychiatric disorders. *European Archives of Psychiatry & Clinical Neuroscience, 243*(3–4), 189–192.

Perri, M., McAdoo, W., Spevak, P., & Newlin, D. (1984). Effect of a multicomponent maintenance program on long-term weight loss. *J Consult Clin Psychol, 52*(3), 480–481.

Powell, T. (1993). Self-help research and policy issues. Special issue: Advances in understanding with self-help groups. *Journal of Applied Behavioral Science, 29*(2), 151–165.

Powell, T., & Cameron, M. (1991). Self-help research and the public mental health system. *American Journal of Community Psychology, 19*(5), 797–805.

Prien, R., & Kupfer, D. (1986). Continuation drug therapy for major depressive episodes: How long should it be maintained? *Am J Psychiatry, 143,* 18–23.

Putnam, D., Finney, J., Barkley, P., & Bonner, M. (1994). Enhancing commitment improves adherence to a medical regimen. *J Consult Clin Psychol, 62*(1), 191–194.

Quackenbush, R. (1991). The prescription of self-help books by psychologists: A bibliography of selected bibliotherapy resources. *Psychotherapy, 28*(4), 671–677.

Rehm, L., (1979). *Behavior therapy for depression.* New York: Academic Press.

Rehm, L., Kaslow, N., & Rabin, A. (1987). Cognitive and behavioral targets in a self-control therapy program for depression. *J Consult Clin Psychol, 55*(1), 60–67.

Rehm, L., Kornblith, S., O'Hara, M., Lamparsky, D., Romano, J., & Volkin, J. (1981). An evaluation of major components in a self-control behavior therapy program for depression. *Behav Modif, 5,* 459–489.

Riordan, R., & Wilson, L. Bibliotherapy: Does it work? *Journal of Counseling & Development, 67*(9), 506–508.

Rosen, L., Targum, S., Teman, M., Bryant, M., Hoffman, H., Kasper, S., Hamovit, J., Docherty, J., Welch, B., & Rosenthal, N. (1990). Prevalence of seasonal affective disorder at four latitudes. *Psychiatry Res, 31,* 131–144.

Rosenthal, N., Levendosky, A., Skwerer, R., Joseph-Vanderpool, J., Kelly, K., Hardin, T., Kasper, S., DePlabela, P., & Wehr, T. (1990). Effects of light treatment on core body temperature in seasonal affective disorder. *Biol Psychiatry, 27,* 39–50.

Rude, S. (1986). Relative benefits of assertion or cognitive self-control treatment for depression as a function of proficiency in each domain. *J Consult Clin Psychol, 54*(3), 390–394.

Rush, A. (1986). Pharmacotherapy and psychotherapy. In L. Derogatis (Ed.), *Clinical psychopharmacology* (pp. 46–67). Menlo Park, CA: Addison-Wesley.

Rush, A. (1988). Cognitive approaches to adherence. In A. Frances & R. Hales (Eds.), *Annual review of psychiatry. Vol. 7* (pp. 625–640). Washington, DC: American Psychiatric Press.

Rush, A., Beck, A., Kovacs, M., & Hollon, S. (1977). Comparative efficacy of cognitive therapy and pharmacotherapy in the treatment of depressed outpatients. *Cognitive Ther Res, 1,* 17–37.

Scogin, F., Hamblin, D., & Seutler, L. (1987). Bibliotherapy for depressed older adults: A self-help alternative. *Gerontologist, 27*(3), 383–387.

Scogin, F., Jamison, C., & Davis, N. (1990). Two-year follow-up of bibliotherapy for depression in older adults. *J Consult Clin Psychol, 58*(5), 665–667.

Scogin, F., Jamison, C., & Gochneaur, K. (1989). Comparative efficacy of cognitive and behavioral bibliotherapy for mildly and moderately depressed older adults. *J Consult Clin Psychol, 57,* 403–407.

Scott, M., & Stadling, S. (1990). Group cognitive therapy for depression produces clinically significant reliable change in community-based settings. *Behav Psychother, 18,* 1–19.

Shaw, B., & Olmstead, M. (1989). *Competency ratings in relation to protocol adherence and clinical outcome.* Paper presented at the Society for Psychotherapy Research (1989, Toronto, Canada).

Shea, M., Glass, D., Pilkonis, P., Watkins, J., & Docherty, J. (1987). Frequency and implications of personality disorders in a sample of depressed outpatients. *J Pers Disord, 1,* 27–42.

Sherbourne, C., Hays, R., Ordway, L., DiMatteo, M., et al. (1992). Antecedents of adherence to medical recommendations: Results from the medical outcomes study. *Journal of Behavioral Medicine, 15*(5), 447–468.

Sluijs, E., & Knibbe, J. (1991). Patient compliance with exercise: Different theoretical approaches to short-term and long-term compliance. *Patient Education & Counseling, 17*(3), 191–204.

Smith, D., & Burkhalter, J. (1987). The use of bibliotherapy in clinical practice. *Journal of Mental Health Counseling, 9*(3), 184–190.

Snaith, P. (1993). What do depression rating scales measure? *Br J Psychiatry, 163,* 293–298.

Spaner, D., Bland, R., & Newman, S. (1994). Major depressive disorder. *Acta Psychiatrica Scandinavica, 89* (376, suppl), 7–15.

Spevak, P. (1982). A multi-strategy approach to the maintenance of personal fitness programs. *Dissertation Abstracts International, 42* (8-B), 3445.

Spevak, P., & Richards, C. (1980). Enhancing the durability of treatment effects: Maintenance strategies in the treatment of nail-biting. *Cognitive Therapy & Research, 4*(2), 251–258.

Spilker, B. (1992). Methods of assessing and improving patient compliance in clinical trials. *IRB: a review of human subjects research, 14*(3), 1–6.

Stein, P., & Motta, R. (1992). Effects of aerobic and nonaerobic exercise on depression and self-concept. *Perceptual & Motor Skills, 74*(1), 79–89.

Stoudemire, A., Frank, R., Hedemark, N., Kamlet, M., & Blazer, D. (1986). The economic burden of depression. *Gen Hosp Psychiatry, 8,* 387–394.

Strober, M. (1984). Familial aspects of depressive disorder in early adolescence. In E. Weller & R. Weller (Eds.), *Current perspectives on major depressive disorders in children* (pp. 38–48). Washington, DC: American Psychiatric Press.

Tannenbaum, L., & Forehand, R. (1994). Maternal depressive mood: The role of the father in preventing adolescent problem behaviors. *Behavior Research & Therapy, 32*(3), 321–325.

Teri, L., & Lewinsohn, P. (1986). Individual and group treatment of unipolar depression: Comparison of treatment outcome and identification of predictors of successful treatment outcome. *Behav Ther, 17,* 215–228.

Terman, M., Botticelli, S., Link, B., Link, M., Hardin, T., & Rosenthal, N. (1989). Seasonal symptom patterns in New York: Patients and population. In T. Silverton & C. Thompson (Eds.), *Seasonal affective disorder* (pp. 77–95). London: Clinical Neuroscience Publishers.

Terman, M., Williams, J., & Terman, J. (1991). Light therapy for winter depression: A clinician's guide. In. P. Keller (Ed.), *Innovations in clinical practice: A source book* (pp. 179–221). Sarasota, FL: Pro Resource.

Thompson, L., Gallagher, D., & Breckenridge, J. (1987). Comparative effectiveness of psychotherapies for depressed elders. *J Consult Clin Psychol, 55*(3), 385–390.

Trick, L. (1993). Patient compliance: Don't count on it! *Journal of the American Optometric Association, 64*(4), 264–270.

Tyler, S., & Brittlebank, A. (1993). Misdiagnosis of bipolar affective disorder as personality disorder. *Canadian Journal of Psychiatry, 38*(9), 587–589.

Uars, X., & Hoyt, M. (1992). The managed care movement and the future of psychotherapy. Special issue: The future of psychotherapy. *Psychotherapy, 29*(1), 109–118.

Udry, E. (1992). Interventions for the anxious and depressed: Suggested links between control theory and exercise therapy. *Journal of Reality Therapy, 12*(1), 32–36.

von Korff, M., Ormel, J., Katon, W., & Lin, E. (1992). Disability and depression among high utilizers of health care: A longitudinal analysis. *Arch Gen Psychiatry, 49,* 91–100.

Walker, E., Katon, A., Harrop-Griffiths, J., Holm, L., Russo, J., & Hickok, L. (1988). Relationship of chronic pelvic pain to psychiatric diagnoses and childhood sexual abuse. *Am J Psychiatry, 145*(1), 75–80.

Warner, R. (1991). Bibliotherapy: A comparison of the prescription practices of Canadian and American psychologists. *Canadian Psychology, 32*(3), 529–530.

Wegner, G. (1993). The information of social networks: Self-help, mutual aid, and old people in contemporary Britain. *Journal of Aging Studies, 7*(1), 25–40.

Weissman, M. (1979). The psychological treatment of depression: Evidence for the efficacy of psychotherapy alone, and in comparison with, and in combination with pharmacotherapy. *Arch Gen Psychiatry, 36,* 1261–1269.

Weissman, M., & Myers, J. (1978). Affective disorders in a U.S. urban community: The use of Research Diagnostic Criteria in an epidemiologic study. *Arch Gen Psychiatry, 35,* 1304–1311.

Weissman, M., & Myers, J. (1980). Psychiatric disorders in a U.S. urban community: The application of Research Diagnostic Criteria to a re-surveyed community sample. *Acta Psychiatr Scand, 62,* 99–111.

Weitzler, K., Strauman, J., & Dubro, A. (1989). Diagnosis of major depression by self-report. *J Pers Assess, 53*(1), 22–30.

Weller, E., & Weller, R. (1990). Depressive disorders in children and adolescents. In B. Garfinkel, G. Carlson, & E. Weller (Eds.), *Psychiatric disorders in children and adolescents* (pp. 3–20). Philadelphia: W. B. Saunders.

Wells, K., Stewart, A., Hays, R., Gurman, M., Rogers, W., Daniels, M., Berry, S., Greenfeld, S., & Ware, J. (1989). The functioning and well-being of depressed patients: Results from the Medical Outcomes Study. *JAMA, 262*(7), 914–919.

Willenbring, M. (1986). Measurement of depression in alcoholics. *J Stud Alcohol, 47*(5), 367–372.

Winstead, D. (1994). Resperidone and clozapine. *Audio Digest, 23,* (10).

Wolbert, L. (1967). *Short-term psychotherapy.* New York: Grune & Stratton.

Wollersheim, J., & Wilson, G. (1991). Group treatment of unipolar depression: A comparison of coping, supportive, bibliotherapy, and delayed treatment groups. *Professional Psychology: Research & Practice, 22*(6), 496–502.

Woody, J. (1990). Clinical strategies to promote compliance. *American Journal of Family Therapy, 18*(3), 285–294.

Youssel, F. (1983). Compliance with therapeutic regimens: A follow-up study for patients with affective disorders. *J Adv Nurs, 8,* 513–517.

Zapotocsky, H. (1992). Psychotherapy of depression. 7th Psychiatric Forum: Actual aspect of depression (1991, Salzburg, Austria). *Psychiatria Danubina, 4*(1–2), 141–143.

Zisook, S., & Shuchter, S. (1991). Depression through the first year after the death of a spouse. *Am J Psychiatry, 148*(10), 1346–1352.

Zoega, T., Barr, C., & Barsky, A. (1991). Prediction of compliance with medication and follow-up appointments. *Nordisk Psykiatrisk Tidsskrift, 45*(1), 27–32.

Zung, W. (1969). A cross-cultural survey of symptoms in depression. *Am J Psychiatry, 126*(1), 116–121.

11

The Managed Care of Anxiety Disorders

DAVID A. GROSS, M.D.
ANDREW ROSEN, Ph.D.

INTRODUCTION TO MENTAL HEALTH CARE IN THE DECADE OF THE BRAIN

The Challenges of Managed Mental Health Care

Health care reform has been fueled by the economics of a triad between technology, business, and geographic mobility. *Technology* has enabled medical advances to prolong life and attenuate the morbidity of disease. However, the price tags attached have become burdensome. For one, the machinery of medicine, including devices, diagnostic apparatuses, and pharmaceuticals, has paralleled the growth and cost of the automobile industrial revolution.

Another simultaneous burden has been created by the psychological impact on the person in the street of the seemingly magical scientific advances made by medicine. Attitudes and belief systems have changed; fatalistic determinism has given way to the free will fostered by organized medicine. The latter refers to the public's perception and expectation that if we can land a person on the moon, transplant hearts, and alter genes, we (the medical community) can do anything if we put our minds to it. All we need to do is to try hard enough. Previously accepted limitations of medical treatment are no longer satisfactory. The public wants more, expects more, and only now realizes that it cannot pay for it. The medical superman fantasy pervades our hospitals, where individuals in the end stages of their disease are kept alive in intensive care units to prolong their lives for months if not weeks. The unconscious wish is for the magic of medicine to do its thing and produce a cure. This attitudinal process may be an even more powerful force than the costly nuts and bolts of equipment because it keeps the pressure on, requiring expensive intervention and a "never say no" mentality. Therein lies the dilemma—an expectation of greatness in an economic environment that will not pay for it.

The second triad member, *business,* is more straightforward and simply stated. The economic forces of a free market society drive a profit motive. The technological breakthroughs described in the preceding paragraph allow for a shift in health care from a labor intensive industry to one dominated by goods (pharmaceuticals), devices (pacemakers, for example) and procedures (diagnostic or therapeutic). What war can do to stimulate the military industrial complex, scientific breakthroughs and progress have done for medicine. Good and bad have emerged from this; managed competition hopes to resolve the bad. Let us hope that managed competition does not lead to costly managed bureaucracies.

Geographic mobility is the final member of the triad. Mass transportation and electronic multimedia communication have irrevocably altered the vocational climate in this country. Americans are no longer staying in one community or even one state. Corporations have multistate locations. Whereas the generalist (the family physician) undertook much of basic medical care in the past, traveling to a specialist is simple these days. Hospitals and specialists have multiplied and populated industrial areas so that travel is rarely needed. Insurance plans have to service members in various areas with different costs and medical needs. The result has been the development of a very sophisticated and effective health care system. But can we afford it? Do we dare not afford it?

The challenge posed to the grassroots clinician can be stated quite simply. We either maintain business as usual and adjust to actuaries and administrators, or we proactively adjust our model to meet the needs of the twenty-first century. The former option most probably will lead to fragmented and inadequate care because of the cost, the dilution of the quality and quantity of mental health professionals, and the clinical inefficiency of a model dictated by numbers and quotas. The latter plan provides an opportunity, a chance to take inventory of what we do and how we do it and to determine what changes are necessary so that we can meet the fiscal and moral needs of the populace.

All participants in the health care reform drama have agreed that there are three mandatory guidelines for any new delivery system: *quality of care, universal access to care,* and *cost containment.* Mental health professionals would add that access to care requires that treatment of psychiatric disease be included in any new system.

The Importance of the Multimodality/Discipline Treatment Plan

It is clear that the greatest fiscal liability risks reside in open-ended psychotherapy and inpatient hospitalization for the mentally ill. The anxiety disorders provide an excellent backdrop for the application of managed mental health care. These disorders lend themselves to discrete treatment protocols once a diagnosis is made.

Judicious pharmacotherapy and time-limited cognitive-behavior therapy are extraordinarily efficacious in the anxiety disordered patient. It is, therefore, possible to tailor a treatment plan for each patient and maximize recovery. Intensive multimodality therapies will be more cost-effective than a prolonged single modality treatment. If the cost savings from rapid return to work, family, and general functioning are factored into this, the benefits are clear.

This approach also takes the mystery out of treatment for our patients. This is made possible through an emphasis upon education and patient participation. Cognitive-behavioral and specific pharmacotherapies permit our patients to actively enter into the therapeutic alliance and honestly take ownership of their illness. Stigma is reduced and wellness emphasized. Placebo response is heightened, and because there is a biological basis for placebo response, (Levine, Gordon, & Fields, 1978), this may be an integral part of treatment.

ANXIETY DISORDERS: PSYCHOLOGICAL PERSPECTIVES

Introduction

The diagnosis and treatment of anxiety has gone through a long, complicated evolution. In 1917, Freud stated, "One thing is certain, that the problem of anxiety is a nodal point, linking up all kinds of most important questions; riddle of which the solution must cast a flood of light upon our whole mental life," (Freud, 1938). This statement reflected his belief that anxiety both reflected major underlying psychological problems and also caused pervasive psychosocial problems. Assessment of the cause of the anxiety symptoms was very complicated and often took many weeks or months. Treatment usually required many hours each week for many months or years. Psychoanalysis as an understanding of the mind and as a treatment method included many schools of thought and approaches. All of these schools had in common a general view that anxiety was a symptom of a much greater psychological difficulty and that the cure of the anxiety symptoms would involve in most cases either a major overhaul of the personality or a remembering and working through of a traumatic childhood event. Suffice it to say that curing anxiety involved a very complicated, long, and ultimately very costly process.

In the 1950s and 1960s other methods were developed to treat anxiety. Following the somewhat problematic past use of barbiturates (for example, phenobarbital), minor tranquilizers such as meprobamate (Miltown), diazepam (Valium), and chlordiazepoxide (Librium) were introduced to aid in the treatment of neurotic anxiety. Unfortunately, these agents were prescribed with limited attention to a treatment plan that included dosage and duration of use. Unfortunately, many individuals became physically and psychologically dependent on these agents and rarely did they receive ongoing psychotherapy to help resolve anxiety or its etiologies. If these individuals eventually did seek psychological treatment they were often not helped to any significant degree, and they frequently would remain dependent upon these medications.

In the 1970s, nonpharmacologic treatment methods were developed that have been proven to be quite efficacious. *Behavior therapy* and *cognitive therapy* models have offered clear models exploring the diathesis of anxiety and also developing more focused and effective treatment methods. These models involve a short-term approach geared to symptomatic improvement without reliance on resolution of unconscious conflicts or personality revision. Outcomes research has revealed very favorable data, suggesting that anxiety disorders can be treated effectively utilizing a focused structured model.

The successful treatment of anxiety disorders requires a careful assessment of the type of anxiety present and a determination of any other psychiatric or medical diagnoses. Very often, a person who presents with the chief complaint of anxiety will have more than one type of anxiety disorder. For instance, a patient may complain of panic attacks and fit the *Diagnostic and Statistical Manual of Mental Disorders, 4th edition* diagnosis of *panic disorder* but also may have an *obsessive-compulsive disorder* about which he or she may not openly complain (DSM-IV, APA, 1994). The person who has *generalized anxiety disorder* may also have a *social phobia* that is just as debilitating, but he or she may not complain about it. It is also very important that the clinician carefully evaluate the presence of other psychiatric problems, including personality disorder and chemical dependency and alcohol abuse. Very often anxiety disorder patients do have addiction problems because these people have discovered that drugs and alcohol can decrease anxiety temporarily. If the clinician does not appreciate this, treatment will not work.

Patients sometimes turn out to have medical problems, such as thyroid dysfunction, which can cause anxiety-like symptoms. Unfortunately, many patients with underlying anxiety disorders have not seen their family physicians in some time; often the psychological dynamics that interfere with their getting help for their psychological problems also shield them from medical scrutiny. However, patients who find their way to an anxiety disorders treatment center often have been medically evaluated several times prior to their initial psychological presentation, including the use of expensive and sometimes intrusive or invasive testing.

Anxiety disorders treatment centers have found that a thorough initial assessment is critical. This writer utilizes the Barlow Anxiety Disorders Interview Schedule-Revised (ADIS-R) (Barlow, 1988). The ADIS-R helps the clinician who suspects the presence of an anxiety disorder determine the type of anxiety disorder and determine the severity of symptoms utilizing a built-in Hamilton Anxiety Scale (Hamilton, 1959). It objectively rates the patient's type of anxiety symptoms as well as depressive symptoms (using the Hamilton Depression Scale) (Lyerly, 1973). In addition to assessing the type of anxiety disorder (panic disorder, agoraphobia, simple phobia, social phobia, obsessive-compulsive disorder, posttraumatic stress disorder, and generalized anxiety disorder), it evaluates the presence of affective disorders such as major depressive episodes, dysthymic disorder, mania and cyclothymic disorder. There is also a screen for alcohol and drug abuse and psychosis, as well as somatoform disorder. The ADIS-R can be administered in one hour and will provide a very thorough assessment of the patient's anxiety problems as well as any other relevant diagnoses. Based on the outcome of the ADIS-R, the clinician can readily formulate a sound treatment plan.

Psychological Treatment Overview

When utilizing a cognitive-behavioral approach for the treatment of anxiety disorders, the clinician generally can expect to see therapeutic gain within six to eight weeks and in general treatment should be completed within 20 weeks. Follow-up care in the form of aftercare support groups and/or individual periodic follow-up sessions can last for up to a year. While the specific treatment plan for each anxiety disorder type may vary significantly, the cognitive-behavior therapy approach has some basic tenets that apply to all anxiety types. The core concept is that all anxiety has three components: (a) physiological, (b) cognitive and (c) behavioral. Utilizing the cognitive therapy approach, the clinician can impact on these three anxiety components, thereby reducing symptoms. Thus, by teaching a patient to do relaxed breathing and progressive muscle relaxation techniques, the clinician can significantly reduce anxiety symptoms such as hyperventilation, shortness of breath, dizziness, palpitations or tachycardia, trembling, sweating, choking, nausea or abdominal distress, numbness or paresthesias, and depersonalization or derealization. By being able to reduce these symptoms, the patient can feel more at ease physically and gain acceptance that he or she actually can control the symptoms voluntarily. Second, the cognitive therapy focuses on helping the patient reduce the catastrophic thinking and excessive worrying and negative self-statements that generate anxiety, mentally and physically. Third, the behavior therapy focuses on issues such as helping the agoraphobic return to such previously avoided activities as driving or going to the supermarket or restaurants. Behavior therapy is also utilized in treating obsessive-compulsive disorder, for instance, by utilizing exposure response prevention techniques.

Panic Disorder and Agoraphobia Treatment

Utilizing David Barlow's panic control treatment program (Barlow, 1989), the clinician can rely on this structured cognitive-behavior therapy program to first educate the patient about panic disorder and agoraphobia in a very clear, comprehensive way. The patient is then taught how to monitor his or her own symptoms in an objective way and how to chart progress. Next, the patient is taught relaxed breathing techniques and progressive muscle relaxation techniques. The patient then is taught how to monitor the self-statements that are the stimulus for anticipatory anxiety and is also taught how to reduce or counteract these self-statements. Next, the patient is helped to get voluntary control over panic anxiety symptoms and finally to overcome the agoraphobia by gradual guided exposure to the feared events or places. Treatment usually requires 20 weeks and is supplemented by an anxiety support group. This model can be applied to individual or group modalities.

Generalized Anxiety Disorder Treatment

Also utilized is David Barlow's treatment program for generalized anxiety disorder treatment (GAD) called "Master of Your Own Anxiety and Worry" (Barlow, 1992). This program emphasizes methods of provoking and learning to control the worry process and associated symptoms of anxiety, incorporating education, cognitive therapy, and behavior therapy. The basic method is to help the patient understand how excessive and needless worrying, which is based on "what if" thinking, causes a person to gradually experience the world as a placed filled with danger and negative, even catastrophic events. The techniques that are offered to help the patient develop a new cognitive map that helps to reduce the what if process and generally see the world for what it is objectively, rather than go through the lens of anxious distortion. A person is helped objectively to assess the likelihood of a particular negative event's happening and to become a better problem-solver instead of a worrier.

Social Phobia Treatment

The cognitive-behavior therapy approach for social phobia involves first helping the patient change the thinking process related to the social anxiety and then behaviorally engaging the various social situations that have provoked the anxiety and overcoming the avoidance and anxiety. For instance, if a patient avoids going to staff meetings because he or she has an intense fear of embarrassing him- or herself by looking nervous, the patient is first helped to identify his or her negative self-statements such as "It would be awful if I looked scared" or "People would really laugh at me if I looked shaky." After identifying these statements, the patient is helped to challenge the accuracy and likelihood of this happening and replacing these negative statements with more rational and likely statements. After the cognitive treatment is well under way, the patient is encouraged to go into the feared or avoided social situations and challenge these negative thoughts. In addition, very often relaxation techniques are taught that help the patient to feel less physiologically anxious. Gradually a person can engage in social situations without significant anxiety.

Obsessive-Compulsive Disorder Treatment

Behavior therapy has been demonstrated repeatedly to be the most efficacious nonpharmacological treatment modality for obsessive-compulsive disorder (OCD). New research has even demonstrated that patients who have pretreatment positron emission tomography (PET) scans with an OCD profile can have their PET scans revert to normal after receiving only behavior therapy. The primary method utilized in behavior therapy for OCD is called exposure and response prevention. Whether it is to reduce obsessions, compulsions, or both, the patient is helped to expose him- or herself to the feared situation and prevent the usual response. For example, if a patient has contamination fears and as a result washes his hands for 10 minutes at a time every time he shakes someone's hand, he will be asked to shake the hands of people in the office, for instance, without washing his own, or maybe even to eat a sandwich without washing. The idea is to show the patient that he can fight off the irrational idea that causes the anxiety that causes the compulsion. Behavior therapy has been a very successful technique for OCD and generally requires only short-term treatment. Then the patient can be instructed to continue to use the learned techniques on his or her own and may need to come for follow-up appointments once in a while.

ANXIETY DISORDERS: PSYCHOPHARMACOLOGIC PERSPECTIVES

When to Use Medication

As the database and technology available to study the human nervous system develops, it has become clear that the subjective experience (signs and symptoms) of anxiety disorders represents the participation of biological events (Klein, 1964). The mind-body dichotomy (Gross, 1981) has been resolved with the conclusion that the mind resides within the brain and the two are one and the same. Human mental activity as expressed in behavior, affect, and thought (language) represents biochemical actions at the synapse and the transmission of electrical energy through neuronal networks. If this represents the usual state of affairs, aberrant manifestations of the mental state must reflect abnormal changes in neuronal chemistry and/or electricity (Gross, 1990).

Although the history of psychiatry and the anxiety disorders is replete with psychodynamic underpinnings, the evolution of the field has produced a more balanced multisystem (biopsychosocial) approach. As it is for many diseases in medicine, biological substrates represent key variables in illness expression. There are several nonmutually exclusive models to explain the development of anxiety disorders utilizing a biopsychosocial approach:

1. **Programmed Genome Model.** This is the biological clock model that assumes that a genetic (biological) cause exists and expresses itself at some particular chronological age. Hence, the age of onset data available for the various types of anxiety disorders (Von Korft, Eaton, & Keyl, 1985).

2. **Permissive Diathesis Model.** This model incorporates a genetic permissive biological factor that in and of itself would not precipitate the development of anxiety states. This factor permits the expression of pathology when an external (e.g., life crisis or trauma) or internal (e.g., coincident viral infection, pharmacologic agents, metabolic derangement) variable is present. Examples abound: (a) the biologically (genetic) predisposed woman who has her first panic attack after receiving novocaine with epinephrine in the dentist's office, or (b) the onset of panic disorder coincident to the development of hyperthyroidism (overactive thyroid leading to autonomic overload) that persists after the thyroid returns to normal with treatment, or (c) panic disorder that can be traced back to a marijuana reaction.

3. **Stress Diathesis Model.** Posttraumatic stress disorder (PTSD) may reveal itself as a psychobiological archetype for this model. Repetitive (or pathologically severe enough) isolated events lead to enduring brain changes that may surface years later in dissociative anxiety states (Post, 1992). The plasticity of the brain (especially the limbic system) is well known and makes this model heuristically very important (Post, 1976). The neuropathological changes that underlie the engrammatic biological effects of such psychological trauma remain to be determined, but the recognition of such changes has represented a major attitudinal advance.

Psychotropic medications are, therefore, an important and sometimes critical component of anxiety disorder therapy. These agents have both palliative (symptomatic relief) and remedial purposes.

Case Example: A 28-year-old woman, a success in business, with incapacitating generalized anxiety disorder whose mental state has interfered with eating and sleeping, discovers that she can begin to return to some level of function with the judicious use of an anxiolytic (antianxiety) agent. Because of symptomatic relief, she has now started focused time-limited psychotherapy dealing with the psychodynamic and cognitive-behavioral foundations of her disorder.

Case Example: A 35-year-old male business executive is about to be demoted because of his inability to attend conferences and make presentations. He is seen in consultation and started on the mono-amine oxydase inhibitor phenelzine, an effective treatment for social phobia.

Case Example: A well-known entertainer has curtailed concert engage-ments and retreated to the safety of a recording studio because of performance anxiety. No underlying nonpsychiatric medical causa-tion was found and a beta blocker trial ensued. Even after the disap-pearance of somatic (autonomic) symptoms, he had to contend with persistent psychic anticipatory anxiety and remained functionally limited. A course of cognitive-behavioral therapy ensued and allowed for complete recovery.

How to Use Medication

The importance of rapid diagnosis and the efficient establishment of a treatment plan, multimodality when appropriate, were reviewed pre-viously. With the decision to pursue a psychopharmacologic trial, the critical variable becomes treatment outcome. Positive response to medi-cation is the goal but there are several factors that can complicate psychopharmacologic intervention.

Medication noncompliance is one of the major problems encoun-tered in evaluating outcome. Noncompliance generally comes from one of two sources: Before a prescription is filled, noncompliance can already have taken a foothold. Patients' attitudes about treatment and illness are the culprit much of the time. Denial of illness, desire to be perfect, "I'll feel better if I just pull myself out of this," "I'm panicking over nothing and need to just stop this nonsense," and "I can't let anyone know I have a mental illness" are all examples. Stigma comes from lack of knowledge and fear. Therefore, writing a prescription is not sufficient. The task is complete only when there exists a doctor-patient alliance and there has been a dose of *pharmacologic psychotherapy.* The latter occurs when the psychopharmacologist spends time with the patient exploring several areas, including:

1. Current attitudes and belief systems regarding anxiety complaints/psychiatric disorders.
2. Past experience (if any) with psychotropic drugs.
3. What does the patient think medication will do or not do?

4. Addiction fears ("Is this going to turn me into a drug addict, Doc?").
5. Medication-induced confrontation of denial ("If I have to take a medication there really must be something wrong with my head").
6. Locus of control issues ("Will this medicine control me and will I ever regain control over myself . . . will I have to take it forever?").

The psychotherapeutic goal is to help patients recognize that by giving themselves permission to be sick and suffer from a biological problem, they can then give themselves permission to recover.

Patient empowerment is a critical component of any managed care initiative. After all, the core alliance in this model is the one with the patient, the provider, and the administrative entity (insurance company, managed care company). The "Sy Syms School"* of service providers would rightly claim that "an educated consumer is our best customer." Our patients need not only to know that they are sick, but to understand the cause of the malady, what course their illness would take without treatment, and how, what, and when medication can be helpful. The ultimate goal is to have a patient state without stigma or guilt that "I am sick, that is okay and a part of life, and treatment is safe and can make me better." That patient will be empowered to call the medication prescribed "my medication" and, therefore, it is worth his or her while to take this medicine responsibly as ordered. These are the patients who tolerate side effects better and become an active part of the treatment team with the clinician. Interestingly, when placebo response plays a role in treatment outcome, these patients seem to maximize this component as well. The clinician's honesty and openness about illness and treatment speeds the development of the therapeutic alliance. Spending the extra time (not extra treatment visits) with the patient covering the above issues always results in a win–win result.

So far, we have touched on the selection of medication based on the type of anxiety disorder and reviewed the art (psychotherapy) of prescribing. The choice of a particular medication trial also depends on a consideration of the balance between therapeutic response and nontherapeutic side effects. A medication can cause patient noncompliance no matter how effective it is in eliciting symptomatic remission when side effects overshadow all gains. We certainly don't want to create symptoms that are as intolerable as the presenting complaints. Side effects can be attenuated by the addition of another agent.

---

*Sy Syms—a clothing retailer that advertises the value of educating customers about the product purchased to improve business.

For example, some of the antidepressants used in the treatment of panic disorder (e.g., selective serotonin re-uptake inhibitors) may be too activating, requiring the addition of a central nervous system depressant, a benzodiazepine, during the day or at night for insomnia. This is, in fact, fairly standard accepted practice. However, one could argue that the need to add on another drug to combat the primary drug side effect must be disconcerting to the patient and adversely affect compliance. Therefore, prudence demands that the psychotropic agent chosen have as benign a side effect profile as possible for the patient. The patient's age, weight, medical problems (especially hepatorenal function, cardio-cerebrovascular status, and central nervous system pathology), other medications taken, and activity limitations (i.e., will medication effect have an impact on job performance or driving) must all be considered.

Each patient deserves his or her own unique prescription of medication based on these variables. A clinician should record whether or not the patient has had past experiences with psychotropic agents and what these experiences were. Commonly, there is a past history of a problematic reaction to another psychotropic agent that had made the patient gun shy to the medication currently being recommended, even if the latter has no chance of causing such adverse effects. Openly discussing with the patient the pros and cons of the agents prescribed actively helps the patient reason through the risk–benefit assessment involved in making this recommendation. This allows patients to feel that they are making the medication decision along with the therapist, and this helps to empower their recovery.

The final necessary component before launching a medication trial requires that the therapist enlist the patient's help in developing an inventory of three to five *target symptoms.* Target symptoms are clearly defined, objective illness signs that the patient can track during the medication trial. Examples include sleep, energy level, ruminative thinking, anticipatory anxiety, avoidant behavior (be specific), loss of appetite, pounding heart, restlessness, and so on. The use of target symptoms also contributes to the patient empowerment noted previously, and it goes a long way to foster the doctor–patient team.

A subjective clinical improvement scale can also be helpful. Ask the patient to use a 0 to 10 scale to rate his or her subjective state of health and develop a ratio with 10 always the denominator. Zero reflects no malady—the patients feels well—and 10 reflects the worst he or she could feel with their illness. Pre-, inter-, and posttreatment ratings can be very enlightening and valuable as therapeutic response is monitored.

The Medication Trial

The cardinal rule in maximizing any psychopharmacologic trial is the provision that the medication must be taken for a therapeutic period at an effective dosage. Steady state plasma (blood compartment) levels are generally reached after five half-lives (a standard way of measuring how long it takes for one half of the drug present to leave the blood stream if no additional drug is administered). The longer the half-life, the longer it takes to reach this steady state. Reaching this level does not ensure maximal medication response because these agents must be available in the central nervous system (CNS) for a necessary period of time to exert their biologic effects. In the case of selective serotonin re-uptake inhibitors (SSRIs) and tricyclic antidepressants (TCAs), long half-lives over 24 hours require ample time for a therapeutic trial. Results often take weeks to become evident and such time constraints create special problems in anxiety sufferers, especially the panic patients. Therefore, it is often necessary to start an antipanic benzodiazepine agent early on in the antidepressant antipanic trial to provide for symptomatic relief. The benzodiazepine can be titrated downward and discontinued at a later date and the antidepressant can then serve as the primary psychotropic. Of course, the benzodiazepines, alprazolam and clonazepam are also used as primary antipanic agents and some would argue obviate the need for antidepressant antipanic agents.

A therapeutic dose of a medication is not always as clear-cut as textbook guideline tables would like us to believe. The effective dose may often be lower or higher than expected. The cost-effective pressures of managed care can set up a common psychopharmacologic trap; the time pressure causes the clinician to escalate the dosage rapidly to reach the desired "therapeutic threshold" (dose) that then results in a prematurely terminated medication trial due to side effects. If the slope of the curve generated by dose increases had been more gradual, many side-effected noncompliant patients would have been medication-tolerant. So start low and go slow. Remember, it is quality of care, not velocity of care. It is easy to see that the time and dollar cost of several medication trials due to side effects far outweigh a successful slow and carefully titrated first trial. Patients want to get well as soon as possible; however, they are usually uneasy and/or ambivalent about the effects of medication and generally are more accepting of a slow and steady approach.

Psychopharmacologists are generally referred the "nonresponders" or "treatment failures." These individuals often turn out to be refractory because of prescribing practices that (a) inadvertently maximize side effect risks; (b) discontinue the trial after too low a dose; or (c) fail to maintain the trial long enough to elicit a response. The upper limits of a dosage range certainly should be influenced by practice guidelines, but also must take into account interpatient variability and the need for carefully escalating dosage until the ratio between side effects and benefits favor the numerator of the risk–benefit fraction. Antidepressant blood levels help guide this process and can often single out the rapid metabolizer.

How long to continue a medication trial is a very reasonable question in light of pharmaceutical expense, side effect costs, and relapse risks. In the treatment of mood disorders, there has been some recent clarification suggesting that for individuals with recurrent depressions, indefinite medication trial at therapeutic dosage is indicated. The risks of relapse and subsequent treatment for refractory depression have triggered this recommendation.

The antianxiety and antipanic pharmaceutical guidelines are not that clear, however. Long-term benzodiazepine use has its drawbacks if sedation, tolerance, and decreased performance are medication effects. Interestingly, panic patients treated with benzodiazepines like alprazolam generally do not have problems with sedation or even medication tolerance (the physiologic need to increase dosage to maintain an effect). When benzodiazepines are utilized for the diminution of neurotic (psychological-conflict driven) or situational (stress diathesis driven) anxiety, tolerance, dependence, and abuse are all potential treatment risks.

The answer to the "how long do I treat?" question is found in the information contained in the following section on the *multidisciplinary team approach*. Although managed care administrative types (the actuaries and other number crunchers) welcome the concept of aggressive pharmacologic intervention, the panic disorder patient warrants a more comprehensive and carefully planned approach. It is true that the mood disorder patient can achieve a fair degree of psychiatric stability with medications alone. Why the difference between the two pathologies—panic disorder and mood disorder—is unclear. A clue may come from the secondary psychological traumatic effects of panic, phobic, or anxiety attacks. Common to all is the incapacitating dread that emanates from perceived *loss of control*. Human beings value maintaining within us the *locus of control*. Anything that weakens or threatens to weaken this control is extraordinary anxiety-provoking. Anticipatory anxiety and avoidant behaviors are the result of such circumstances.

Medication produces symptomatic relief. However, medication does not necessarily return the locus of control to the patient. Instead, the act of taking medication may acquire greater significance and symbolically embody the control locus. This psychological paradigm may sound familiar, for the chemically dependent addict demonstrates a similar psychology. Therefore, we do not want the locus of control to reside within the medication alone. On the other hand, avoiding a pharmacologic trial is no solution because of the valuable and proven efficacy of this treatment modality. The multidisciplinary and multimodality model takes these issues into consideration and allows for the development of a truly efficient and effective treatment plan.

THE MULTIDISCIPLINARY TEAM

Essential to the success of any managed care mental health delivery service is the system's input process. Access requires an effective communication net and the ability to rapidly obtain a diagnostic assessment. As will be highlighted in this section, the use of a multidisciplinary team providing panic anxiety disorder treatment is strongly recommended. At first glance, this model might appear to be incompatible with the cost saving requirements of the managed care philosophy. However, it is quality of care impacting on short- and long-term outcome that is critical. What the team may cost in professional salary expense is more than compensated for by the adequacy of treatment response. Patients refractory to treatment will be encountered less frequently in this model. The treatment goal is to address the critical pathological variables that have resulted in the presenting complaints. The biopsychosocial model in the general systems approach is more suited to this undertaking.

Returning to the assessment phase, it becomes evident that this entry point to clinical care is the place where we must "make it or break it," where outcome measures are often determined and it is paramount that the odds for success must be in our favor. This is accomplished by making sure that the senior member(s) of the team actively participate(s) in the diagnostic assessment. This person or group of people must be comfortable with the biopsychosocial model and be able to develop a treatment plan based upon a differential diagnostic approach. Differential diagnosis is integral to the medical model and requires that a hierarchy of possible diagnoses and etiologies be developed. This list helps guide treatment and alert the treating clinicians to the complexities of the case. By providing different possibilities, the diagnostician indicates that certain entities must be *ruled out* (R/O). For example, a childhood sexual abuse survivor presents with symptoms in young adulthood that are compatible with social phobia. The presence of early trauma, hypervigilance, and possible flashback experiences warrant that "R/O posttraumatic stress disorder" be added to the differential diagnosis. Let us assume that our patient has also noted unexplained weight loss, heat intolerance, and persistent jitteriness, all signs of hyperthyroidism and a possible anxiety disorder *medical mimic*. This, too, would be added to our differential diagnosis list as an R/O and guide the ensuing evaluation and treatment.

The senior clinician mentioned above must be able to perform the critical portions of the diagnostic assessment in *one visit*. Gone are the days of allowing several (usually up to four) evaluation sessions. This does not mean that the workup must be completed in one session. However, the acuity level and the differential diagnostic assessment must be accomplished within the first session. Further testing (e.g., Millon Personality Inventory or thyroid profile laboratory studies) may be required, and depending upon the level of acuity, treatment can be initiated based on the preliminary data base. For example, the acuity of the aforementioned panic patient would necessitate judicious use of an antipanic/anxiety benzodiazepine while laboratory testing proceeds to investigate the R/Os. Referral for the institution of a cognitive-behavioral panic protocol would then follow. Rapid symptomatic relief avoids the loss of work and functional absence from family responsibilities, while generally providing fast recovery as the patient gains greater confidence in the fact that help is possible.

The multidisciplinary anxiety disorder team generally consists of a psychiatrist, a psychologist (doctoral level), and Master's level clinicians. The senior clinician (M.D. and/or Ph.D.) providing the initial assessment and treatment plan may undertake an appropriate segment of care. If the senior member of the team does not participate directly in treatment, overall supervision of the case should still be this individual's responsibility. Weekly treatment planning conferences are a must, as are routine chart review and outcome measurement.

The multidisciplinary team allows for the provision of a multimodality treatment plan, bearing in mind that close utilization review is a must. It is important that the treatment plan differentiate elective from essential therapeutic interventions. Let us take, for example, the treatment of panic disorder with agoraphobia. Treatment goals, simply put, are to return this individual's functional capacity to an acceptable level initially, and to full capacity at the end of recuperation. This means that the practical outcome of treatment involves work, family, and home. Now it could be argued that clinical attention should be paid to the secondary psychological sequelae that result from developing or experiencing a panic disorder. The impact upon self-esteem, self-confidence, identity, marriage and family relationships can be significant. Does this mean that the multidisciplinary treatment plan include individual, couples' and/or family therapies? Not at all. If the assessment and treatment phases are carefully designed, the aforementioned clinical variables can be attended to. This may require a shift from the more traditional dyadic psychodynamic therapeutic model.

Traditionally, the psychiatric patient enters into a one-to-one relationship with minimal involvement of outside family or significant others. In the model being presented here, the initial assessment is obtained both from patient and significant others. The significant others (with patient's permission) are invited to participate actively in the evaluation phase. This accomplishes several things: (a) it allows for more comprehensive and sometimes more objective data base, (b) the stigma of mental health services is ameliorated and both patient and significant others come to view mental illness as an objective illness like any other medical problem; and (c) the diagnostic and treatment process allows for the education of patient and others, fostering therapeutic alliance, compliance, outcome measurement, and treatment response. This interaction is truly psychotherapeutic and beneficial to all concerned parties, including the clinician. It is also recommended that significant others participate in outcome measurement of treatment response.

REFERENCES

American Psychiatric Association (1994). *Diagnostic and Statistical Manual of Mental Disorders,* 4th edition. Washington, DC: American Psychiatric Association.

Barlow, D. H. (1988). *Anxiety Disorders Interview Schedule—Revised,* Albany; Graywind Publications.

Barlow, D. H. (1989). *Mastery of Your Anxiety and Panic.* Albany; Graywind Publications.

Barlow, D. H. (1992). *Mastery of Your Anxiety and Worry.* Albany; Graywind Publications.

Brawman-Mintzer, O. & Lydiard, R. B. (1994). Psychopharmacology of anxiety disorders, in Psychiatric Clinics of North America Annual of Drug Therapy. Jefferson, J, Greist, J. A. Eds., 1: 5179, Philadelphia; W. B. Saunders.

Engel, G. L. (1968). A life setting conducive to illness: The giving up given up complex, *Bull. Menninger Clin.,* 32: 355–365.

Extein, I. Gold, M. S. (1986). *Medical mimics of psychiatric disorders.* Washington, DC; American Psychiatric Association.

Freud, S. (1938). *Basic Writings of Sigmund Freud.* New York; Modern Library, Random House.

Klein, D. F. (1964). The delineation of two drug-responsive anxiety syndromes, *Psychopharmacologia,* 51: 397–408.

Gross, D. A. (1981). Medical origins of psychiatric emergencies: The systems approach, *Intl. Journal of Psychiatry in Med.,* 1.

Gross, D. A. Anticonvulsant use in mood disorders: The clinical relevance of the temporal lobe-limbic-hypothalamic checklist. Paper presented at the American Academic of Clinical Psychiatrists, Boston, Oct., 1990.

Hamilton, M. (1959). The assessment of anxiety states by rating. *British Journal of Psychiatry.* 32: 50.

Kupfer, D. J., Frank, E., Perel, J. M., et al. (1992). Five year outcome for maintenance therapies in recurrent depression, *Arch. Gen. Psychiatry,* 49: 769–773.

Levine, J. D., Gordon, N.C., Fields, H.L. (1978). The mechanism of placebo analgesia. *Lancet 2:* 654–657.

Millon, T. (1983). Millon Clinical Multiaxial Inventory Manuals, Ed. 5, Interpretive Scoring Systems, Minn.

Post, R. M. (1992). Transduction of psychological stress into the neurobiology of recurrent affective disorder, *American Journal of Psychiatry,* 149: 999–1010.

Post, R. M., Kopanda, R. T. (1976). Cocaine, kindling and psychosis. *American Journal of Psychiatry,* 133: 627–634.

Schweitzer, E, Rickels, K, Weiss, S, et al. (1993). Maintenance drug therapy of panic disorder: I. Results of a prospective placebo controlled comparison of alprazolam and imipramine. *Arch. Gen. Psychiatry,* 50: 51–60.

Von Korft, M. R., Eaton, W. N., & Keyl, P. M. (1985). The epidemiology of panic attacks and panic disorder: Results of three community surveys. *American Journal of Epidemiology,* 122: 970–981.

12

Treating Alcohol Problems in a Managed Care Environment

JUDITH A. LEWIS, Ph.D.

The advent of managed care has called into question virtually all of the assumptions about client needs and treatment modalities that have formed the basis of traditional approaches to alcohol-related problems. Many treatment providers initially responded to newly implemented utilization review and cost containment processes by expressing the fear that they would no longer be able to provide the intensive, long-term services that some clients needed. As one experienced practitioner put it, "For addicts in publicly supported treatment programs, *managed care* just means *how to manage without care*" (D. Deitch, personal communication, 1994). This fear has some basis in fact because managed care protocols do encourage brief, focused interventions at the expense of strategies aimed toward the total life change that some patients require. If adequate care for clients with multiple special needs is assured, however, managed care may also provide the opportunity for a sorely needed revamping of alcohol treatment methods.

In recent years, treatment for people with alcohol-related problems has been plagued by reliance on myths that are widely accepted but that have little or no empirical support. Many treatment providers, as well as the general public, have accepted without question the notions that the effects of alcoholism are uniform across cases, that confrontation and lecturing are effective strategies, that inpatient care is always preferable to outpatient care, and that the client alone is accountable for his or her ability to improve when provided with the usual treatment package. The fact that this set of assumptions is unsubstantiated has had little effect on common practice. "The negative correlation between scientific evidence and application in standard practice remains striking, and could hardly be larger if one intentionally constructed treatment programs from those approaches with the *least* evidence of efficacy" (Miller et al., 1995).

Perhaps managed care can succeed where the dissemination of empirically derived data has fallen short! The managed care environment creates pressure to identify the services that an individual needs rather than to provide a set of high-cost services to all alcohol-affected clients. As Table 12-1 shows, the practice of subjecting clients to uniform treatment programs that lack empirical validation is unlikely to survive in the managed care environment. In contrast, the strategies that are adaptive in a managed care environment include comprehensive assessment processes, individually tailored treatments, use of empirically supported modalities, attention to cost-effective options, and provider accountability. These approaches coincide with alcohol treatment's cutting edge.

ASSESSMENT AND DIAGNOSIS

Utilization management systems, whether they use preadmission or concurrent reviews, leave treatment providers little choice but to justify

TABLE 12-1
Adaptations to the Managed Care Environment

	Nonadaptive in Managed Care Environment	*Adaptive in Managed Care Environment*
ASSESSMENT/ DIAGNOSIS	Scientifically unsubstantiated diagnoses.	Comprehensive assessments.
TREATMENT PLANS	Uniform goals and treatments.	Goals and treatments tailored to individual needs.
MODALITIES	Untested modalities.	Empirically based modalities.
COST	Unquestioned use of high-cost options.	Selection of cost-effective options when appropriate for client.
ACCOUNTABILITY	Client responsible for treatment failures.	Treatment provider accountable for documenting outcomes.

a client's treatment plan with detailed assessment results. Traditionally, treatment providers tended to oversimplify the processes of diagnosis and assessment when alcohol problems occurred. The diagnosis of alcoholism was frequently proffered on the basis of generalities about appropriate or inappropriate drinking behaviors. The notion that there could be a simple dichotomy between alcoholic and nonalcoholic individuals failed to recognize the complexity of alcohol-related issues.

> What is usually called "alcoholism" is a multivariate syndrome. Drinkers vary in terms of consumption, physical symptoms, patterns of drinking behavior, life consequences of drinking, personality, social environment, gender, culture, and a variety of other factors. Given the differences among individuals, no one treatment plan—and no one label—could possibly be appropriate for all clients. (Lewis, Dana. & Blevins, 1994, p. 3)

In the absence of a comprehensive assessment, even the DSM-IV criteria for differentiation between alcohol abuse and alcohol dependence make these diagnoses only marginally more useful. As long as the focus remains solely on the presence or absence of an alcohol-related problem, individual differences are masked and people tend to be subjected to uniform levels of care that they might not need. "An either/or diagnosis leads inexorably to a generalized, diffuse treatment package that at worst may be ineffective and at best may meet the needs only of individuals with serious, chronic, long-standing substance abuse disorders" (Lewis et. al., 1994, p. 4).

Because alcohol abuse tends to be associated with a variety of psychosocial problems, effective assessment requires attention to all of the client's major concerns. If the assessment process takes note of the client's goals, resources, and deficits in several domains, it can form the basis for designing a treatment plan with the potential for effectiveness. For instance, use of the Addiction Severity Index (McLellan, Luborsky, Woody, & O'Brien, 1980) helps to lead the way toward treatment planning by assessing seven separate areas: medical status, employment status, drug use, alcohol use, legal status, family/social relationships, and psychological status. Based on a structured interview format, the instrument yields severity ratings from 0 (no treatment necessary) to 9 (treatment needed to intervene in life-threatening situation) for each area. Because this tool is helpful both for treatment planning and for outcome assessment, some managed care systems, such as that of the Illinois Department of Alcoholism and Substance Abuse (1994), have begun requiring that providers use it.

Several alcohol-specific assessment devices are also conducive for tailoring treatment to individual needs. The Comprehensive Drinker Profile (Miller & Marlatt, 1984) is a structured interview that addresses multiple issues related to alcohol and its interactions with other aspects of the client's life. Information is gathered concerning basic demographics, family and employment status, history and patterns of alcohol use, alcohol-related problems, severity of dependence, social aspects of use, associated behaviors, relevant medical history, and motivations for drinking and treatment. Unique to this instrument is a series of card sorts allowing the client to identify typical drinking situations, life problems, and alcohol-related effects. These self-reports help to target both treatment plans and behavioral strategies.

The cognitive and behavioral factors underlying effective behavioral strategies are also addressed in two instruments developed by Annis: the Inventory of Drinking Situations (Annis, 1982a) and the Situational Confidence Questionnaire (Annis, 1982b). The Inventory of Drinking Situations helps the client identify situations associated with drinking, placing these situations in eight categories: negative emotional states, negative physical states, positive emotional states, testing of personal control, urges and temptations, interpersonal conflict, social pressure to drink, and pleasant times with others. The resulting profile helps the client identify high-risk situations and develop plans for coping with them. The Situational Confidence Questionnaire asks clients to imagine themselves in a number of drinking situations and to indicate their degree of confidence in being able to handle each situation without drinking. This instrument helps clients design a hierarchy of drinking situations so that they can begin by handling tasks about which they feel confident and then progress gradually to situations about which they feel less confident. Ideally, the assessment process should be sufficiently comprehensive to make all of the individual's treatment needs readily apparent.

TREATMENT PLANNING

Treatment providers who employ comprehensive assessment procedures are able to provide help that is tailored to the individual needs of their clients. In any case of alcohol abuse or dependence, one of the goals of treatment should of course be the reduction or elimination of alcohol use. If long-term maintenance of new behaviors is to be expected, however, the treatment plan should also address other areas of life functioning, including legal and financial issues, mental and physical health, family stability, career development, and social functioning. Effective case management clearly requires that the traditional chasm between alcohol treatment and mental health treatment be bridged so that coexisting disorders are addressed within one unified treatment plan.

TREATMENT MODALITIES

In a landmark effort, Holder, Longabaugh, Miller, and Rubonis (1991) reviewed a large number of controlled studies, limiting their analysis to studies that used randomized clinical trials to assess the effects of specific modalities on alcohol-related outcomes. Holder and his colleagues developed a weighted index for each of 33 modalities by subtracting the number of negative from the number of positive results. They also took into account the number of positive findings for each modality. When they separated treatment modalities into qualitative categories based on the evidence for their effect, they were able to identify six modalities as having "good evidence of effect" (p. 522). These modalities included the following: (a) social skills training, (b) self-control training, (c) brief motivational counseling, (d) behavioral marital therapy, (e) the community reinforcement approach, and (f) stress management training.

In addition to their empirical support, these promising modalities share another commonality. Each of these methods uses a brief intervention designed to help clients take control of their own long-term recovery. Clients and their families develop the skills, and even the technology, that they will need to maintain positive behaviors and prevent relapse. Clients who succeed in developing these competencies are unlikely to need intensive, long-term treatment but may, instead, benefit from the provision a series of brief, focused services over time. Although these modalities should not become a new standard package for treatment of alcohol-related problems, they should become part of the repertoire of a provider who deals with alcohol-related issues in his or her practice, possibly replacing the untested methods that are likely to lose their predominance in the managed care environment.

Social Skills Training

Social skills training can play a key role in treating alcohol-affected clients because of the impact that these skills have on the maintenance of new behaviors. "The importance of this general approach lies in the fact that effective social skills can give clients important tools to be used in their recovery, whereas deficits in this area can place recovering clients in jeopardy" (Lewis, 1994, p. 51). Clients can learn to cope with specific situations that might normally place them at risk for drinking. Moreover, they can use their newly acquired skills to develop the kinds of social support networks that are associated with healthy functioning.

Monti, Abrams, Kadden, and Cooney (1989) developed a group program offering alcohol-dependent clients training in the following interpersonal skills: (a) starting conversations, (b) giving and receiving compliments, (c) nonverbal communication, (d) "feeling talk" and listening skills, (e) assertiveness, (f) giving criticism, (g) receiving criticism about drinking, (h) drink refusal skills, (i) refusing requests, (j) close and intimate relationships, and (k) enhancing social support networks. The training techniques used by Monti and his colleagues include the use of skill guidelines, role-played modeling, behavior rehearsal, and practice exercises. The long-term impact of this strategy can go way beyond what might be expected of such a modest, time-limited approach.

Self-Control Training

Self-control training provides an efficient mechanism for helping clients select and reach their own goals. Alcohol-affected individuals have been taught successfully to analyze and monitor their drinking behaviors and to use self-reinforcement and stimulus-control methods on their own. Typically, clients identify the situations that normally place them at risk for abusive drinking. Whether they identify these situations by monitoring their day-to-day behaviors, by recalling their past behaviors, or by using Annis's Inventory of Drinking Situations, they can begin to address methods for coping more effectively in the future.

For example, Sanchez-Craig, Wilkins, and Walker (1987) achieved successful outcomes in a short-term outpatient program that prepared clients to use cognitive or behavioral coping strategies that fit their own styles and goals. Cognitive strategies included self-statements such as reappraisals or reminders about their commitment to change. Behavioral methods included alternative behaviors or use of skills such as relaxation or assertiveness. In any self-control training program, clients need to have a large enough repertoire of alternative coping skills available so that they have choices when dealing with difficult challenges. Clients learn to plan for anticipated situations and to engage in repeated rehearsals of the coping strategies they will need. These self-control training methods are applicable whether the individual client's goals involve complete abstinence or moderation.

Brief Motivational Counseling

Miller and Rollnick (1991, p. 31) point out that "relatively brief interventions of one to three sessions are comparable in impact to more extensive treatments for alcohol problems" and that brief interventions are "substantially more effective than no treatment in altering problem drinking." Like the other research-supported modalities, brief motivational counseling appears to work for clients because they become encouraged about the possibility of making changes independently.

Unlike the confrontational intervention, for which Holder and his colleagues found no evidence of effect, motivational interviewing is based on a realistic approach to client motivation. "Research has generally failed to support a trait view of alcoholics as poorly motivated, prone to particular defense mechanisms (e.g., denial), inherently resistive, or possessing a characteristic personality" (Institute of Medicine, 1990, p. 533). The assumption that alcohol-affected people must be harshly confronted in order to break down their denial is now being exposed as a myth to be replaced by the principle that motivation can best be engendered through the kinds of positive and supportive relationships that therapists normally expect to have with their other clients.

Motivational interviewing, as described by Miller and Rollnick (1991), provides an alternative to the highly directive style that is commonly used with substance abuse clients. This motivational strategy is based on the concept that the denial that is often assumed to be characteristic of addicts may in fact result from the way we tend to interact with these clients. When clients are pressed to admit that their alcohol use is the underlying cause of all of their problems, their resistance becomes entrenched. Motivational interviewing circumvents this impasse by avoiding labels and placing decision-making responsibility in the hands of the client. A comprehensive assessment is done, but the decisions about how to use the data are explored with the clients rather than imposed on them. In general, the step-by-step process of the motivational interview involves an initial exploratory stage in which self-motivational statements are elicited, an assessment stage in which the results of a comprehensive assessment are shared with the client, and a period of confirmation in which the client decides whether he or she is committed to change. Only after commitment has been made are client and therapist ready to negotiate alternatives for behavior-change methods.

The concept of the motivational interview may appear simplistic at first glance because it describes basic procedures and assumptions that would be familiar to any therapist. In fact, however, there has been a tendency, even among experienced therapists, to concentrate on the differences between addicts and other members of the client population.

What motivational interviewing does is to overcome the myth that substance abuse clients are so different from others that the usual principles of human behavior fail to apply to them. As long as we assume that people with alcohol or drug problems are unable to make responsible choices and must therefore be told what to do, we will be forced to deal with defensiveness and denial. If we recognize the unassailable truth that behaviors are based on individuals' choices—not therapists' wishes—we are more likely to see motivated clients (Lewis, 1992, p. 31).

Behavioral Marital Therapy

As Lawson (1994, p. 228) points out, "Given the vast amount of research on the problems of children of alcoholics, the intergenerational transmission of addictions, and the problems of the alcoholic family system, it is impossible to ignore the role of the family environment in the etiology and perpetuation of addictions." Given the fact that drinking behaviors are embedded in family systems, it is not surprising that couple and family therapy have found a place among the more promising modalities for treating alcohol-related problems. Within this general category, behavioral couple therapy has been studied most intensively and yielded the most positive results.

Several studies have shown promising results in using behaviorally based couples counseling with alcohol-affected clients in early recovery (O'Farrell, 1992). A study of the Program for Alcohol Couples Treatment (McCrady, Noel, Abrams, Stout, & Nelson, 1986) compared three treatments. Each couple studied was randomly assigned to one of three treatments: (a) minimal spouse involvement; (b) alcohol-focused spouse involvement, which trained spouses in skills for dealing with alcohol-related situations; and (c) alcohol behavioral marital therapy, which added the use of behavioral therapy to increase positive activities and to teach communication and negotiation skills. All three treatments led to decreases in alcohol use, but the behavioral family therapy also led to more stability and satisfaction in the couples' marriages. O'Farrell, Cutter, and Floyd (1985) also studied behavioral marriage therapy in their program, Counseling for Alcoholics' Marriages (CALM). Their study showed that a combination of behavioral skill building with a focus on the couple relationships brought about positive results both for marital adjustment and for drinking-related outcomes. In a study comparing individual counseling with short-term couples group therapy, Bowers and Al-Rehda (1990) found that clients in each treatment group showed reductions in drinking immediately after treatment but that clients in the couples therapy group showed significantly lower alcohol consumption at follow-up. Based on the trend toward positive results in studies of couple-oriented therapy, O'Farrell (1991) suggested that couples-based interventions can be used effectively to stimulate the alcoholic's commitment to change, to stabilize both the marital relationship and drinking behaviors during early recovery, and to maintain improvements during long-term recovery. Like the other promising modalities identified by Holder et al. (1991), couples therapy has the potential to use a short-term, focused intervention as the basis for the client's long-term, independently managed recovery.

Community Reinforcement Approach

Since the 1970s, the Community Reinforcement Approach (CRA) has been one of the most stringently evaluated alcohol treatment approaches available (Azrin, 1976; Mallams, Godley, Hall, & Meyers, 1982). This multifaceted program may now be more appropriate than ever before because its design addresses the transition from treatment to community environments. The brief strategies that work in the managed care era must provide opportunities for the natural environment to build on the treatment provider's work, encouraging the client's continued progress after the formal phase of treatment has been concluded. Success in this arena is the strength of the Community Reinforcement Approach, which "acknowledges the powerful role of environmental contingencies in encouraging or discouraging drinking and attempts to rearrange these contingencies such that sober behavior is more rewarding than drinking behavior" (Smith & Meyers, 1995, p. 251).

CRA, from its beginnings in an inpatient setting for chronic alcoholics, has evolved into a broad spectrum approach appropriate for both inpatient and outpatient settings and for clients seeking abstinence or moderation. The components of the program include the following (Smith & Meyers, 1995):

- **Functional analysis** of drinking and nondrinking behaviors.
- **Sobriety sampling** (negotiating with clients to commit to abstinence for a specified period of time, whether their ultimate goal is abstinence or moderation).
- **Behavioral compliance** program with Disulfiram as an option.
- **CRA treatment plan,** using a "Goals of Counseling" form based on the client's goals in ten life areas: drinking/sobriety, job or educational progress, money management, social life, personal habits, marriage/family relationships, legal issues, emotional life, communication, and general happiness.
- **Basic skills training** in communication, problem solving, and drink refusal.
- **Job club** focused on the skills needed for finding and keeping employment.
- **Social/recreational counseling** to help clients change peer groups and develop alcohol-free social outlets.
- **Marital therapy** focused on attaining couple-oriented goals in ten "marriage happiness" categories: household responsibilities, raising children, social activities, money management, communication, sex and affection, job or school, emotional support, partner's independence, and general happiness.
- **Relapse prevention training** using an early warning system and focusing on action plans.

All of these components are available for clients who need them. Because of CRA's emphasis on assessment and treatment planning, the program is tailored to meet the individual client's needs and goals.

Stress Management Training

In their identification of *stress management training* as one of the modalities showing good evidence of effect, Holder and his colleagues (1991) defined this term to include a variety of relaxation, systematic desensitization, and cognitive techniques that can be used for reducing personal tension and stress. The relevance of this modality for alcohol treatment lies in the fact that alcohol-affected individuals tend to use drinking routinely as their primary means of coping with stress. If alternate methods for dealing with either major stressors or daily hassles have not been learned, the client is of course at high risk for relapse.

Therapists frequently use relaxation training to help substance abuse clients reduce general tension, cope with anxiety-provoking situations, and diminish the intensity of cravings that might otherwise lead to relapse. Relaxation training is also used as the basis for systematic desensitization when clients have difficulty with intrusive anxiety in high-risk situations. After developing a rank-ordered hierarchy of anxiety-provoking situations normally associated with drinking, the client who has become adept at maintaining the relaxation response can gradually work his or her way through the imagined situations. Following desensitization, the client can move on to a hierarchy of real-life situations.

Cognitive strategies can also be used to help clients deal with their reactions to stressors. Alcohol-affected individuals frequently interpret situations as stressors and make assumptions that lead directly to relapse (for example, assuming that a drink is necessary in order to become sufficiently relaxed to give a speech or participate in a job interview). With cognitive restructuring, alcohol-affected individuals can mediate arousal through recognition of their typical thought patterns.

Of course, clients need to learn a variety of ways for intervening more effectively with environmental demands. They can cope with stress by altering the stressors themselves through problem solving, by altering their interpretations of the stressors through cognitive restructuring, or by altering their physiological responses through relaxation methods. The client who is able to implement these skills may be in a good position for preventing the "relapse chain" (Washton, 1989, p. 118) that often follows the onset of stress among addicted individuals.

COSTS

The intent of most utilization management programs is "to ensure that each patient is certified for the most appropriate level of service that the available clinical information indicates" (Silverman, 1994, p. 91). The likely impact of this process is that the numbers of alcohol-affected clients served in inpatient facilities will plunge, while outpatient and partial hospitalization programs will grow. Just as alcoholism treatment providers have erred in the direction of overemphasizing inpatient modalities, decision makers in the managed care environment might risk clients' well-being by certifying levels of care that are less costly but also less appropriate to an individual's needs. If objective clinical criteria are used to decide on the individual's treatment setting, changes in the continuum of care might be positive.

Miller (1985) says that "the absolutely consistent testimony of . . . controlled studies . . . is that heroic interventions—those in longer, more intensive residential settings—produce no more favorable outcomes overall than treatment in much simpler, shorter, and less expensive settings" (p. 2). As long as we bear in mind that "overall" does not mean "universal" and that severely impaired clients continue to need "heroic interventions," we can use this opportunity to provide more balanced options for all alcohol-affected individuals. In general, clients should receive treatment based on the least intrusive possible alternative. For clients who have adequate personal and social resources, outpatient treatment is preferable to inpatient care. If the life-disrupting effects of hospitalization can be avoided, clients maintain their employment and social ties, retain a sense of responsibility and self-efficacy, and have the chance to try out new behaviors in real-life situations.

Fortunately, the treatment modalities that have the strongest evidence of effectiveness tend also to be among the lowest in cost. Holder and his colleagues (1991) actually went beyond their review of the clinical effectiveness of empirically supported modalities to consider cost effectiveness as well. Taking into account the settings in which services could be delivered, the authors estimated the costs of each modality. Modalities were placed in cost categories including minimum, low, medium-low, medium-high, and high. The interesting finding of this exercise was that the modalities with strong evidence of effectiveness tended to be low in cost, while high costs tended to be identified for the modalities with the least evidence of effectiveness.

> The selection of a more expensive treatment is not likely to yield any more effective results. . . . Brief intervention in the "minimum" cost category, behavioral self-control training and stress management training in the "low" cost category, and social skills training, marital behavioral therapy and community reinforcement in the "medium-low" cost category are desirable modalities in terms of predicted effectiveness and costs. On the other hand, chemical aversion therapy, residential milieu and insight psychotherapy are in the "high" cost category, while also categorized as having "no evidence of effectiveness." (Holder et al., 1991, p. 529)

To put it bluntly, "as costs increase there is less evidence of demonstrated effectiveness" (Holder et al., 1991, p. 529).

ACCOUNTABILITY

If there is any one factor that underlies every policy and every procedure of managed care it is accountability. The time when providers could ignore outcome measurement in deference to their own faith in their therapeutic models is gone and cannot be expected to return. This circumstance is especially difficult for alcoholism specialists, many of whom felt comfortable with the assumption that treatment failures could be explained by their clients' denial, resistance, and failure to "work the program."

Outcome evaluation for alcohol treatment has also been negatively effected by overly simplistic, dichotomous measurements. Traditionally, follow-up measures have been designed merely to determine whether the client was drinking or abstinent. A multivariate conceptualization of alcohol problems brings the recognition that drinking behaviors are actually continuous variables and that a number of further outcome criteria need to be used in addition to measures of substance use. Emrick and Hansen (1983) suggested that the alcoholism field could be improved if providers and researchers could agree on a number of core indexes to be used in treatment evaluation studies. They suggested that outcomes be measured in terms of the following criteria: (a) treatment completion, measured by discharge status; (b) recidivism, measured by self-reports, collateral information, and agency records; (c) mortality, measured by time from treatment admission to day of death; (d) treatment use, measured by self-reports and records; (e) physical health, measured by such data as the number of days the patient experiences medical problems; (f) drinking behavior, defined as the number of days the patient is abstinent, drinks moderately, or drinks heavily and measured through multiple avenues; (g) other substance use, also measured by multiple avenues; (h) legal problems, measured through self-reports, collateral information, and official records; (i) vocational functioning, defined by such criteria as employment status and number of days worked; (j) family/social functioning, defined in terms of the patient's satisfaction and measured by self-report; and (k) emotional functioning, measured through the use of psychological instruments.

The suggestion made by Emrick and Hansen has finally come of age. We have entered an era when outcome evaluation has become the province not just of researchers but also of treatment providers across the continuum of care.

In the final analysis, both treatment providers and managed care programs must be accountable.

Companies characterized by fairly administered managed care, a willingness to settle for reasonable profits, an interest in delivering a quality product, and maintenance of an interest in the well-being of the patient are stimulating a welcome change in the delivery of addiction services. . . . Better and more comprehensive evaluations are being done, unnecessary hospitalizations are being avoided, treatment planning is comprehensive, and treatment for all of the problems needing attention—including psychiatric disorders requiring medication—is being given. The process has forced the field to develop a spectrum of services previously unavailable when there was no economic incentive to provide care in lower-cost settings. All these advantages and progress exist, however, only when dealing with ethical managed care organizations. (Miller, 1994, pp. 98–99)

It is undoubtedly time for alcohol treatment modalities to change, but the direction these changes will take is not assured. Whether alterations in treatment methods bring about improvements in client well-being depends on the ability of all stakeholders in this process to work collaboratively toward a shared vision.

REFERENCES

Annis, H. M. (1982a). *Inventory of Drinking Situations.* Toronto: Addiction Research Foundation of Ontario.

Annis, H. M. (1982b). *Situational Confidence Questionnaire.* Toronto: Addiction Research Foundation of Ontario.

Azrin, N. (1976). Improvements in the community-reinforcement approach to alcoholism. *Behavior Research and Therapy, 14,* 339–348.

Bowers, T. G., & Al-Redha, M. R. (1990). A comparison of outcome with group/marital and standard/individual therapies with alcoholics. *Journal of Studies on Alcohol, 5*(4), 301–309.

Emrick, C. D., & Hansen, J. (1983). Assertions regarding effectiveness of treatment for alcoholism: Fact or fantasy? *American Psychologist, 38,* 1078–1088.

Holder, H., Longabaugh, R., Miller, W. R., & Rubonis, A. V. (1991). The cost effectiveness of treatment for alcoholism: A first approximation. *Journal of Studies on Alcohol, 6,* 517–540.

Illinois Department of Alcoholism and Substance Abuse (1994). *Managed care system for substance abuse services in Illinois: Recommendations and workplan.*

Institute of Medicine. (1990). *Broadening the base of treatment for alcohol problems.* Washington, DC: National Academy Press.

Lawson, A. (1994). Family therapy and addictions. In J. A. Lewis (Ed.), *Addictions: Concepts and strategies for treatment* (pp. 211–232). Gaithersburg, MD: Aspen.

Lewis, J. A. (1992, Winter). Applying the motivational interviewing process. *The Family Psychologist, 8*(1), 31–32.

Lewis, J. A. (1994). Treating people with alcohol problems. In J. A. Lewis (Ed.), *Addictions: Concepts and strategies for treatment* (pp. 47–58). Gaithersburg, MD: Aspen.

Lewis, J. A., Dana, R. Q., & Blevins, G. A. (1994). *Substance abuse counseling: An individualized approach (2nd ed.).* Monterey, CA: Brooks/Cole.

Mallams, J. H., Godley, M. D., Hall, G. M., & Meyers, R. J. (1982). A social-systems approach to resocializing alcoholics in the community. *Journal of Studies on Alcohol, 43,* 1115–1123.

McCrady, B. S., Noel, N. E., Abrams, D. B., Stout, R. L., & Nelson, H. F. (1986). Comparative effectiveness of three types of spouse involvement in outpatient behavioral alcoholism treatment. *Journal of Studies on Alcohol, 47,* 459–467.

McLellan, A. T., Luborsky, L., Woody, G. E., & O'Brien, C. P. (1980). An improved diagnostic instrument for substance abuse patients: The Addiction Severity Index. *Journal of Nervous and Mental Disorders, 168,* 26–33.

Miller, S.I. (1994). Drugs and alcohol: The clinician's view. In R. K. Schreter, S. S. Sharfstein, & C. A. Schreter (Eds.), *Allies and adversaries: The impact of managed care on mental health services* (pp. 91–99). Washington, DC: American Psychiatric Press.

Miller, W. R. (1985). *Perspectives on treatment.* Paper presented at the 34th International Congress on Alcoholism and Drug Dependence, Calgary, Alberta.

Miller, W. R., Brown, J. M., Simpson, T. L., Handmaker, N. S., Bien, T. H., Luckie, L. F., Montgomery, H. A., Hester, R. K., & Tonigan, J. S. (1995). What works? A methodological analysis of the alcohol treatment outcome literature. In R. K. Hester & W. R. Miller (Eds.), *Handbook of alcoholism treatment approaches: Effective alternatives (2nd ed.)* (pp. 12–44). Boston: Allyn & Bacon.

Miller, W. R., & Marlatt, G. A. (1984). *Manual for the Comprehensive Drinker Profile.* Odessa, FL: Psychological Assessment Resources.

Miller, W. R., & Rollnick, S. (1991). *Motivational interviewing: Preparing people to change addictive behavior.* New York: Guilford Press.

Monti, P. M., Abrams, D. B., Kadden, R. M., & Cooney, N. L. (1989). *Treating alcohol dependence: A coping skills training guide.* New York: Guilford Press.

O'Farrell, T. J. (1991). Using couples therapy in the treatment of alcoholism. *Family Dynamics of Addiction Quarterly, 1*(4), 39–45.

O'Farrell, T. J. (1992). Families and alcohol problems: An overview of treatment research. *Journal of Family Psychology, 5,* 339–359.

O'Farrell, T. J., Cutter, H. S. G., & Floyd, F. J. (1985). Evaluating behavioral marital therapy for male alcoholics: Effects on marital adjustment and communication from before to after therapy. *Behavior Therapy, 16,* 147–167.

Sanchez-Craig, M., Wilkins, D. A., & Walker, K. (1987). Theory and methods for secondary prevention of alcohol problems: A cognitively based approach. In C. W. Cox (Ed.), *Treatment and prevention of alcohol problems* (pp. 287–331). New York: Academic Press.

Silverman, C. (1994). Drugs and alcohol: The managed care view. In R. K. Schreter, S. S. Sharfstein, & C. A. Schreter (Eds.), *Allies and adversaries: The impact of managed care on mental health services* (pp. 85–91). Washington, DC: American Psychiatric Press.

Smith, J. E., & Meyers, R. J. (1995). The community reinforcement approach. In R. K. Hester & W. R. Miller (Eds.), *Handbook of alcoholism treatment approaches: Effective alternatives (2nd ed.)* (pp. 251–266). Boston: Allyn & Bacon.

Washton, A. M. (1989). *Cocaine addiction: Treatment, recovery, and relapse prevention.* New York: Norton.

13

Consultation with Health Care Organizations

LEN SPERRY, M.D., Ph.D.

Until recently hospitals, clinics and other health care organizations (HCOs) were considered so different from business or work organizations in mission, accountability, and productivity that many wondered if they really should be considered work organizations. Things have changed dramatically, so that today many health care organizations now proudly proclaim that they are "in the business of providing health care." HCOs have worked diligently to become more businesslike in their operation particularly in an era when health care cost containment is a national priority. Nevertheless, there remain unique differences between the worlds of for-profit corporations and HCOs. Comparing a high tech manufacturing corporation with a high tech academic medical center illustrates this point. Typically, the high tech manufacturing organization might have a structure that is lean and responsive, and governed by leadership that is precise and predictable. And, typically, the high tech academic medical center will have a structure of loosely coupled units and division, and leadership that resembles the director's efforts in improvisation theater!

Whether an organization is a for-profit business corporation or an HCO, the waves of change are battering both, with little end in sight. Change requires adaptation and, in some cases, transformation in mission, structure, culture, and leadership style. Organizations don't change easily of their own doing, and often need expert assistance. While profit and not-for-profit corporations have dramatically increased their utilization of a full range of consultants in the past few years, there is a growing awareness that HCOs also will need to increase their utilization of consultants in the coming years. This chapter describes the need HCOs have for consultation, the components of the consultation process, differences between consultation and clinical services, and the consultation process operative in HCOs. Extensive case material illustrates the consultation process in common HCO situations and settings.

THE NEED FOR CONSULTATION IN HCOs

Here are some reasons why HCOs need the services of psychologically trained consultants:

1. The rate of change experienced by HCOs is faster than in other kinds of organizations. The concept of managed care illustrates this point. In the past ten years managed care has gone through three generations of change and is ready to evolve further. The first generation of managed care was *managed access,* wherein costs were managed by limiting access to treatment. Managed access was marked by precertification, high copayment rates, nonclinical reviewers, and limited numbers of providers. The second generation of managed care was characterized by *managed benefits.* Managed benefits emphasized utilization review, discounted fee-for-service networks, and cost containment over clinical care. The third generation involves *utilization management* with quality-based networks of providers and hospitals. The focus is on providing the most appropriate care in the most appropriate setting with the emphasis on treatment planning and quality management. Today, most HCOs reflect this generation, but the fourth generation, *managed outcomes,* which is an integrated behavioral health care system, is already on the horizon (Grant, 1995). The basic point here is that each of these first three generations required both patients and, clinicians to accommodate to these changes, in a very short period of time. Clinicians had to relinquish or repress many of their values and beliefs about the nature and process of therapeutic change, as well as practice styles that may have taken years to acquire and refine.
2. While mental health clinicians are asked to treat clients who are suffering from the effects of major changes in their lives—

including merger syndrome, downsizing, or job loss—mental health clinicians are experiencing these same stressors, and probably , as or more intensely than are their clients. In fact, Fox (1995) the former president of the American Psychological Association states that some psychotherapies are experiencing posttraumatic stress disorder as a result of the strain of managed care. Similarly, Sussman (1995) has edited a book entitled *A Perilous Calling: The Hazards of Psychotherapy Practice* that details the emotional, relational, and legal hazards that clinicians now face.

3. While mental health clinicians have the intrinsic capacity to function as consultants to both HCOs and other organizations, their individually focused training actually is an impediment to functioning in this role. Though not as vehemently as in the past, some clinicians also harbor an antipathy and distrust of organizational processes. Functioning in the role of consultant requires viewing behavior from a systems perspective and formulating and strategizing change in categories such as morale and cohesion, roles and communications, and norms and standards, rather than in terms such as ego defense mechanisms or dysfunctional cognitions. Nevertheless, clinicians who are able to learn to think organizationally and can translate some of their clinical skills to organizational settings could become highly effective change agents and consultants to organization. And since such clinician/consultants have first-hand experience in HCOs, they stand to be the consultants of choice as internal or external consultants to HCOs.

In short, HCOs are changing and evolving at a dizzying rate. Such speed is bound to wreak havoc with organizations that are not structured to accommodate those changes. Personnel within organizations can and do experience considerable distress and suffering. And, finally clinicians have considerable potential to understand the change process in the organizations in which they work, and can with further training function effectively as internal and external consultants to HCOs and other organizations.

CASE EXAMPLE: THE NEED FOR HCO CONSULTATION

A medium-sized behavioral health care corporation with 110,000 subscribers approached a psychiatry practice group about contracting psychiatric services, and it accepted the offer. Apparently, the psychiatry group that had been working with the corporation declined to review its contract. The managed care corporation already employed 23 full-time masters-level clinicians who were deployed at three sites, and they had a contract with a nonprofit psychiatric hospital for inpatient treatment. Although the new psychiatry group was well regarded in the community, none of its members had any formal training or experience in a capitated Health Maintenance Organization (HMO) or any training in organizational consultation. The managed care corporation had shown a modest profit in only one of the previous three years, and so was receptive when the new psychiatry group stipulated in the 12-month contract agreement that they would evaluate and modify policies about psychotherapist–psychiatrist relations and practice patterns should they consider it advisable.

During the first two months of the contract the group kept moderately busy becoming acquainted with medication-monitored patients. While they saw patients back-to-back at 20-minute intervals, group members noted that some other psychotherapists were standing around the coffee machine or had their office doors open, suggesting that they were not in session. A review of utilization data showed that therapists were averaging only 12 billable hours per week while the psychiatrists were averaging 31 hours. Further review of data indicated that 104 patients had been referred to other clinics outside the capitated programs. Presumably this was because the type of therapy provided by these therapists was considered to be inappropriate for those clients. The three clinic sites advertised that they provided brief therapy to families and individuals. One social worker completed an evaluation on all new referrals at each clinic site. Those clients not considered to be candidates for brief therapy were referred to the psychiatrists for medication evaluation or to outside psychotherapists. A review of case loads revealed a bimodal distribution among the therapists' use load: Fifty-five percent of patients were seen for five or fewer sessions, and 45 percent were considered to be "chronic patients," and of those, 40 percent were seen weekly for three or more years. There was a weekly case conference at each clinic, but the group of psychiatrists that preceded this one wanted to be present only for the last 20 minutes, when patients who were on medication were reviewed. There was no other formal contact between medical and nonmedical therapists.

Over the next three months the new psychiatry group became increasingly angry and discontented with the apparent inequality of work loads, referral only of patients taking medication, all-night call, and assuming responsibility for all emergencies, day or night. On the other hand, the therapists had regular 40-hour work weeks, no afterhours responsibilities, and minimal billable hours. During the sixth month the head of the psychiatry group confronted the clinic director, a social worker, and the financial officer of the managed care corporation with data on the previous five months. A set of demands included an expectation of at least 28 billable hours a week for therapists, a reduced number of patients referred outside the system, and a cap of 70 percent of medication-only patients referred to the psychiatry group. The demands were accepted and implemented to some extent. For the next month and a half things seemed more efficient, but relations were less cordial between the therapists and the psychiatry group. In the ninth month the psychiatry group insisted that each therapist share night call responsibilities with the psychiatrists. This demand was met with considerable consternation by the therapists. Finally, by the start of the eleventh month things settled down sufficiently so that relations between the groups were reasonably civil. Utilization review data was encouraging for the financial officer and the psychiatry group. The psychiatry group had been asked to renew its contract but waited until the middle of the twelfth month before signing. The efforts of the psychiatry group to produce change had been effective, but the time and emotional price paid was high for all parties involved.

This case illustrates some of the difficulties involved in effecting change in an organizational system, specifically an HCO. Had either the psychiatry group or the managed care corporation drawn on the expertise of an internal or external consultant, the process might have been much less painful. It would likely have been considerably shorter, lasting only a few months rather than nearly a year. While the psychiatry group's effort were ultimately successful, the risk they assumed in making demands was high and could have backfired. The expertise of a psychologically informed consultant would have greatly reduced the risk while increasing the probability that the expected changes would be realized.

In short, then, HCOs face the same degree and intensity that other work organizations face. Consultants can facilitate the process of both planned and unplanned change. Given that HCOs are qualitatively different from other organizations, the more consultants are familiar and respectful of these differences, the more outcomes are likely to be efficacious and rewarding for all parties involved in the change process.

THE PROCESS OF CONSULTATION

The process of organizational consultation will be described briefly in this section, and illustrated in the next section. First, four models of consultation will be delineated. Next, five organizational domains or problem areas that plague work organizations will be described. The five domains of an organization serve as convenient targets for organizational diagnosis and intervention. Finally, the matter of differentiating the consulting role from the clinical role of the psychotherapist will be addressed, along with a brief discussion of the advantages and disadvantages of rendering consultation as either an internal or an external consultant.

CONSULTATION MODELS

Four models relevant to consultation with HCOs are reviewed here: mental health consultation, clinical consultation, organizational consultation, and the training consultation models (Sperry, 1993).

Mental Health Consultation Model

For Caplan (1970), consultation is viewed as a process of interaction between two professionals wherein the consultant assists in dealing with the psychological aspects of a current work problem. He distinguished four types of mental health consultation. *Client-centered case consultation* is equivalent to the clinical consultation model discussed in the next section. It focuses on cases, and the goal is to diagnose the problem and recommend a solution. Most psychiatric and psychological consultation referrals done in HCOs are of this type. For instance, a hospital administrator may request a psychiatric evaluation of a junior administrator suspected of substance abuse. In *consultee-centered case consultation,* the focus is on the case, yet the primary goal is increasing the competence of the consultee. For example, a psychologist consults with a group of charge nurses to increase their understanding of alcoholism and how its early signs can be recognized. *Program-centered administrative consultation* focuses on an organizational program or project. The primary goal is to assist the consultee in planning, implementing, or evaluating a project, such as when the psychiatric consultant is asked to help the EAP director develop a hospital-wide depression awareness program. Finally, in *consultee-centered administrative consultation,* the focus is on a program; however, the primary goal is to help the administrator function more effectively by increasing his or her expertise. Caplan (1970) discusses consultee-centered case consultation in the most detail and emphasizes its teaching or liaison function.

Clinical Consultation Model

Based largely on the medical model, the clinical consultation model is most familiar to and the one most used by consultation-liaison psychiatrists. The clinical model conceives of problems in terms of a patient's disease or dysfunction, whether the "patient" is a health care executive, a work team, or the entire HCO. The primary goal is the diagnosis and remediation of the problem, and success is defined by the remediation of symptoms and the restoration of normal function. A complete and comprehensive diagnostic workup is the hallmark of this model. Levinson's diagnostic approach, as described in *Organizational Diagnosis* (1972), exemplifies the clinical model.

Levinson's case study outline is a rigorous and time-intensive method of analyzing the patient. The case study report involves four major sections: (a) genetic data, (b) organizational structural and process data, (c) interpretive data about current organizational functioning and attitudes and relationships, and (d) an analysis and conclusion section that includes both genetic and dynamic formulations with prognostic conclusions and recommendations. Levinson's approach blends psychoanalytic theory with systems theory. Unlike the mental health consultation model, the liaison function is limited in Levinson's approach.

Training Model of Consultation

The training model of consultation is the most common form of consultation that is currently utilized by HCOs. Prearranged and organized consultant-led seminars, lectures, and workshops that are information-centered rather than diagnostic and treatment-focused exemplify this model. The consultant who presents a workshop on stress among health care personnel is utilizing this model. This model conceives of consultee problems in terms of deficits in knowledge or skills. The goal of this type of consultation is to provide the knowledge or skill training needed. Representative of this approach is the *Annual Handbook for Group Facilitators*, edited by J.E. Jones and J.W. Pfeiffer each year since 1972. This publication and *Instrumentation in Human Relations Training*, also edited annually by Jones and Pfeiffer since 1975, provide user-friendly lectures, background theory, training exercises, and short self-scoring instruments for use by consultees in seminars and workshops.

Organizational Consultation Model

Unlike the previous models, the basic assumption of the organizational consultation model is that problems arise because the corporation's personnel lack the knowledge, skills, or values to function at optimum levels of effectiveness. It *clearly* is not based on the medical model. Organizations—work teams, departments, or entire HCOs—are viewed as clients rather than as patients, and the process—the *how*—is considered as important as the context—the what. The behavior of individuals, teams, and organizations tends to be cyclical or repetitive, and often counterproductive (Blake & Mouton, 1976). Thus, the primary goal of consultation is to identify and change ineffective cyclical behavior. Another important goal is to help individuals better deal with the complexities of organizational life in order to enhance their effectiveness.

Schein (1987) describes three types of organizational consultation: technical expertise, doctor or clinical, and process. Both *technical expertise* and *clinical* types of consultation focus on what needs to be done. With the *expertise* type, the consultee retains a consultant who can provide knowledge or skill to solve a previously determined problem. With the *doctor* type, the consultee retains a consultant both to diagnose and to prescribe appropriately. With the *process* type, the consultant is retained to help the consultee focus on process—as compared to content—events, on how problems can be solved, rather than on the content of problems. Here the consultant is a facilitator and catalyst rather than a problem solver.

The organizational consultant is either an internal or an external consultant who applies organizational and behavioral science knowledge to managing change and increasing the organization's effectiveness. The consultant utilizes a variety of interventions, such as organizational diagnosis, team building, executive seminars, strategic planning, career and developmental counseling, and so on, to achieve specific goals. Representative writings on this model are by Blake and Mouton (1985), Lippitt and Lippitt (1978), and Schein (1987).

While clinicians can easily assume the role of mental health consultant as defined by Caplan (1970), the current kinds of problems and concerns faced by HCOs, as organizational entities are not effectively addressed by this model. Rather, the models of training, clinical, and particularly organizational consultation are more compatible with the changes taking place in the structure and culture of HCOs. Accordingly, the process of the organizational consultation model will be emphasized in the following sections.

PHASES IN THE CONSULTATION PROCESS

Models of consultation, particularly models of organizational consultation, are usually described in terms of several steps or phases (Doughtery, 1990; Gallessich, 1982; and Lippitt & Lippitt, 1978). Seven phases are briefly delineated here. These seven phases represent the typical process of organizational consultation.

1. **Preliminary exploration and contract negotiation.** The consultant and the consultees—that is, the people with whom the consultant works directly in the client organization—explore the organization's needs in relation to the consultant's competencies, interests, and values. The task is to determine whether there is sufficient **fit** to justify working together. If there is, a tentative contract begins to evolve, possibly even resulting in a written contractual agreement.

2. **Entry.** The consultant now officially enters the organization, begins to get acquainted with individuals, work teams, divisions, and so on, and to explore their problems and concerns. Similar to the engagement phase in psychotherapy, the task is to get sufficiently inside the organization to understand its general nature, establish open communication, and develop sufficient rapport and acceptance before continuing further.

3. **Diagnosis and formulation.** Similar to the psychiatric evaluation and formulation process, the task here is to gather and interpret sufficient data from interviews, observations, instruments, and review of appropriate records, to formulate a descriptive, explanatory, and prognostic statement of the actual problem (Sperry, Gudeman, & Blackwell, 1992). This diagnostic process includes examining the context of the problem and the organization systems affecting it.

    There are five areas of organizational problems or dysfunctioning most commonly noted among HCOs. They are power/authority, norms/standards, morale/cohesion, goals/objectives, and roles/communications. These will be described in the next section.

4. **Feedback and setting and planning the intervention.** In this phase, the consultant meets with the consultee and provides feedback on the problem formulation and the proposed goals and feasibility of the intervention alternatives. Sometimes it is concluded that there is no realistic solution, or that the goals can be reached without further help from the consultant, or that consultation

would require skills and demands outside the consultant's expertise or availability. If there is mutual agreement to proceed, the goals and intervention alternatives are discussed and negotiated in terms of time and money, barriers to be anticipated, and roles and responsibilities of consulted and consultant.

5. **Implementation of intervention.** Next, the agreed-on strategy is implemented.

6. **Evaluation of outcomes.** An evaluation of the degree to which goals have been achieved is conducted and discussed. The evaluation provides feedback for further decisions.

7. **Termination of consultation.** Termination may come at any phase in the process. Usually it comes at the end of the process after sufficient positive change has been noted. Termination plans may include follow-up sessions to reinforce the change and reduce relapse. These plans may include temporary task forces, the engagement of an internal consultant, or on-site visitation or telephone follow-ups by the contracted consultant (Gallessich, 1982).

FIVE TARGETS FOR ORGANIZATIONAL DIAGNOSIS AND INTERVENTION

The problems areas that form the basis for organizational diagnosis and intervention reflect five domains of organizational functioning. The first involves the exercise of power/authority, while the second relates to morale/cohesion. The third is centered on problems arising from norms/standards of conduct, and the fourth is any issue involving goals/objectives of the organization. Blake and Mouton (1976, 1983) have contended that all organizational problems can be subsumed in one of these four domains. Goodstein (1978) disagrees, and contends that the domain of roles/communication is an additional necessary and distinct domain of organizational functioning.

Power/authority, morale/cohesion, standards/norms, goals/objectives, and roles/communication are actually interdependent phenomenon. This means that initiating a change in one domain subsequently will result in changes in the other domains as well. For instance, a reduction of a manager's unilateral use of authority may increase morale/cohesion among staff members In short, the focal target is the domain of the organization causing or exacerbating a particular problem or concern. Though these five domains are interdependent, it is important that the consultant identify the underlying problem and domain so that interventions can be focused effectively. It is equally important for the consultant not to confuse surface problems with underlying problems.

1. Power/Authority:

Power refers to the capability of having an effect, and authority refers to the right to exercise power. Power/authority issues revolve around whether power and authority are used effectively in both formal and informal manners within the organization. Power/authority issues can arise over the ways power and authority are in fact used or over the ways their use is perceived by those who are not in positions of power within the organization. *Power/authority issues* are the most common focal target, outnumbering others by a frequency of about three to one (Blake & Mouton, 1983).

2. Morale/Cohesion:

Morale is a state of high, positive mental energy among members of an organization. Cohesion refers to the degree to which members of a group experience a positive sense of togetherness and unity. *Morale/ cohesion issues* concern how members perceive the organization and its direction, as well as the degree to which members see themselves as part of a "team."

3. Standards/Norms:

Standards are the criteria organizations use for measuring quality. Norms are the rules that govern appropriate behavior by members of all or some part of the organization. *Standard/norm issues* are frequently raised when an organization is forced to cope with internal and/or external changes. Standards and norms are usually difficult to change.

4. Goals/Objectives:

Goals are the aims and purposes of an organization, and objectives are those things that are accomplished when goals are met. *Goal/objective issues* are frequently related to standards and norms issues and typically arise when goals and objectives are either poorly defined or have not been achieved. Goal/objective issues frequently surface during investigation of standards/norms issues.

5. Roles/Communication:

Roles are expected behavior patterns attributed to a particular position in an organization. The structure of an organization specifies the reporting relationship of all roles within a given organization. Roles, along with the polices and procedures for communication, are essential in achieving the organization's task and goals. Communication is the transmission of information and understanding among individuals in various roles in the organization. *Role/communication issues* arise as roles become less clear and boundaries blur, particularly with the roles of manager and subordinate.

When compared with power/authority, other focal targets might seem less important, but such a conclusion would be unwarranted. Expecting that all organizational problems can be solved by imposing an intervention targeted at the power/authority domain is a mistake that novice consultants often make. When a surface problem is mistaken for an underlying problem the intervention that is implemented often will backfire. For example, a consultant may diagnose a clinic group's practice style as disorganized and unpredictable, and then plan an intervention to impose order via the power/authority domain. But, in due time, the group's response to this action may engender an additional set of problems, this time clearly reflective of power/authority issues. Had the consultant accurately diagnosed the underlying problem as one of standards/norms, and provided the clinic staff a structured format for discussing the situation so that constructive standards/norms would emerge without excusing power/authority dynamics, a quicker and more effective solution could have been reached without the painful side effects.

Blake and Mouton (1983) report an actual consultation with a grocery chain that further illustrates the failure to identify the underlying target problem and the subsequent failure of the intervention. The consultants assisted the organization to change its structure so that the corporate office could provide its outlets with a fuller range of marketing and distribution services. This change involved the standards/norms for operating the organization's structure. In hindsight the consultants were stunned by their failure to recognize power/authority as the underlying problem. Because power/authority was not the focus of the intervention strategy, the intervention did not produce the expected outcomes. However, had the intervention been initially directed at the power/authority focus, the consultants might then have shifted to a focus on standards/norms as a second phase of the consultation. The point of this discussion is that skill in identifying the basic focal target(s) is one of the important competencies of the effective consultant.

DIFFERENCES BETWEEN CLINICAL AND CONSULTING SERVICES

In a sense, the worlds of the clinician and of the consultant are quite different. This is particularly true with regard to roles and tasks. Consultant roles can be viewed as a continuum ranging from directive to nondirective (Lippitt & Lippitt, 1978). In a directive role the consultant acts primarily as an expert, whereas in a nondirective role the consultant is primarily a process consultant (Schein, 1987) who facilitates the consultee's expertise. The most common role that consultants take on is that of expert or technical adviser (Gallessich, 1982). In this case the consultee needs knowledge, advice, or a service that the consultant can provide on request.

The nondirective and process role has some similarity to psychotherapy. Although there are similarities between consulting and psychotherapy, there are also differences. Comparing psychotherapy and consultation makes clear the role and task differences between the clinician and the consultant.

In most forms of psychotherapy, the clinician functions more in a process-oriented and nondirective role. Although the consultant may assume various roles, such as expert, advocate, trainer, fact finder, and sounding board, during the course of a single consultation, the clinician's range of roles tends to be quite limited. Nevis (1987) used the metaphor of "working by sitting down" to describe the work of the clinician or psychotherapist, and "working by standing up" to describe the consultant's work.

The clinician tends to perform his or her service on the clinician's turf, where the usual supports and rules of the clinician prevail. But in consultation, the consultant works on the client's turf, often without the usual supports. Unlike the clinician, the consultant usually must negotiate the rules of the game.

Psychotherapy consists of primarily private events in which the clinician has low public visibility. In consultation, public events prevail and they are evaluated by many people, and the consultant may be highly visible.

In psychotherapy, the patient's values are generally close to those of the clinician, whereas in consultation, the consultee who hires the consultant may be the only one in the system with values similar to those of the consultant.

In psychotherapy, the patient is seen as owning a problem, even if he or she is confused about its nature. In an organizational context, it is often unclear what the problem is and who owns it. Whereas psychotherapy emphasizes intensive, interpersonal contact between clinician and patient, consultation usually involves contact among various parts of the system, usually with less intense interpersonal content.

Nevis (1987) noted that patients expend considerable effort in proving themselves to clinicians, whereas in consultation, clients expect consultants to prove themselves. In short, consultation tends to be a process that is less formal, less scheduled, and more complex in terms of agenda and roles than psychotherapy or other clinical services (Sperry, 1996).

INTERNAL AND EXTERNAL CONSULTANTS: ADVANTAGES AND DISADVANTAGES

An individual employed by a corporation that calls upon him or her to function in the consultant's role is called an internal consultant. External consultants, on the other hand, establish either a case-by-case contract or an ongoing retainer relationship with a given organization. There are advantages and disadvantages to each situation.

There are a number of advantages to being an internal consultant, not the least of which are a regular salary and benefits plan. Also, an internal consultant might be hired with no formal training or organizational experience and through on-the-job training become highly skilled. Another important advantage is that the internal consultant has actual membership in the corporation and is usually seen by the client as "one of us." The external consultant, on the other hand, has only quasi-membership and does not have the image of an insider. The internal consultant knows the organization's history and its typical problems, patterns, and attempted solutions. This consultant can identify the key decision makers and the power and politics of the system without needing to engage in the arduous diagnostic process in which the external consultant must engage.

There are some disadvantages to the internal consultant's role. One is that it is more difficult to have credibility as an expert in the corporation. Steele (1982) referred to this as "the prophet without honor in his own land." Similarly, by being viewed as an insider, the consultant may be taken for granted. Furthermore, the internal consultant can easily become enmeshed and find it difficult to remain objective, or he or she may even become controlled by the setting because of the need for job security. Also, by being close to one group, the consultant may be perceived as not being objective, which will allow for scapegoating and stereotyping. This consultant may have difficulty advocating a position that alienates peers. Finally, his or her recommendations are less likely to be taken seriously by peers.

The external consultant has the advantage of being more impartial and less constrained by peer pressure. The external consultant can more easily assume an advisory role, particularly to top management, which may be quite problematic for an internal consultant. External consultants, particularly those offering technical advice, may not be involved in the implementation of their recommendations. They usually do not have the administrative control of the consultee, but provide information and experience from a broader resource base. The external consultant has an ascribed status and is usually perceived to possess more special power in the organization than would the internal consultant. Accordingly, it is much easier for the external consultant to provide consultation and coaching to senior executives. The primary disadvantage of external consultants is the increased effect required to become familiar with the organization and to understand the intricacies that the internal consultant would know well.

It is becoming more common for medium-sized and large HCOs to establish an ongoing relationship with a consulting firm, usually on a retainer basis. Often this means that for a contracted annual fee, an external consultant is available to provide a given number of days of consultation per month, either on site or in the consultant's office. Even when an HCO utilizes either a full time internal consultant or the services of one or more clinicians who are occasionally asked to function in the role of internal consultant, external consultation may be sought for specific concerns. Such concerns might be outside the internal consultant expertise or involve a delicate issue, such as consultation with a senior executive (Sperry, 1996).

COMMON CONSULTATION ISSUES IN HEALTH CARE ORGANIZATIONS

Case 1: Implementing a New Treatment Outcomes System

A social worker with previous program evaluation experience was asked to assist the medical director of a large outpatient psychiatry clinic to implement a new provision in their capitation agreement: an accountability system for monitoring a treatment outcome. Previously the clinic had only a patient satisfaction survey administered quarterly, as a measurement of outcomes. Neither the clinic staff nor the capitation manager felt that this survey provided useful feedback.

The consultant arranged meetings with the capitation manager, the clinic director, and four clinicians to clarify the new system's purpose and the expected specifications and budget parameters. She then proceeded to evaluate the commercially available outcomes systems and chose one that most closely approximated the specifications that the group wanted. Provision for purchasing and implementing the system were arranged.

At the same time the consultant scheduled a series of meetings to inform the clinic and support staff about the reasons for replacing the old system with the new one, and how the outcome measures system worked. It was demonstrated using two actual cases from the clinic. Because the system provided regular feedback every fourth session from the clinician to the case manager, the consultant facilitated the staff in processing their concerns about this intrusion in their previous independent practice style, which had involved little oversight by clinic management or the capitation source. This half-day meeting served to allay clinicians' fear of breaching patient-therapist confidentiality, the intrusion of case management, and the inconvenience of a change in routine. After one year the consensus by staff was that the system was working and was effective.

This consultation illustrates how an internal consultant was able to utilize technical expertise (clarifying the clinic's need and evaluating different systems), training (demonstrating the system to the staff), and process consultation (working through the staff's concerns about the impact of the system on their practice style). This consultation could also have been provided by an external consultant. But given that the internal consultant was well-regarded by the clinic staff and that she would be utilizing the new system herself, it is more likely for there to be greater acceptance of the system and less resistance than if an external consultant had been retained.

Case 2: Bringing Harmony to a Deeply Divided Staff

Discontent and increasingly high turnover among the psychiatry staff of a large staff-model HMO led the Chief Operating Officer (COO) to retain the services of a health care consulting firm. The consultants proceeded to interview all of the remaining psychiatrists, some key administrators, and a cross-section of other clinicians. Telephone survey data on psychiatrists who used to work there was also collected. The data was analyzed and presented to the COO with a recommendation. Essentially, it was reported that the status and role of the psychiatry staff had incrementally changed over the past four years from one in which psychiatrists served as team lenders with broad discretion to provide a full range of clinical services and to supervise the psychology and social work members of their team. Currently, psychiatrists were relegated to functioning as medical and medication consultants, while a social worker or psychologist assumed the role of case manager/team leader. Some psychiatrists felt that nonmedical clinicians were insistent that psychiatrists sign off on their cases without even seeing the patient, and in some instances to request that the psychiatrist sign off on medication changes that these nonmedical therapist were advocating. Morale among the psychiatrists had plummeted, and the prospects of even more psychiatrists quitting was high.

The consultant formulated the problem as principally one of power/ authority and role/communications, and secondarily, as one of morale/ cohesion. Initially, the consultant met with the COO and presented the formulation and recommendations to revise the reporting relationship among clinical personnel. The consultant emphasized the psychiatry staff's concern about both legal liability and ethical principles regarding both medication and signing off, and the liability and malpractice implications of these practices. It was agreed that the COO would meet with the entire staff to discuss these matters. The consultants would be present at the meeting to provide input and to support the COO, but the meeting was to be lead by the COO. At the meeting the COO reviewed changes in the past five years of the HMO's history. He then proposed a new experiment regarding reporting relationships and the rationale for it. In the experiment, which would begin immediately and be evaluated in six months, all clinical staff would have dual reporting relationships. They would report to their team's case manager for fiscal and administrative matters regarding their patients, and for clinical matters they would report to the team's psychiatrist. Furthermore, role expectations for all clinicians were clarified and articulated, particularly regarding medical malpractice and ethical standards. Because the consultants had assessed that the staff had a high level of trust and respect for the COO, they predicted that his recommendations would be accepted, not only because the rationale was reasonable, but also because the change was an experiment that would be reviewed in six months. The clinic staff did, indeed, implement these changes.

This case illustrates a technical-expertise intervention (data collection and advisement of the COO) for power/authority and role/communication problems in an HCO. By advising the COO to conduct the meeting and to frame the proposed changes in terms of legal and ethical necessity instead of turf war, unnecessary conflict was avoided. Finally, framing the changes as an experiment, which would be reviewed after a short time, further reduced the potential for splitting and negative catharsis, while increasing morale and cohesion among the staff, particularly among the psychiatrists.

Case 3: Consultation Involving Staff Safety

An organizational psychology firm specializing in workplace violence was engaged by the Director of Human Resources (HR) of a skilled nursing care facility after both clinical and support staff raised concerns about their safety and that of their patients. Apparently, a former boyfriend of a nursing assistant had been stalking her for over a month. Recently, he had been seen waiting for her in the parking lot. The day before the firm was hired the man had been roaming the halls of the facility brandishing a pistol and saying, "I'll get her." Fortunately, the stalked employee had left earlier that day to keep a dental appointment, and the stalker left upon learning this. Nevertheless, staff and patients who had seen the man with a gun were extremely distressed. The two consultants quickly ascertained that the facility had a security department but no safety-violence policy, nor programming for the aftermath of a violent episode. The consultation took two forms: immediate attention to the crisis situationn and a program to prevent violence in the future. The consultants met with the nursing assistant to assess her need for protection and crisis counseling. They also met with the HR director, the director of nursing, and the director of security to formulate a strategy for dealing with the stalker. The goal was to ensure that proper security measures were in place to protect the facility, its employees, and its patients. Next, the consultants assisted the HR director in establishing a work safety committee made up of four employee representatives plus the directors of safety, nursing, and HR. Their task was to develop and implement a safety-violence policy. The consultants provided examples of policies used by other nursing facilities, and assisted the group in tailoring a policy to their unique circumstances. In addition, education programs to teach staff to respond to threatening situations were planned and implemented, as was a violence aftermath program of group stress debriefing intervention and individual crisis counseling. The consultants contracted to provide counseling services for staff and patients and their families for violence-related issues beginning with the recent episode.

This consultation was quite straightforward and illustrates how the external consultants provided clinical and technical expertise and process consultation that converged on the problem of morale/cohesion— here, on the high degree of fear and threat engendered by the stalker.

Secondarily, this consultation focused on the goal/objectives domain of safety policy and programs. While an external consultant provided these services, one or more knowledgeable staff clinicians could have assumed the consulting role.

Case 4: Decreasing Dissatisfaction and Increasing Strategic Focus Among Clinicians

A social worker in a small behavioral health care network was asked to be an internal consultant to improve the network's effectiveness in service delivery. Dissatisfaction had been expressed by clients and referral sources about the increasing time lag between referral and initial appointment. Some complained the certain clinicians were inflexible in their practice style and were committed only to longer-term psychotherapy. The consultant was charged with defining the network's problem areas and prescribing strategies for managing them effectively.

The social worker had previous experience consulting to community health centers, in addition to having considerable clinical experience. She began by informing all network providers of the nature of the consultation. Interviews and surveys were utilized to gather data from administration, providers, and present and former clients. Information was collected, with the guarantee of confidentiality, on matters such as the network's mission, culture, practice styles, and staff relations. Based on the analysis of data the consultant concluded that there was minimal consensus about the network's mission, which led to a lack of understanding of the functioning of the network and roles of different clinical and administrative staff members. The result was overall dissatisfaction and factionalism, particularly among clinicians.

She prescribed a review and modification of the mission statement and practice styles. Furthermore, she recommended that a three-year strategic plan be developed and suggested that all staff be involved in this process. Subsequently, the consultant facilitated the mission statement review and the strategic planning design. Out of this came an updated mission statement and set of guidelines for case loads, practice style, and indications and contraindications for longer-term versus time-limited psychotherapeutic services.

This case illustrates a situation in which the consulting focus was primarily on goals/objectives and secondarily in norms/standards. Specifically, this intervention established practice guidelines for case load, practice style, and similar issues by and for the network's clinicians. Because the clinicians themselves were thoroughly involved in the process, they owned the practice guidelines. The case also illustrates how both technical expertise—data collection by survey and interviews—and process—mission and strategic planning—consultation modes were utilized.

CONCLUDING COMMENT

All work organizations are being radically affected by the mounting changes occurring in our society. In some ways, HCOs are experiencing these changes, and demands for change, even more painfully than other organizations. Consequently, HCOs are in great need of assistance, and psychologically trained consultants can assist HCOs in adapting to these changes. These consultants may be either internal or external. These services may be provided by inhouse HCO psychologists, social workers, or psychiatrists who have sufficient training and confidence to allow them to shift from the clinical to the consulting role.

REFERENCES

Blake, R., & Mouton, J. (1976). *Consultation.* Reading, MA: Addison-Wesley.

Blake, R., & Mouton, J. (1983). *Consultation: A handbook for individual and organizational development, (2nd ed.)* Reading, MA: Addison-Wesley.

Blake, R., & Mouton, J. (1985). *The Managerial grid III.* Houston, TX: Gulf.

Caplan, G. (1970). *The theory and practice of mental health consultation.* New York: Basic Books.

Dougherty, A. (1990). *Consultation: Practices and perspectives.* Pacific Grove, CA, Brooks/Cole.

Gallessich, J. (1982). *The profession and practice of consultation: A handbook for consultants, trainers, and consumers of consultation services.* San Francisco, CA: Jossey-Bass.

Goodstein, L. (1978). *Consulting with human service systems.* Reading, MA: Addison-Wesley.

Grant, B. (1994). Organizational change in your own back yard. *Academy of Organizational and Occupational Psychiatry Newsletter 3,*(2), 1.

Levinson, H. (1972). *Organizational diagnosis.* Cambridge, MA: Harvard University Press.

Lippitt, G., & Lippitt, R. (1978). *The consulting process in action.* San Diego, CA: University Associates.

Martin, S. (1995). Fox identifies top threats to professional psychology. *APA Monitor,* 26(3), 44.

Schein, E. (1987). *Process consultation: Lessons for managers and consultants, Vol 2.* Reading, MA: Addison-Wesley.

Sperry, L. (1993). *Psychiatric consultation in the workplace.* Washington, DC: American Psychiatric Press.

Sperry, L. (1996). *Corporate consulting and therapy.* New York: Brunner/Mazel.

Sperry, L., Gudeman, J., & Blackwell, B. (1992). *Psychiatric case formulations.* Washington, DC: American Psychiatric Press.

Steele, F. (1982). *The role of the internal consultant.* Boston, MA. CBI Publishing.

Sussman, M. (Ed.). (1995). *A perilous calling: The hazards of psychotherapy practice.* New York: John Wiley.

Taylor, R., & Taylor, S. (Eds.). *The AUPHA manual of health services management.* Gaithersburg, MD: Aspen.

APPENDIX A

Glossary of Managed Care Terms and Definitions

This glossary of terms has been compiled from several sources including *Charter Medical's Clinical Documentation for Managers,* the *Managed Healthcare Handbook Glossary of Terms,* and the *Psychiatric News.*

AAPCC: Adjusted Average Per Capita Cost. The Health Care Financing Administration's (HCFA's) best estimate of the amount of money it costs to care for Medicare recipients under fee-for-service Medicare in a given area. The AAPCC is made up of 122 different rate cells; 120 of them are factored for age, sex, Medicaid eligibility, institutional status, and whether a person has both Part A and Part B of Medicare; the two remaining cells are for individuals with end-stage renal disease.

Access to Care: An estimated 37 million Americans are without health insurance, and millions more are believed to be uninsured. Lack of access is the defining moral and ethical problem with the current system of health delivery and financing; lack of access to mental health services is even more pervasive.

Accrual: The amount of money that is set aside to cover expenses. The accrual is the plan's best estimate of what those expenses are, and (for medical expenses) is based on a combination of data from the authorization system, the claims system, the lag studies, and the plan's prior history.

ACR: Adjusted Community Rate. Used by Health Maintenance Organizations and Competitive Medical Plans with Medicare risk contracts. A calculation of what premium the plan would charge for providing exactly the Medicare-covered benefits to a group account, adjusted to allow for the greater intensity and frequency of utilization by Medicare recipients. The ACR includes the normal profit of a for-profit HMO or CMP. The ACR may be equal to or lower than the APR (see below), but can never exceed it. This is also known as ASO (Administrative Services Only).

ACS Contract: See ASO contract.

Actuarial Assumptions: The assumptions that an actuary uses in calculating the expected costs and revenues of the plan. Examples include utilization rates, age and sex mix of enrollees, cost for medical services, and so on.

Actuary: An expert in the mathematics of life insurance, annuities, and accident and health insurance. Usually involved in the calculation rates, reserves, dividends, statistical studies, and the annual statement.

Admission Review: Review that is conducted subsequent to the admission.

Adverse Selection: The problem of attracting members who are sicker than the general population, specifically, members who are sicker than was anticipated when developing the budget for medical costs.

All-Payer System: A plan to impose uniform prices on medical services, regardless of who is paying. President Clinton is exploring the possibility of at least a temporary all-payer structure.

Alternative Programming: Alternative services developed by providers, which can replace traditional, standardized inpatient treatment programs. These are attractive to employers and payors due to lower costs. Some examples include: intensive outpatient programs, partial hospitalization, short-stay inpatient programming, and so on.

Anniversary Date: The date each year when an insurance contract becomes effective.

APR: Average Payment Rate. The amount of money that HCFA could conceivably pay an HMO or CMP for services to Medicare recipients under a risk contract. The figure is derived from the AAPCC for the service area, adjusted for the enrollment characteristics that the plan would be expected to have. The payment to the plan, the ACR, can never be higher than the APR, but may be less.

ASO Contract: A contract between an insurance company and a self-funded plan where the insurance company performs administrative services only and does not assume any risk. Services usually include claims processing, but may include other services such as actuarial analysis, utilization review, and so on.

At Risk/Risk Sharing: Any reimbursement agreement other than fee for service is considered at risk in some way. The more variables a provider takes into consideration (price risk, volume risk, actuarial risk, and so on), the greater the risk. A discounted fee-for-service agreement represents the least risk to a provider while reimbursements such as capitation and percent of premium represent the greater financial risk.

AWP: Average Wholesale Price. Commonly used in pharmacy contracting.

Beneficiary: A patient or member of a particular benefit plan. This term includes the concept of dependents.

Board Certified: A term used to describe a physician who has passed examinations given by a medical specialty group and as a result has been certified as a specialist in an area of practice. Board certification generally denotes a degree of competency across national standards that is higher than the minimal standards to practice as defined by individual state licensure.

Bundling of Services: Grouping related items and services into bundles and establishing a price for it—for example, chemical dependency, open heart surgery. This is also known as all-inclusive per diem.

Capitation: A specific population is assigned to a provider, and the provider is paid a flat payment each month for each member of the population. In return for this per capita payment, the provider assumes the obligation and the risk to provide all medical services required by plan members as defined by their benefit plan.

Carrier: Insurance company (primary insurer).

Carve-Outs: A benefit strategy in which the employer separates (carves out) the mental substance abuse portion of health care benefits from others and hires an MMHC company to manage or provide these benefits through its networks. Affords the employer with specialized management for this portion of the overall benefits package.

Case Management: Medical management of a patient's individual condition and needs (as opposed to a standardized program). This involves management of the patient's entire course of treatment through the continuum, including aftercare. The case manager works closely with the treating therapist, additional treatment team professionals, family and/or patient in the development and ongoing management of a treatment plan that is an alternative to the current acute level of care.

Certification: Certification denotes the process of patient-specific, individualized review and determination based on clinical data provided by the attending physician. Elements of the review process include: diagnosis, severity of illness, intensity of treatment, and level of care. The certification decision establishes the medical necessity and appropriateness of treatment within the clinical criteria as it applies to the benefit design.

Channeling: Methods of steering patients toward discounted services or providers. Some examples include: EAP (when required as a point of entry to the system), toll free numbers, and financial incentives or disincentives, such as a sufficient spread in the in-network/out-of-network reimbursement (90%/70%).

Chemical Dependency: Substance abuse; alcohol or drug abuse.

Claim adjudication: A claims department review to determine patient eligibility, provider status, the existence of certification, and the amount of appropriate payment. Claims are adjudicated and forwarded to a third- party payor (insurance company) for payment.

Closed Panel: A managed care plan that contracts with physicians on an exclusive basis for services, not allowing members to see physicians outside of the limited exclusive panel of providers for routine care. Examples include staff and group model HMOs, but could apply to a large private medical group that contracts with an HMO.

CMP: Competitive Medical Plan. A federal designation that allows a health plan to obtain eligibility to receive a Medicare risk contract without having to obtain qualification as an HMO. Requirements for eligibility are somewhat less restrictive than for an HMO.

COA: Certificate of Authority. The state-issued operating license for an HMO.

COBRA: Consolidated Omnibus Reconciliation Act. A portion of this act requires employers to offer the opportunity for terminated employees to purchase continuation of health care coverage under the group's medical plan. Another portion eases a medical recipient's ability to disenroll from an HMO or CMP with a medical risk contract.

Coinsurance: The ratio by which the member's/covered insured's share of medical claim expenses is determined. It is generally limited to a maximum fixed dollar liability for the insured. The provision in a member's (or insured's) coverage limits the amount of coverage by the plan to a certain percentage, commonly 80%. Any additional costs are paid by the member out of pocket.

Community Rating: The rating methodology required of federally qualified HMOs, and required of HMOs under the laws of many states. The HMO must obtain the same amount of money per member for all members in the plan. Community rating does allow for variability by allowing the HMO to factor in differences for age, sex, mix (average contract size), and industry factors; not all factors are necessarily allowed under state laws, however.

CON: Certificate of Need. The requirement that a health care organization obtain permission from an oversight agency before making changes or adding services. Federally qualified HMOs are exempt from having to obtain a CON.

Concurrent Review: Review of inpatient status by utilization review or payor during hospitalization to verify appropriate length of stay and the medical necessity of services being provided.

Continued Stay Review: Conducted subsequent to the initial review. The purpose of these periodic reviews is to obtain further certification based on medical necessity, appropriateness of treatment, progress, and discharge planning.

Contractuals: The difference between the provider's charges billed to the contracted payor and the amount paid by the payor. The contract or agreement generally requires that this amount be adjusted from the patient's balance and cannot be collected from the patient.

Coordination of Benefits (COB): An agreement using language developed by the National Association of Insurance Commissioners that prevents double payment for services when a subscriber has coverage from two or more sources. It is a process to coordinate multiple active insurance policies. This sharing of medical expenses through primary and secondary insurers determines how the charges related to a medical claim will be settled. One organization has primary responsibility for payment and the other has secondary responsibility for payment.

Copayment (or copays): Refers to the amount of money that a beneficiary is responsible for paying per visit; copayment is usually either a flat dollar amount or a percentage of a fee schedule (and varies from contract to contract). That portion of a claim or medical expense that a member (or covered insured) must pay out of his or her own pocket. Usually a fixed amount, such as $5 in many HMOs.

Cost Containment: Containing costs of health care, or at least slowing their annual rise.

Cost of Services Ratio (COS Ratio): The ratio between the cost incurred by managed care entity that is directly related to service delivery, and the amount of revenue taken in. A COS ratio of 75% or more is common in MMHC operations, and excludes administrative or overhead costs.

Cost Shifting: When dwindling access meets rising costs, the result is a shift in costs from those who cannot pay for their care to those who can and do. Many uninsured people, for instance, access the health system at a very expensive level—namely, the emergency room. The costs of that care get shifted onto paying patients.

Current Procedural Terminology (CPT) Codes: Sets of five-digit codes frequently used for billing professional services.

DAW: Dispense as Written. The instruction from a physician to a pharmacist to dispense a brand-name pharmaceutical rather than a generic substitution.

Deductible: An insurance term that refers to the amount of monetary liability that an individual assumes during a particular period or for a given occurrence. It is that portion of a subscriber's (or member's) health care expenses that must be paid out of pocket before any insurance coverage applies. Deductibles are generally fixed-dollar amounts, while coinsurance is usually a percentage. Deductibles are not allowed in federally qualified HMOs (and often not allowed under state HMO regulations), although copayment requirements can achieve exactly the same result. Common in insurance plans and PPOs.

Delegated Review: Future trend of managed care to assign the responsibility of review to the provider that has demonstrated a willingness to deliver appropriate services and length of stay. In other words, the provider reviews itself.

Detoxification (Detox): A medical regimen to systematically reduce the amount of a toxic agent in a patient's body, provide reasonable control of active withdrawal symptoms, and avert a life threatening medical crisis, which is conducted under the supervision of a physician.

Discounted Fee-for-Service Rate: Provider discounts full charges for services rendered. Typically covers room, board, and ancillaries, but not physician fees. Ancillary services include services such as lab work, pharmacy, and activity therapy, that are normally provided during the course of inpatient treatment with the hospital. Providers that accept discounted charges risk the possibility that the discounted prices will not cover variable cost and make an adequate contribution to overhead. This is called price risk.

Disenrollment: The process of termination of coverage. Voluntary termination would include a member quitting because he or she desires to do so. Involuntary termination would include leaving the plan because of changing jobs. A rare and serious form of involuntary disenrollment is when the plan terminates a member's coverage against his or her will. This is usually only allowed (under state and federal laws) for gross offenses such as fraud, abuse, nonpayment of premium or copayments, or a demonstrated inability to comply with recommended treatment plans.

DRG: Diagnosis-Related Groups. A system of classifying any inpatient stay into groups for purposes of payment. DRGs may be primary or secondary, and an outlier classification also exists. This is the form of reimbursement that HCFA uses to pay providers for Medicare recipients. Also used by a few states for all payers, and by some private health plans for contracting purposes.

DSM-IV: Diagnostic Statistical Manual, Fourth Edition. This is the current edition of the nationally recognized classification/labeling system used to identify psychiatric and substance abuse diagnoses.

Dual Choice: Sometimes referred to as Section 1310 or Mandating. The portion of the federal HMO regulations that require any employer with 25 or more employees residing in the HMO's services area, who pays minimum wage, and who offers health coverage, to offer a federally qualified HMO as well. The HMO must request it.

Dual option: The offering of both an HMO and a traditional insurance plan by one carrier.

Elective: Those services that are not considered to be an emergency and could be delayed by the patient to a later time with no ill effects.

Eligibility: A condition defined by provisions of a group policy that states the requirements members of the insured group must satisfy to become insured with respect to themselves and their dependents.

ELOS: Estimated length of stay for full course of treatment.

Emergency: Those services required to provide an immediate diagnosis and treatment of a medical condition of sudden and unpredictable onset. Such conditions must be marked by acute symptoms of sufficient severity so that, in the absence of emergency medical attention, could reasonably be expected to jeopardize the patient's life, they cause severe impairment in bodily functions, or cause serious dysfunction of bodily parts.

Employee Assistance Programs (EAP): Counseling service that provides short-term assessment counseling and refers employees to appropriate services. This counseling and assessment process is generally viewed as a prevention service that performs triage and refers employees entering the mental health/addictive disease treatment system. Employee participation in these programs have been voluntary for the most part. Generally, there are two types of EAPs:

> • *In-House EAP:* Clinical staff employed by the company who perform short-term assessment counseling and referral service on behalf of the company. Levels of service vary greatly depending upon the company. These individuals typically work very closely with other regional/national EAPs and/or directly with local providers. J.C. Penney Company is an example of a company with an in-house EAP that has combined traditional EAP, PPO, and Utilization Management services in house. In this case, the in-house EAP negotiated a nonexclusive PPO with providers and, through its corporate staff, performs precertification and case management procedures.

> • *National/Regional/Local EAP:* Historically, these companies provide services to employers on a per capita fee for service basis. Fees typically cover both the employees and their dependents and are usually expressed as a certain amount per employee per month. Services typically include utilization reporting, management reports, policy and procedure development on mental health/addictive disease issues, supervisory training, employee orientations, and/or educational material.

Enrollee: An individual who is eligible for benefits under a health care plan. Frequently used in connection with indemnity insurance.

EOB: See Explanation of Benefits.

EPO: Exclusive Provider Organization. An EPO is similar to an HMO in that it uses primary physicians as gatekeepers, often capitates providers, has a limited provider panel, uses an authorization system, and so on. The main difference is that EPOs are generally regulated under insurance statues rather than HMO regulations.

ERISA: Employee Retirement Income Security Act. One provision of this act allows self-funded plans to avoid paying premium taxes or comply with state-mandated benefits, even when insurance companies and managed care plans must do so. Another provision requires that plans and insurance companies provide an Explanation of Benefits (EOB) statement to a member or covered insured in the event of a denial of a claim, explaining why a claim was denied and informing the individual of his or her rights of appeal.

Exclusions by Contract: Conditions or services that are not covered under the beneficiary's medical plan.

Experience Rated Premium: A premium calculation method that takes into account the actual utilization of the group rather than the combined utilization of all groups.

Explanation of Benefits (EOB): A statement mailed to a member or covered insured explaining why a claim was or was not paid. The statement contains the minimum legally required information relating to the amounts paid on a given claim and an explanation of any amounts not paid. Sending an EOB (or practitioner voucher), usually with the check, is sometimes a contract requirement and sometimes done only as an informational courtesy.

Favored Nations Discount: A contractual agreement between a provider and a payor stating that the provider will automatically provide the payer with the best discount it provides anyone else. Common between Blue Cross and participating providers.

Fee for Service: Medicine, the old fashioned way. Patients pay doctors and hospitals for each service rendered. President Clinton says that this method gives doctors an incentive to perform unnecessary services.

FEHBP: Federal Employee Health Benefits Program. The program that provides health benefits to federal employees. See OPM.

Fiduciary: Under ERISA, any person or entity that exercises discretionary control over the administration of a benefit plan. Self-insured employers can delegate this responsibility to MMHC or Utilization Review firms concurring Mental Health and Substance Abuse benefits.

First Level Appeal: This is an appeal by a treating therapist, Utilization Review coordinator or beneficiary, either in writing or via phone, in response to a non-certification decision rendered by the Utilization Review entity.

FTE: Full-Time Equivalent. The equivalent of one full-time employee. For example, two part-time employees are ½ FTE each, for a total of one (1) FTE.

Group HMO: Delivers services at one or more locations through a group of physicians with which the HMO has a contract to provide care. An example is Kaiser Permanente.

HCFA: Health Care Financing Administration. The federal agency that oversees all aspects of health financing for Medicare and also oversees the Office of Prepaid Health Care.

HCXFA 1500: Standard outpatient billing form for providers.

HIPCs: The abbreviation for "health insurance purchasing cooperatives." An essential component of managed competition, HIPCs would purchase a menu of accountable health plans—or organized systems of care—for groups of businesses and individuals. As envisioned by proponents of managed competition, these cooperatives would allow for universal coverage and could offer insurance at lower rates by spreading risk over a larger pool of insured individuals.

HMO (Health Maintenance Organization): HMOs are an organized system of health care delivery and financing. These organizations are at risk, since payment for services is on a fixed prepaid basis based on the number of enrolled members (a predetermined amount per member per month). HMOs can be classified into four types of organizational structures or models that are determined primarily by their relationship with physicians. These are:

- *Group HMO:* Delivers services at one or more locations through a group of physicians with which the HMO has a contract to provide care.

- *Mixed Model HMO:* A managed care plan that mixes two or more types of delivery systems. This has traditionally been used to describe an HMO that has both closed panel and open panel delivery systems.

- *Network HMO:* Delivers services through two or more group practices or IPAs with which the HMO has contracts to provide care.

• *Staff HMO:* Delivers services at one or more locations through a staff of physicians who are salaried employees of the HMO.

HMO Act of 1973: Amended in 1988. This law allowed HMOs to become federally qualified by meeting various standards. Once so designated, the HMO has the right to ask any local employer of twenty-five or more employees to offer it as a health care benefit option. HMOs were required to charge the same community rate to all employers, pooling all employers together for risk purposes. In 1988, Congress amended the Act. The right of HMOs to put themselves on the benefit menu of local employers was scheduled to expire in 1995. HMOs were allowed to adjust premiums by actual employer group experience, no longer adhering to a community rating system. Caps were placed to provide services through non-HMO physicians, charging extra fees when members utilize such services.

Hospital Days: A measurement of the number of days of hospital care a population uses in a specific period of time. Usually reported in days per 1000 lives per year.

IBNR: Incurred But Not Reported. The amount of money that the plan should accrue for medical expenses that it knows nothing about yen These are medical expenses that the authorization system has not captured and for which claims have not yet hit the door.

ICD-9-CM: International Classification of Diseases, 9th Revision, Clinical Modification. The classification of disease by diagnosis, codified into 4-digit numbers. Frequently used for billing purposes by hospitals.

Independent Physician (or Practice) Association (IPA): Individual community physicians or healthcare providers who contract with a variety of health care plans or individual providers to provide services in return for a single capitation rate. Such services may include health care, utilization review, and so on.

Independent Practitioner Organization (IPO): Similar to an IPA, an IPO is an organization of providers—usually physicians. The primary differences between an IPA and an IPO are that most IPAs contract with one single HMO, while an IPO may contract with multiple types of plans, and IPOs generally do not assume risk.

Initial Review: The initial or first review, during which an estimated length of stay (ELOS) is established for the case being reviewed. The reviewer grants the provider an initial length of stay based on the severity of the illness and the intensity of the treatment at that point in time. The reviewer then selects a date for the first continued stay review to discuss progress towards the treatment goal identified.

Integrated Health Plans: A type of benefit plan in which all employees are enrolled into a single managed care system for all health care services. Members may have options to utilize non-network providers, but at an increased cost.

Leg Study: A report that tells managers the age of the claims being processed and how much is paid out each month (for that month and for any earlier months), and compares those totals to the amounts of money that had been accrued for expenses each month. The most powerful tool available to determine if the plan's reserves are adequate to meet all expenses. To avoid financial difficulties, it is imperative that lag studies be performed, and performed properly.

Length of Stay: The amount of time an individual spends in the hospital per admission, averaged for group numbers.

Level of Care: The intensity of professional medical care required to achieve the treatment objectives for a specific episode of care.

Lives: The number of people insured by a particular insurance plan.

LOS/ELOS/ALOS: Length of Stay/Estimated Length of Stay/Average Length of Stay. Refers to a hospital stay.

MAB: Medical Advisory Board is a selected panel of experts in mental health/ substance abuse treatment who act as advisors/consultants.

MAC: Maximum Allowable Charge (or Cost).

Managed Care or Managed Mental Health Care (MMHC): Refers to any of a variety of systems and strategies aimed at marshalling appropriate clinical and financial resources to ensure needed care for consumers. It features increased structure and accountability for providers and the overall coordination of care, while eliminating duplicative or unnecessary services.

Managed Competition: Originally formulated by the so-called Jackson Hole Group, an informal group of economists, policymakers and providers, the managed competition model views problems in today's system as stemming from perverse market incentives that cause patients to seek more and more services, and induce physicians to provide ever more costly services. Managed competition would restructure the system so that care is provided by "accountable health plans" or organized systems of care competing with one another on the basis of cast and outcome.

Mandated Benefits: Minimal benefit levels established by statutes enacted by state legislatures. These vary from state to state and can add to overall health care costs. ERISA exempts employers who are self-insured from these mandates. Other exceptions have been made for basic, low cost insurance products that can be offered to the uninsured segment of the workforce.

MCE: Medical Care Evaluation. A component of a quality assurance program that looks at the process of medical care.

Medical Reimbursement Account: An increasingly popular feature of new employer sponsored health benefit plans designed to assist employees with the increased cost-sharing associated with these plans. The employee annually sets aside pre-tax dollars into the medical reimbursement account that may be used for expenses such as copayments, payments deductibles, eyeglasses, well baby care, or child care expenses. Employers sometimes contribute to the accounts.

Medical Loss Ratio: The ratio between the cost to deliver medical care and the amount of money that was taken in by a plan. Insurance companies often have a medical loss ratio of 96% or more; tightly managed HMOs may have medical loss ratios of 75% to 85%, although the overhead (or administrative cost ratio) is concomitantly higher. The medical loss ratio is dependent on the amount of money brought in as well as the cost of delivering care; thus, if the rates are too low, the ratio may be high, even though the actual cost of delivering care is not really out of line.

Medical Necessity and Appropriateness of Services: Services that are: (a) required for the diagnosis or care and treatment of medical condition; (b) appropriate and necessary for symptoms, diagnosis or treatment of a medical condition; (c) generally accepted standard of medical practice recognized in the medical community; (d) performed in the least costly setting or manner appropriate to treat the patient's medical condition; and (e), not primarily for the convenience of the patient, the patient's family, the physician, or another Provider.

Member: An individual who is eligible for benefits under a health care plan, particularly an HMO or other prepaid system.

Member Months: The total of all months that each member was covered. For example, if a plan had 10,000 members in January and 12,000 members in

February, the total member months for the year-to-date as of March 1 would be 22,000.

MIS: Management Information System. The common term for the computer hardware and software that provides the support—data, management information, and so on—for managing the plan.

Mixed Model HMO: A managed care plan that mixes two or more types of delivery systems. This has traditionally been used to describe an HMO that has both closed panel and open panel delivery systems.

MLP: Midlevel Practitioner. Physician's assistants, clinical nurse practitioners, nurse midwives, and so on. Nonphysicians who deliver medical care, generally under the supervision of a physician, but for less cost.

NAHMOR: National Association of HMO Regulators.

NAIC: National Association of Insurance Commissioners.

National Health Board: More than one model for health reform, including the managed competition model, has envisioned a central governing body that would define a basic benefits package, provide consumer information about health care, and negotiate rates with physicians.

Network or Provider Network: A group of providers, organized, accredited, and administered by a MMHC firm. Members agree to practice in an effective, cost-conscious manner utilizing the MMHC firm's clinical guidelines or standards. Members also agree to discounted fee arrangements. In turn, they are eligible for referrals, through their MMHC firm, of members of employer groups contracting with the firm. Providers agree to the MMHC firm's quality management program. The network may include both inpatient and outpatient providers. It is increasingly important for providers to join networks in order to allow access to their services by large numbers of potential patients. This requires providers to become familiar with goal-oriented, solution-focused therapies, to manage practices efficiently, and to develop innovative practice styles in order to compete successfully for referrals.

Network HMO: Delivers services through two or more group practices or IPAs with which the HMO has contracts to provide care. An example would be SHARE or Health America.

OBRA/SOBRA: Sixth Omnibus Reconciliation Act Of 1985. Portions of this act created quality review organizations (QROs) and empowered QROs and peer review organizations (PROs) to monitor quality of care for Medicare recipients enrolled in HMOs or CMPs, provided for civil monetary penalties for plans that failed to provide proper care, and restricted the types of physician incentives that a managed care plan may use when providing care for Medicare recipients. Also made disenrollment from HMOs and CMPs far easier for Medical recipients.

OHMO/OPHC: Office of Health Maintenance Organizations (old name)/Office of Prepaid Health Care (new name). The federal agency that oversees federal qualification and compliance for HMOs and eligibility for CMPs. Was once part of' the Public Health Service, now is part of HCFA.

Open Enrollment Period: The period when an employee may change health plans. Usually occurs once per year. A general rule is that most managed care plans will have approximately half of their membership up for open enrollment in the fall, for an effective date of January 1. A special form of open enrollment is law in some states. This yearly open enrollment requires an HMO to accept any individual applicant for coverage (persons not coming in through an employer group), regardless of health status, and only charge them the standard community rate. Such special open enrollments occur for one month each year.

Open Panel: A managed care plan that contracts (either directly or indirectly) with private physicians to deliver care in their own offices. Examples would include a direct contract HMO and an IPA.

OPM: Of Personnel Management. The federal agency that administers the FEHBP. This is the agency that a managed care plan contracts with to provide coverage for federal employees.

Organized Systems of Care: Also known as accountable health plans, organized systems of care are an essential component of managed competition. Under that model, these systems of care would be induced to provide quality, low-cost medical treatment by being forced to compete with other systems in a regional market, on the basis of cost and outcome.

Out-of-Pocket Maximum: The maximum amount an insured person will have to pay for a covered health care expense. Often this amount is $500, $1000, or more, or a percentage of annual salary. Usually calculated on a yearly basis.

PAR: Preadmission Review; also referred to as precertification. While this function is used in virtually all types of managed care plans, the term is most commonly applied to plans that utilize telephone-based nurses to review cases, assign expected lengths of stay, and issue an authorization number.

PAS Norms: The common term for Professional Activity Study results of the Commission on Professional and Hospital Activities. Broken out by region; the Western region has the lowest average length of stay (LOS), so it tends to be used most often to set an estimated LOS. Available as *LOS: Length of Stay by Diagnosis,* published by CPHA publications, Ann Arbor, MI.

PCP: Primary Care Physician. Generally applies to internists, pediatricians, family physicians, general practitioners, and occasionally to obstetrician/gynecologists.

Peer Review: Internal or external case review of treatment and/or length of stay between the treating clinician and another designated clinician.

Per Case Rate: Occasionally providers are asked to contract with managed care companies on a per case basis. Providers are paid an average flat price per discharge. This is similar to the Medicare DRG system although the patient categories can be defined differently. With a Variable Per Case rate, the per case rate decreases as volume from a particular contract increases over the contract period.

Percent of Premium: In these contracts, the managed care company agrees to give a predetermined percentage of its monthly premium to the provider to cover the total cost of medical services for a defined population. Since payment to the provider depends both on the number of enrollees and on the premium charged to subscriber, the provider is exposed to an actuarial and marketing rise, in addition to all other risks, and should include stop-loss provisions.

Per Diem Rate: Reimbursement based on a set rate per day rather than on charges. Represents the most common form of payment sought by managed care companies today. Providers are asked to aggregate individual services into average daily rates. Typically covers room, board, ancillaries, but not physician fees. However, there is a growing trend on the part of managed care companies to include physician fees in the negotiated per diem rate. With a Variable Per Diem rate, the per diem rate decreases as volume from a particular contract increases over the contract period. Also see Bundling of Services.

PMPM: Per Member Per Month. Specifically applies to a revenue or cost for each enrolled member each month.

PMPY: The same as PMPM, but based on a year.

Point-of-Service Plan: A plan where members do not have to choose how to receive services until they need them. A common example is a simple PPO, where members receive coverage at a greater level if they use preferred providers than if they choose not to do so. Less common examples include an HMO Swing-out, a Point-of-Service HMO, an Out-of-Plan Benefits Rider to an HMO, or a Primary Care PPO. These are plans that provide a dramatic difference in benefits (100% coverage vs. 60%) depending on whether the member chooses to use the plan (including its providers and compliance with the authorization system) or go outside the plan for services.

PPA: Preferred Provider Arrangement: Same as a PPO, but sometimes is used to refer to a somewhat looser type of plan in which the payer (that is, the employer) makes the arrangement rather than the providers.

PPO (Preferred Provider organization): A plan that contracts with independent providers at a discount for services. The panel is limited in size and usually has some type of utilization review system associated with it.

Practice Guidelines: Recommended therapies and procedures for the treatment of specific disorders so as to achieve optimum results as efficiently as possible. They are not rigid standards, but rather offer supportive guidance to clinicians. Many MMHC organizations use such guidelines for quality assurance or accountability purposes. Practice guidelines are developed from the clinical literature, professional societies, and/or through other clinician input forums.

Practitioner/Therapist: Individual clinical provider of services.

Preadmission Review (PAR): Also known as precertification for admission. A common function in various managed care systems. This term is also commonly used to denote a participating facility, one that is contracted with a managed care entity to participate in its utilization management activities, including preadmission review.

Precertification: A process of contacting the designated utilization management company on behalf of the beneficiary to obtain authorization for treatment. Precertification is generally required by most benefit plans and must take place prior to the provision of any treatment, or reimbursement could be effected. See Certification.

Primary Care Physician (PCP): Usually internists, family physicians, general practitioners, and pediatricians. Some managed care plans require PCP screening and referral of members in need of mental health or substance abuse treatment services.

Provider: professional who delivers clinical services to a managed care member. Facility provider refers to hospital or other institutional entities.

Provider Relations Manager: A coordinating position, found in some HMOs, which has responsibility for the recruitment and credentialing of PCPs or other providers. Provider relations is a function in all managed mental health care systems that utilize Provider Networks.

PTMPY: Per Thousand Members Per Year. A common way of reporting utilization. The most common example is hospital utilization, expressed as days per thousand members per year.

Quality Assurance: Established standards of good care that are periodically evaluated to determine how well a hospital's physicians and clinical staff live up to those standards. Minimum program components include: inspection of training & credentials, precision of documentation, appropriateness of ordered tests, and effectiveness of treatment ordered. A Q.A. program should determine the effectiveness of clinical patient care as evidenced by patient outcome.

Rates: Rates are determined by a variety of factors: market share, competition, exclusivity, channeling, and so on, and can be an amount per unit of service, per case, per day, or a predetermined monthly premium amount. Listed below are the various types of rates, in order from lowest degree of provider risk to the highest degree of provider risk: fee for service, discounted fee for service, variable discounted fee for service, per diem, per case, variable per diem or per case rate, capitation, and percent of premium.

Rationing: Also known as priority-setting, rationing, of health care is the inevitable result of limited resources meeting unlimited needs. Critics of the current system argue that care is rationed today, on the basis of ability to pay. The State of Oregon has established the only system of explicit rationing—or priority setting—of health services for defined population, namely, Medicaid patients.

RBRVS: The resource-based relative value scale was developed as a reformed fee schedule for physicians treating patients on Medicare. The RBRVS system, which was intended to favor cognitive over procedural services, has implications for system-wide reform, because it could be adopted as a model for physician reimbursement by insurance companies.

Readmit: An inpatient admission that occurs within 30 days of discharge from a previous inpatient acute care episode.

Reasonable and Customary Charge: Also known as usual, customary and reasonable charge (UCR). The maximum amount an insurer will consider as eligible for reimbursement. A claim cost control device.

Rehabilitation Treatment: A program structured to provide the resources necessary to rehabilitate a patient to a drug-free lifestyle. The program generally incorporates a step model, disease model, educational and family component. The program utilizes A.A./N.A. structure and provides an aftercare program. (Note: substance abuse treatment regimes can be provided across a variety of levels of care.)

Relapse: An inpatient case readmitted more than 30 days but less than 1 year from the last discharge date from an inpatient acute care episode.

Retrospective Review: Review of discharged or completed patiently services by Utilization Review or payor to determine appropriateness of length of stay or services rendered.

Second Level Appeal: Conducted after the first level appeal, the second level appeal is initiated by the treating therapist, Utilization Review manager, or beneficiary. It is a request to review the patient's medical record to determine if the original Utilization Review decision will be upheld or changed.

Self-Insured or Self-Funded Plan: A health plan in which the risk for medical cost is assumed by the company rather than an insurance company or managed care plan. Under ERISA, self-funded plans are exempt from certain requirements such as premium taxes and mandatory benefits. Self-funded plans often contract with insurance companies or third-party administrators (TPAs) to administer the benefits.

Single-Payer System: A centralized health-care payment system, with the government footing all the bills. Canada has perhaps the best-known single-payer system. There, people go to the doctors and hospitals of their choice and bill the government according to a standard fee schedule.

Small Group Insurance Reform: This would be an interim measure to address the fact that many of the uninsured are self-employed or work in very small companies. A popular reform option is to allow for community rating—as opposed to experience rating—so that individuals in small groups can get health insurance at premiums adjusted for a larger market.

Staff HMO: Delivers services at one or more locations through a staff of physicians who are salaried employees of the HMO. An example would be Group Health Associates.

Stop Loss: Stop loss provision (or stop loss limit) is the maximum out-of-pocket dollar amount that a beneficiary is responsible for, per calendar year, before the plan pays 100% for covered services. A form of reinsurance that provides protection for medical expenses above a certain limit, generally on a year-by-year basis. This may apply to an entire health plan or to any single component. For example, the health plan may have stop loss reinsurance for cases that exceed $100,000: After a case hits $100,000, the plan receives 80% of expenses in excess of $100,000 back from the reinsurance company for the rest of the year. Another example would be the plan providing a stop loss to participating physicians for referral expenses over $2,500: When a case exceeds that amount in a single year, the plan no longer deducts those costs from the physician's referral pool for the remainder of the year. In general, this phrase is used to refer to insurance that a plan purchases to protect itself against catastrophic losses that could cause financial burden.

Subrogation: The contractual right of a health plan to recover payments made to a member for health care costs after that member has received such payment for damages in a legal action.

TEFRA: Tax Equity and Fiscal Responsibility Act. One key provision of this act prohibits employers and health plans from requiring full time employees between the ages of 65 and 69 to use Medicare rather than the group health plan. Another key provision codified Medicare risk contracts for HMOs and CMPs.

Third Party Administrators (TPA): An entity that represents purchasers of healthcare who may be involved directly or indirectly, with Negotiations of contracts on behalf of one or more clients. In some areas of the country TPAs may conduct quality assurance and/or audits, as well as perform administrative functions (e.g., claims processing, membership, and so on) for a self-funded plan or a start-up managed care plan.

Triple Option: The offering of an HMO, a PPO, and a traditional insurance plan by one carrier.

UB82 Form: Universal billing form for inpatient hospital billing.

UCR: Usual, Customary, and Reasonable. A schedule of charges for medical services that are generally considered acceptable for claim payment. UCR rates can differ from one geographic area to another. A method of profiling prevailing fees in an area and reimbursing providers based on that profile. One common methodology is to average all fees and choose the 90th percentile. Sometimes this is used synonymously with a fee schedule when the fee schedule is set relatively high.

Underwriting: In one definition, this refers to bearing the risk for something (for example a policy is underwritten by an insurance company). In another definition, this refers to the analysis of a group that is done to determine rates, or to determine if the group should be offered coverage at all.

URC: Utilization Review Coordinator. Also referred to as a Utilization Review Nurse (UR nurse) or Utilization Management Coordinator (UMC).

Utilization Management Companies: Perform precertification, concurrent review, and/or case management services on behalf of employers. These companies will review clinical data to determine the medical necessity of treatment or services, and identify the most efficient and cost-effective method of treating the patient. It is estimated that approximately 95% of employers use some form of utilization management. Utilization management is performed by almost every type of managed care company in the market today.

Utilization Review: The review (and sharing) of clinical information to first determine and then ensure the medical necessity of treatment and the provision of effective, quality care through the most cost effective means. Can be an internal or external case review. See Certification.

•*Concurrent Review:* Review of inpatient status by Utilization Review or payor during hospitalization to verify appropriate length of stay and the medical necessity of services being provided.

•*Delegated Review:* Future trend of managed care to assign the responsibility of review to the provider that has demonstrated a willingness to deliver appropriate services and length of stay. In other words, the provider reviews itself.

• *Precertification:* A process of contacting the designated Utilization Management company, on behalf of the beneficiary, to obtain authorization for treatment. Precertification is generally required by most benefit plans and must take place prior to the provision of any treatment, otherwise reimbursement could be affected.

• *Retrospective Review:* Review of discharged or completed patient services by Utilization Review or payor to determine appropriateness of length of stay or services rendered.

Variable Discounted Fee for Service Rate: Provider discounts its full charges for services rendered, but the level of discount applied to full billed charges increases commensurate with the number of individuals utilizing provider services during a contract year. Sometimes referred to as volume discounting. Note: Sliding Scale is a variable percentage discount based upon amount of revenue or volume.

Wraparound Plan: Commonly used to refer to insurance or health plan coverage for copays and deductibles that are not covered under a member's base plan. This is often used for Medicare.

APPENDIX B

Sample Guidelines for the Review of Outpatient Mental Health and Substance Abuse Cases *

GUIDELINES FOR THE PRECERTIFICATION OF OUTPATIENT PSYCHOTHERAPY

- If the employee/dependent of a client who requires preauthorization of outpatient psychotherapy call for preauthorization, that person is to be advised to go ahead with an initial visit and then to have the clinician call to authorize further visits.

- When the provider calls after the first visit, use the following Guidelines For Certification of Outpatient Psychotherapy.

GUIDELINES FOR CERTIFICATION OF OUTPATIENT PSYCHOTHERAPY
(Cases must be reviewed with the clinician or authorized personnel)

Diagnosis

- The identified patient must have DSM-IV diagnosis on Axis I or Axis II.

Level of Functioning

- Do symptoms significantly interfere with daily functioning? How?

Providers

- Treating clinicians must be state licensed for the independent practice of psychotherapy ...

---

*From *Cigna: Level of Care Guidelines for Menal Health and Substance Abuse.* (First Edition), 1991. Cigna Corp., Philadelphia, PA.

or

• ... the service may be delivered in a state licensed clinic/facility by an unlicensed but qualified clinician under the supervision of a state licensed psychologist or psychiatrist.
• Clinicians must practice within the scope of their licensure or education.

Note: In network-based delivery systems CIGNA credentialing and contracting standards supersede the above.

Treatment plan
(All of the following must be met)

• Provider must have identifiable treatment goals that are consistent with resolution of the presenting problem or diagnosis.
  • The frequency of visits is appropriate to the diagnosis and the treatment plan.
  • More than 1 (one) visit per week requires an identifiable need such as the patient is potentially a danger to self or another, but does not require an inpatient stay.
• An inpatient stay may be avoided by frequent/intense outpatient psychotherapy.
• A medication evaluation by a psychiatrist if appropriate.
• Family therapy is part of the treatment plan of an adolescent or child. This does not require the patient to be present at all sessions but does require that the focus of the sessions is the child or the adolescent.
• The patient is generally motivated and cooperating in treatment.

If any of the above requirements are not met, refer to a physician/peer advisor for review.

Authorization/certification

• To be certified, cases must meet guidelines for diagnosis, provider and treatment plan.
• Five (5) to eight (8) visits may be authorized before another review occurs.

CONTINUED VISIT REVIEW GUIDELINES

To receive certification for continued visits in outpatient treatment, all of the following must be met:

• The identified patient continues to be generally motivated and participating actively in the therapy process.

• Symptoms, behaviors or problems still require ongoing treatment.

• There appears to be progress with the treatment where progress could be reasonably expected. (In some cases there may be no progress, but the outpatient visits stabilize the patient enough to prevent hospital admission.)

If any of the above requirements are not met, refer to a physician/peer advisor for review.

Authorization/Certification

• For continued visit certification, cases must meet the above guidelines.

• Five (5) to eight (8) visits may be authorized before another review occurs.

GUIDELINES FOR DISCHARGE FROM OUTPATIENT TREATMENT

Any of the following constitute appropriate guidelines for the discontinuation of out patient treatment:

• The patient has reached treatment goals.

• The problem that brought the patient into therapy no longer has the potential to interfere with day-to-day functioning.

• The patient requires inpatient treatment.

• The patient is generally uncooperative/noncompliant.

If any of the conditions is present, refer to a physician/peer advisor for review.

PHYSICIAN ADVISOR REFERRAL

In addition to the above guidelines for referral to a physician/peer advisor, a referral should also be made if:

• Therapy has gone beyond 20 visits.

• The frequency of visits is greater than 8 visits per month.

• Sessions are longer than 60 minutes for individual psychotherapy.

• Sessions are longer than 90 minutes for family psychotherapy.

- Sessions are longer than 120 minutes for group psychotherapy.
- It appears that therapy may be for educational purposes, communications enhancement, or other problems that are not for the direct treatment of a mental or emotional disorder as listed in DSM-IV-R, Axis I or Axis II.
- Continued outpatient treatment is due to legal requirements or environmental pressures (An example of an environmental pressure is when a person is required to participate in therapy as a condition of returning to work when there is no clinical necessity for continuing treatment).

APPENDIX C

How to Write Treatment Planning Reports for Axis II Disorders

INTRODUCTION

DSM-IV Axis II Diagnosis. An Axis II diagnosis, by itself, is generally not a covered benefit in most managed care contracts. An Axis I diagnosis accompanied by an Axis II diagnosis, however, is often a covered benefit. Patients with Axis I and Axis II diagnoses may require longer treatment. Drs. David Rice and Ira Polonsky provide three examples of these categories. (See D. Rice and I. Polonsky, 1993, *How to Write Treatment Planning Reports for Managed Care Companies, Part II: Axis II Disorders,* Oakland, CA: Corporate Health Plan.)

DEPENDENT PERSONALITY DISORDER (301.6)

Relevant History

Mrs. S. is a 33-year-old woman who works as a cashier in a supermarket. She has been married once and has a 10-year-old daughter from that marriage. Since her divorce, she has been in two relationships, each of which ended when the man left her. Each of these men had a problem with alcohol and after each relationship, Ms. S. felt "crushed." She has begun a new relationship soon after the previous one ended and has never lived just with her daughter for more than six months. For the past year, she has been involved with a man who works as a truck driver for the same supermarket. He drinks regularly and uses cocaine occasionally. Ms. S. does not use chemicals regularly, although she sometimes drank and used drugs at the urging of her boyfriend. Although she has never been physically beaten by a man, Ms. S. reports that she has been verbally abused in the past, though not by her current boyfriend.

Mrs. S. was the middle of three children. Her parents had continual money problems and were often working or worrying about not having enough money. Ms. S. said she was the "typical middle child" who got "lost in the shuffle." When she is not working, she spends most of her time cooking or cleaning for her boyfriend and daughter. She does not like to make plans on her own in case her boyfriend wants to do something. She has no close women friends.

Presenting Problem

Ms. S. said her boyfriend would like her to have a child. Ms. S., though, is worried about what might happen to her if she has another child and her boyfriend then leaves her. She said she was also afraid he might leave her if she didn't get pregnant. She has been getting headaches and has been crying a lot. Her boyfriend has responded to her crying by withdrawing. Because her job has a 1 to 3 session EAP program, she decided to ask a counselor what she should do. She said she is getting tired of starting a new relationship every few years and would like to find a man she can depend on, preferably one who didn't drink or use drugs.

Symptoms and Behavior

1. Difficulty making decision about having another child, even though boyfriend uses drugs and withdraws from her emotionally.
2. Tries to please others. Rarely takes the initiative.
3. When a relationship ends, starts up new one quickly. Hates being without a man.
4. Drinks or uses drugs occasionally, even though she doesn't like to, at boyfriend's urging.

Treatment Objectives

1. Have her continue in therapy for more than 3 EAP sessions.
2. Raise self-esteem. Learn that she is able to handle more things on her own.
3. Learn that she can get help from other people, if she needs help, without doing things she doesn't want to do.
4. Develop women friends.
5. Develop assertiveness skills.
6. Find some activities outside of work that she like to do.

Treatment Strategies

1. Do not take either a nondirective or an authoritarian approach. A nondirective approach will evoke too much anxiety, and an authoritarian role will encourage dependency. A balance between the two different styles is essentials.

2. Set clear limits on calls after hours or extra visits. In setting limits, take a very supportive but firm approach.

3. Point out the discrepancy between her strengths (she works, she is raising her daughter) and her thoughts about herself ("I can't make it by myself. I need a man to take care of me.")

4. Use cognitive therapy technique to unravel her all-or-nothing thinking: if she isn't with someone, she'll be all by herself and will fall apart.

5. Refer to group therapy.

6. Refer to a codependency group.

7. Refer to an assertiveness training class.

PASSIVE-AGGRESSIVE PERSONALITY DISORDER

Relevant History

Mr. P.-A. is a 38-year-old man who works as a case worker in a county social service agency. He has never married and reported he was not close with his parents, whom he described as demanding and who "still treat me as a child." He said he had entered the social work profession because he wanted to "help people," but that he had become more and more dissatisfied with all the rules and regulations of the agency. He said that over the years, he had a number of ideas about how to deliver services better, but that his supervisors never listened to him. When not at work, Mr. P.-A. was on a number of sports teams (softball, bowling, volleyball). He prided himself on being in shape and wanting to win. He thought that if his teammates worked as hard as he did, his teams would be more successful. However, he never voiced this opinion. When teammates asked him to do something a little differently (e.g., perhaps play deeper in outfield, or hit softer serves) he usually had a number of reasons why their ideas were not good. He had never gotten close with any of his teammates because, he said, "If you get close to people, they'll try to use you."

Presenting Problem

Mr. P.-A. came to therapy because his supervisor had put him on probation for not following agency guidelines, for being chronically late with reports, and for being argumentative when told to do something. Mr. P.-A. said that the supervisor's allegations were technically accurate with regard to late reports, but that his supervisor was singling him out unfairly because everyone in the agency was behind in their reports. He also said that he felt his supervisor did not see all the good things he was doing in his job. Mr. P.-A. did acknowledge, however, that he felt "a little depressed and nervous" about his job situation. He said he could not talk to his supervisor because his supervisor had a "bad temper."

Symptoms and Behavior

1. Difficulty meeting work deadlines.
2. Inability to assert himself with his supervisor.
3. Blames other people for his problems. Believes his supervisor and other people are unreasonable. Does not see how his behavior effects his predicament.
4. Believes he has good ideas that others just don't recognize.
5. Argumentative when asked to do something both at work and outside work.

Treatment Objectives

1. Minimize therapist becoming an authority figure and patient reacting passive-aggressively to therapy.
2. Becoming more assertive. Become less fearful or verbal disagreements.
3. Learn how to evaluate other people's behavior more accurately (for example, is patient's supervisor actually treating the patient unfairly?)
4. Learn to evaluate his behavior with other people more accurately (i.e., is the patient's response to his supervisor's behavior effective?)
5. Blame others less for his problems and see more clearly how his point of view (as well as his behavior) contributes to his problems.
6. Become less pessimistic.

Treatment Strategies

1. Engage patient in treatment, including rules of therapy (fees, times). Make patient a partner in establishing goals and agreeing to rules.
2. Emphasize the difference between patient's feelings about a situation (e.g., the supervisor is trying to get him) and the situation has job to do and patient has a job to do).
3. Give homework to look at specific interactions between patient and supervisor, patient's assumptions about those interactions, and the effect of patient's behavior on his supervisor.
4. Refer to an assertiveness training group. Use role playing techniques. Find alternative ways to respond to supervisor that will be more effective.

5. Patient is likely to make payments late and to miss or be late for appointments. Make a clear contract with specified consequences for late payments or missed appointments. When the patient is late, discuss the meaning and consequences of his behavior.

AVOIDANT PERSONALITY DISORDER (301.82)

Relevant History

Ms. R. is a 35-year-old single woman who works as a chemist for a large corporation where her job involves developing materials for new products. She was well thought of at work and reported a high degree of job satisfaction. She lived alone and had lived alone ever since she entered graduate school. She said that although she had had a few opportunities, she had never dated. She had a few woman friends whom she saw every 2 to 3 weeks for dinner or a movie. She claimed she was rarely bored and that her hobbies or reading and following the political situation kept her busy outside of work.

She came from a middle-class family and was the youngest of two daughters. Her sister had been more outgoing, and Ms. R. had been the shy and studious one. She thought her mother liked her sister more, although she emphasized that her parents treated both children the same. She said that her father had high standards and had often criticized her as a child when she, supposedly, hadn't done her best. She defended her father's behavior, though, because he knew she was smart and just wanted her to realize her potential. Ms. R. now lived in a different city from her parents and sister and had little contact with them, except for a perfunctory phone call every other Sunday.

Presenting Problem

Ms. R. came to therapy because a new man at work, whom she liked, had asked her out and she had refused by making up a nonexistent conflict. She said she wanted to know why she had done that. She said she was happy with her life, but also recognized that something was missing. She said she had read some books about therapy and though therapy could maybe help her. She said she knew she "didn't like to fail." When asked to discuss this fear of failure in more detail, Ms. R. had little to say.

Symptoms and Behavior

1. Scared to accept a date with a man she likes.
2. Few friends; no close friends.

3. No interest or hobbies that involve other people.

4. Fear of other people's reactions if she were to fail at something.

5. Despite above-average intelligence, low level of awareness of her own psychological functioning (she knows that something is missing in her life and that she fears failure, but she can't elaborate).

Treatment Objectives

1. Go out with the man at work whom she likes.

2. See her few friends more often. Talk with them more about herself.

3. Do some things where she might meet people (for example, join a hiking club or enroll in an adult education class).

4. Learn to identify some of her feelings and thoughts about herself in more detail. Recognize that she is afraid of being rejected and that is why she avoids other people so much. Link her fears of rejection to the way her parents raised her.

5. Recognize how she puts herself down and how she assumes other people will reject her. Have experiences that show her that her assumptions are often inaccurate.

6. Learn to accept that even if she feels scared, she can still function with other people and doesn't have to withdraw.

7. Be more assertive.

Treatment Strategies

1. Use her ability to analyze and logically evaluate data to examine her own behavior. Have her make lists of her assumptions about what will happen if she talks to other people. Use role playing.

2. List a hierarchy of social situations: talk to the man at a coffee break, have lunch with the man in the office, go out to lunch, go out for dinner, spend a day together. Ask a woman friend to the movies and talk with her more openly, ask a woman friend to go on a day trip. List local clubs and activities she could join and/or attend where she would interact with either people. Give homework to do these things.

3. Discuss what happened when she did the homework: were her predictions of rejection and failure met? Discuss ways to deal with uncomfortable feelings (recognize them, write them down). Link fear of rejecting with earlier childhood experiences so she can see connection.

4. If patient does not do homework, discuss what happened. Use therapy session to bring up her anxiety or uncomfortable feelings and fears.

Discuss where these came from and how her avoidant behavior is not allowing her to find that part that is missing from her life.

5. Encourage her assertiveness, both during the therapy sessions and in what she does outside of therapy. Break assertiveness down into small pieces (asking questions, making phone calls). Give homework to be more assertive. Discuss results.

6. Be aware that the patient is very sensitive to rejection and is uncomfortable with closeness. Be consistent in the length of your sessions. If you miss an appointment due to illness, or when you go on vacation, be especially clear about informing the patient.

Name Index

Subject Index

WIDENER UNIVERSITY
WOLFGRAM
LIBRARY
CHESTER, PA